What People are saying

Bernie Clark's *Yinsights* is one of the best yoga resources now available, no matter what your preferred style of practice. It is really three books in one: It is a scientific explanation of yoga and how it works. It is a practical handbook on how to get started. And it is a guide to developing mindfulness during practice. It is the book we will use in our own training programs.

Paul Grilley

Yin Yoga is a practice much needed in today's difficult, divisive times. It offers us a way to leave behind our ideas of how we should be, and return to our true selves, where all lasting healing takes place. Bernie Clark has written a wonderfully detailed account of the history, philosophy, and practice of Yin Yoga. *YinSights* is written with compassion and deep understanding, and I recommend it not only for those interested in Yin Yoga, but for all yoga practitioners.

Biff Mithoefer – author of The Yin Yoga Kit

YinSights is an intelligently written, extensively researched, and comprehensive study of the system of Yin Yoga that Paul Grilley and Sarah Powers teach.

Master Paulie Zink

I love the *YinSights* book … I am in yoga teacher training. I have a love for Yin Yoga and want to teach this form of yoga. The book is a great resource for me; being a newbie, as it breaks down each pose giving the meridians affected, counter poses, etc. Invaluable for a new teacher trying to put a class together. Thanks again for this wonderful resource!!!!

Jann McGinnis, training yoga teacher

YinSights is a comprehensive guidebook for both curious students and dedicated teachers of Yin Yoga. Bernie is thoughtful and thorough as he arranges the immense body of knowledge, which influences the practice of Yin Yoga. He manages to weave threads of historical foundation, theoretical elucidation and practical application into a tapestry rich in spiritual tradition. This work could only come into being authentically through the efforts of a passionate spirit who has dedicated his life to the journey and has experienced some harmony along the way – thank you Bernie. I hope this lovely book finds its way into the hands, heads, hearts and bodies of many people… that they may experience a glimpse of what we know to be true and real.

Marla Erickson - creator of Yoga Inspired Functional Fitness

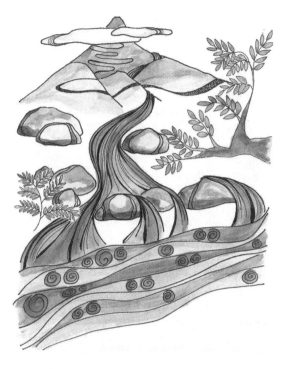

Yang Mountain – Yin River

Welcome to YinSights
A Journey into the
Philosophy & Practice of Yin Yoga
By Bernie Clark

– Foreword by Sarah Powers –

ISBN 978-0-9687665-1-4
Library of Congress Control Number: 2007902489
First Printing – August 2007
Second Printing – November 2007
Third Printing – June 2016
Printed in the U.S.A.

*Do your work without attachment and with being
balanced in success or failure.
Balance is called yoga.*

Bhagavad-Gita

Yin balances Yang

A lesson from the Dao-de-ching

Warning & Disclaimer

Please Note! Before embarking on this practice, please make sure you are able to do so: check with your doctor, or health care professional, before starting any yoga practice. The guidance given in this book is not meant to replace medical advice and should be used only as a supplement if you are under the care of a health care professional. While care has been taken in compiling the guidance in this book, we cannot take any responsibility for any adverse effects from your practice of yoga. When you are not sure of any aspect of the practice, or feel unwell, seek medical advice. For more information on precautions before practicing yoga, please check the section called *Before You Practice*.

YinSights

Table of Contents
Part One – Physiology and Philosophy

Chapter Ten: The Buddhist View of Mind   **183**

Chapter Eleven: The Western View of Mind   **215**

Part Two – Practice

Chapter Fourteen:
Yang Counterposes and Yin Flows   329

Preface to the print version of YinSights

YinSights was originally envisioned as an online resource to help students and teachers learn more about the philosophy and practice of Yin Yoga. As an online resource, the document allows the reader to link to other resources by simply clicking on the Web links embedded within the text. It is also easy to jump from one place in the document to another. This, unfortunately, is not possible in a print version. We have attempted to keep some of the links in the print version; however, they can only be typed and are offered as footnotes. An e-book is also easy to update and keep current, which again is not possible for a printed book – short of publishing a new version on a regular basis. Unfortunately some of the links listed in this book will be out of date by the time you try them. A little searching on your own may help you rediscover where the page has gone.

Also, due to the nature of the Internet, readers can jump into and out of the book at any point, so many key concepts were deliberately repeated at many places within the book. This is especially noticeable for the warnings about the possible dangers of the practice. We could have removed these duplications from this print version; however, most of them stayed. The reason? Repetition builds familiarity. When we see something once, we hardly ever remember it. When we see it twice, it seems familiar but is again forgotten. By the third time, we start to remember it. For this reason, we retained the original duplication we put into the Web version. If this is annoying to some readers, please breathe deeply … pause and smile slightly … and move on.

Despite the advantages of the electronic version of YinSights, there are several drawbacks to that format: it is not comfortable to curl up at night with a computer, and it is not easy to lay a computer on the floor beside you and flip to the page you want to study as you do your practice. It is also difficult to read an electronic book when you are traveling: laptop batteries do run down. So, due to many requests, I decided to transform the e-book YinSights into a traditional print version.

The two versions of YinSights, the print version and the e-book, are not identical. The differences will grow over time. The Web-based version has more images and will be continually updated, while the print version is, by its very nature, static. However, both versions are available, so the reader is encouraged to check the online version of YinSights occasionally to see what is new. We do expect to add new Yin Yoga asanas and flows over time. And as new research relating to Yin Yoga is conducted and released, this too will be documented. You can continue to find YinSights online at www.YinYoga.com.

One final note, on the use of gender-specific pronouns in this book: although yoga in India was predominantly a male practice, today, in the West, by far the greatest numbers of practitioners are women. Yoga has benefited greatly from this infusion of feminine sensibilities. In recognition of this fact, whenever the opportunity demands the use of the cumbersome phrases "he or she" or "his or hers," I have chosen to simplify the wording and use just the feminine pronoun. Hopefully, any of my fellow men who are traumatized by this choice will get over it quickly. The term "yogi" is defined to be "a person who practices yoga" and so is gender neutral. When we wish to specifically refer to a male practitioner, the term "yogin" is used, and for a female practitioner, "yogini" is used.

Acknowledgements

I have many people to thank for helping to make this project become a reality, and for assisting me on my own journey down the Yin River. Firstly, for introducing me to yoga, I must acknowledge and express my gratitude to my first teacher, shakti mhi, of the Prana Yoga & Zen Centre in Vancouver, Canada. I am also very grateful to Saul David Raye, my Thai Yoga Therapy teacher, for introducing me to the subtle energies within us, and for giving me my first taste of Yin Yoga. The day after I attended my first Yin Yoga class, conducted by Saul, I came across Sarah Powers' video, *Yin and Vinyasa Yoga*, and resolved to meet this woman. To Sarah I owe a great debt; her combination of yoga knowledge and dharma truths has inspired me greatly. Through Sarah I met Paul Grilley, to whom I am also deeply indebted. Paul shone a light, and illuminated for me a totally new aspect of yoga. Paul taught me so much about anatomy, and helped me realize just how unique each person is, inside and out. Paul also fired within me a desire to learn more about what is really going on within us when we practice yoga.

To all my teachers, and all their teachers, my thanks.

I also wish to acknowledge the support of my family and friends and their assistance in creating this book. My thanks to Jessica Clark, for her design of the www.YinYoga.com Web site, the layout of this book, her patience in teaching me Illustrator and Photoshop, and for her help in "prettying up" the illustrations. To Ryan Clark, for his computer skills, for creating the Web page and the html templates for the online version of the book, and for patiently answering all my questions. To Violette, for contributing many of the illustrations. To

Louise, for the original Web-book cover art: Yang Mountain – Yin River. To Professor James Clark, for the initial proofreading of the entire manuscript, for offering invaluable suggestions, and for acting as my science editor, especially in the sections on energy. I also need to thank the good folks at BookSurge for their invaluable editing services and printing the book. For the index I want to thank Pilar Wyman. (A book without a good index is not worth reading!) My gratitude also goes to Stewart, Julie, and Roberta for their encouragement. I also wish to thank the models for many of the pictures, especially Lindsay and Stephanie. And lastly, my special thanks to a good friend, Diana Batts, for her encouragement and support, for patiently posing for most of the pictures in the book, for proofreading the early manuscripts, and for being my traveling companion on our ride down the Yin River.

Finally, my blessings and thanks to all the students who have allowed me the honor of teaching them; one really learns when one attempts to teach. Indeed, my students have been my greatest teachers.

Lokah samasta sukhino bhavantu.
May all beings everywhere be happy.

Foreword

In the winter of 2005, Paul Grilley and I taught a Yin and Vinyasa Yoga and Buddhist Mindfulness Meditation Teacher Training in Napa California. In order for the students to receive their certificates of completion for the course, we assigned a paper, a kind of thesis about the course. Paul and I each took half of the entries home post training to read. I got a call from Paul exhorting me to read Bernie Clark's paper, he said, "It's one of the best I have *ever* read." It was.

While that particular paper is not included in this book, it portended what is. Bernie has written a beautiful, thorough, humorous, and insightful book not only on Yin Yoga, but about the broader umbrella of Yoga in general, and further, the value of combining an eastern spiritual perspective with western scientific rigor.

It's not Bernie's intention here to write the definitive history of the many schools of thought he outlines, but he nevertheless manages to present not only an ambitious (and to my mind successful) map for further exploration, but also reflections on how that map could be looked at. One minute he writes on the basic praxis and theory of Buddhism, the next on the western view of the mind, as postulated by Carl Jung.

This book is a wonderful place to begin to grapple with these topics. A quick glance at the chapter headings gives a clue of the breadth of what's offered: Prana, Bioelectricity, Chakras, Cognitive Therapy, Meridians, Bones and Cartilage … there is something interesting here for just about everyone, whether one is initially drawn to these subjects or not.

To love one's subject, and to realize the value that any subject has to change human understanding and behavior for the better, requires intelligence, dedication, and a facility for communicating that potential. Bernie proves here that he has that facility.

During the course of the trainings and retreats of mine that Bernie has attended, he has proven himself to be a thoughtful and dedicated student and teacher. He's doing it again here as a writer.

May this book create a bridge of understanding and dedicated practice and be a vehicle for extending the possibility of true freedom.

With Metta,
Sarah Powers
June 2007

Introducing YinSights

Acommon metaphor for the spiritual journey is climbing a mountain. We all start somewhere near the base of the mountain. Craning our necks to look up, we are inspired by its magnificence. Often the peak of the mountain is obscured, hidden

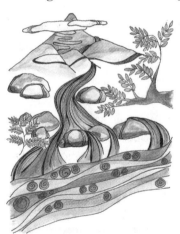

Yang Mountain – Yin River

by the clouds of ignorance, and we are not sure where we are headed. The paths are varied, and there are many ways to begin the long climb. Along the way, guides appear who know this or that particular part of the path, but we meet very few people, if any, who have actually been all the way to the top. We are told that, once we reach that lofty summit, called "Samadhi," everything will become clear to us. We will be able to look out and see the entire world in a way we could never have imagined. We will be able to look at where we have come from, and see that all paths, as different and varied as they may be, lead to this one peak.

However, a peak is a small place. Not many can fit here, and no one can actually remain at this Summit of Samadhi. Even the most accomplished yogi must descend from time to time.

This metaphor is very *yang* in nature. It requires a lot of effort to climb a mountain, especially the Yang Mountain. People who do this we call *yangsters*. It is hard work. Yang refers to things that are higher and brighter, to actions that are more forceful and dynamic. For many people, yang is their favorite way to live, and the only way they know how to live. But … it is not the only way. Yin always exists as a complement to yang. Yin refers to things that are lower and calmer, to actions that are passive and yielding. The spiritual practice has another metaphor that may be more appealing to many of us: the flow of a great river, the Yin River. Here we find the *yinsters*.

The journey we are about to embark upon is a yin journey: it is a trip down the Yin River, toward the universal ocean. At the dock, the Buddha is waiting, inviting us to board a ferryboat. The river will carry us; all we need to do is pay attention and steer. Occasionally we will have to manage a few rapids: no activity is ever completely yin, or completely yang. Even if we are climbing the Yang Mountain, there will be yin times to rest and admire the view. As we float down the Yin River, there will be yang bursts of activity and times when we need to make decisions. Occasionally the river will be broad and slow, and we will have time to investigate many interesting sights: these are our *yinsights*. At other times, the river will narrow and our pace will quicken. We will have less time to investigate the waters around us.

Along this journey down the Yin River, side trips will beckon to us: broad lakes and other rivers will appear. We will have the option to explore these new waters, or linger in one area for a more thorough investigation. Perhaps we will take up these options right away, or perhaps we will note them for some future investigation. The trip overall will be leisurely. As we journey, we will meet many other travelers. The river is broad and, unlike the tiny peak of the Yang Mountain, the Universal Ocean we are heading toward can accommodate everyone. We will, hopefully, come to appreciate the yin side of life, the easy pace of the river, and the breadth of our discoveries.

The journey begins with the very question that may have brought you to the pier of departure: *What is Yin Yoga?* Once you board our little ferryboat, your question will be addressed. The first part of the journey will show you some of the history of yoga in general and of Yin Yoga in particular. This will become a theme throughout the journey: many of our discoveries will apply, not just to the tributaries of Yin Yoga, but also to the broader, grander river of yoga. We will pass through waters where we will see our body reflected through different eyes, through different models. We will see ancient and modern views of our body mind. As we explore these views, we will also see the benefits yoga practice has for our body mind.

The Universal Ocean awaits us at the end our journey, but before we catch sight of these vast waters, we will see how to practice Yin Yoga. We will find some simple principles to guide our practice. A description of many of the most commonly used Yin Yoga postures, or asanas, will be provided, along with some suggested ways to build these postures into flows, and into a complete yoga practice. Around the final bend will be an exploration of how to move energy through physical practice, breath work, and meditation.

How, where and when the journey will end ... will depend upon you.
The journey will begin with our first yinsight:
What is Yin Yoga?

Chapter One: What is Yin Yoga?

What is Yin Yoga? This question is asked a lot by students who have been practicing yoga for a while but have never come across this particular challenging style. Simple answers such as "It is the balancing practice for your yang style of yoga" or "It is yoga for the joints, not the muscles" are not overly satisfying. If students haven't heard of Yin Yoga, they won't know what a yang style of yoga is. And isn't all yoga good for the whole body, including our joints? To really answer the question and get to know Yin Yoga requires a fuller explanation. This part of our journey provides a deeper look into Yin Yoga and begins with an explanation of what it is, how it evolved, and its benefits for the whole body mind.

Yin Yoga has the same goals and objectives as any other school of yoga; however, it directs the stimulation normally created in the asana portion of the practice deeper than the superficial or muscular tissues (which we are calling the yang tissues). Yin Yoga targets the connective tissues, such as the ligaments, bones, and even the joints of the body that normally are not exercised very much in a more active style of asana practice.

Suitable for almost all levels of students, Yin Yoga is a perfect complement to the dynamic and muscular (yang) styles of yoga that emphasize internal heat, and the lengthening and contracting of our muscles. Yin Yoga generally targets the connective tissues of the hips, pelvis, and lower spine.

While initially this style of yoga can seem quite boring, passive, or soft, yin practice can be quite challenging due to the long duration of the poses. We can remain in the postures anywhere from one to twenty minutes! Yin and yang tissues respond quite differently to being exercised. You need to experience this to really know what Yin Yoga is all about. After you have experienced it, even just once, you will realize that you have been doing only half of the asana practice.

> **Please Note!** Yin Yoga is **not** restorative yoga. Like all yoga practices, if the tissues you are targeting for exercise are damaged in some way, please give yourself a chance to heal before resuming your regular practice.

Let's start delving deeper into the study. Just around the bend we will start to understand the nature of yin and yang and see how they are applied in life and in our body.

Yin and Yang

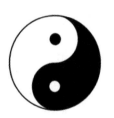

Patterns define our lives. Look around you right now; look carefully and you will notice the patterns surrounding you. Look up; you will see things that are high. Look down; you will see things that are low. Listen; you will hear things close by, and you will hear things far away. You will hear loud or obvious noises. You may hear soft, subtle sounds. Bring your attention inward; you may feel the tip of your nose (especially now that you just read the words "tip of your nose") or the top of your head. Now you may be feeling the tips of your toes. Up, down … near, far … louder, softer … these are just some of the adjectives we can choose to describe the patterns of life, of existence. All patterns are formed by contrasts. The pattern on a chessboard is formed by the contrast of dark and light. The pattern of your life, when reflected upon, has displayed a contrast of good times and bad. For the Daoist, harmony and health are created when conditions arise where the contrasting aspects are in balance.

Balancing is not a static act. Imagine the typical depiction of weighing scales: two plates held by a common string suspended at a point halfway between them. When two equally weighted objects are placed upon the scales, there is a slight swaying motion, like a pendulum. If one side is too heavy, the scales tip and balance is lost. When both sides are equal, there is still a slight oscillation around the middle position. This rebalancing is the returning to wholeness and health.

The ancient Chinese called this middle point "the Dao."[1] The Dao is the tranquility found in the center of all events. The center is always there even if we are not always there to enjoy it. When we leave the center we take on aspects of *yin* or *yang*.

Yin and yang are relative terms: they describe the two facets of existence. Like two sides of one coin, yin cannot exist without yang; yang cannot exist without yin. They complement each other. Since existence is never static, what is yin and what is yang are always in flux, always changing.

Yin	Yang
Dark	Light
Cold	Hot
Passive	Active
Inside	Outside
Solid	Hollow
Slow	Rapid
Right	Left
Dim	Bright
Downward	Upward
Substance	Function
Water	Fire
Matter	Energy
Mysterious	Obvious
Female	Male
Moon	Sun
Night	Day
Earth	Heaven
Even	Odd
Dragon	Tiger

The observation that everything has yin or yang attributes was made many thousands of years ago in ancient China. The terms existed in Confucianism and in the earliest Daoist writings. The character yin refers to the shady side of a hill or stream. Yang refers to the sunny side. Shade cannot exist without light: light can only be light when contrasted to darkness. And so we see how, even in the earliest uses of these terms, patterns are observed.

Darkness and light are just two of the many aspects separating yin and yang. Yin is used to describe things that are relatively denser, heavier, lower, more hidden, more yielding, more feminine, more mysterious, and more passive. Yang is used to describe the opposite conditions: things that are less dense, lighter, higher, more obvious or

---

[1] Tibetans have called it the *Rigpa*.

superficial, more masculine, and more dynamic. The table on the previous page shows a more complete, but not complete, comparison. There is no limit to the relative contexts in which yin and yang can be applied.

Yin Contains Yang

Look again at the symbol for yin and yang at the beginning of this section; do you see the white dot within the dark paisley swirl? Even within the darkness of yin, there is found a lightness of yang. And vice versa: within the white swirl is a black dot; within yang is always found yin. In the context of temperature we say that hotter is yang and cooler is yin: but slightly hot is yin compared to extremely hot. And extremely hot is yin compared to hotter yet, which would be yang. In the other direction there is cool and there is cold. Yang would be cool relative the yin of cold.

In our yoga practice there are very active asana workouts, which we may call yang, but even within these relatively yang practices we can find relatively yin aspects; watching our breath mindfully while we flow through a vigorous vinyasa[2] is just one example.

Yin Becomes Yang

Just as we can detect yin elements within the yang aspects, we can also notice how yin becomes yang, and yang can transform into yin. These transformations may be slow and subtle, or they may be devastatingly quick. The seasons roll slowly by; they change imperceptibly. The yang of spring and summer transforms day by day into the yin of fall and winter. It is not possible to pick the exact moment at which one season becomes another, astronomical observations notwithstanding. But the transformation may also come quickly: the eye of a hurricane quickly brings calm, and just as quickly the eye moves on and the other half of the storm strikes.

In our own life we often experience both the slow transformations of yin into yang, and yang into yin, and the quick

---

[2] A *vinyasa* is a sequence of postures or asanas that flow smoothly from one to the next. It literally means to place in a special way.

changes. We wake up in the morning; yin becomes yang. Sometimes our awakening is slow, leisurely; this is a slow transformation. Sometimes we wake with a start and jump out of bed, perhaps because we realized we overslept. When we work long hours for many weeks or months in a row (a very yang lifestyle), our body may seek balance by suddenly making us too sick to work (a very yin lifestyle), or it may gift us with a severe migraine to slow us down. Yang is quickly transformed into yin.

Yin Controls Yang

In this last example, we can see that if we stay too long in an unbalanced situation, the universe acts to restore balance. It throws us to the other side: our health may suffer; our lives may change. If we do not heed the need for balancing yin and yang, this transition can be devastating; a heart attack could be the balancing force applied to us. These imbalances are often referred to as either a "deficiency" or an "excess." We can have an excess of yin or a yin deficiency; we can have an excess of yang or a yang deficiency. The cure is to apply the opposite energy to control the excess or deficiency.

In the Eastern world of the Daoists and yogis,[3] the need for balance is well known and understood.[4] In the West, the concepts of yin and yang are more foreign. We don't think in these terms; our lifestyles rarely reflect a need for balance. We seek it only when the universe forces us to pay attention. Fortunately, the idea of yin and yang is becoming more widely known here in the West. Let's look now at how these terms can be applied to our own bodies.

---

[3] The term "yogi" is defined to be "a person who practices yoga" and so is gender neutral. When we wish to specifically refer to a male practitioner, the term "yogin" is used, and for a female practitioner, "yogini" is used.

[4] The yogis have similar words for yin and yang, *tha* and *ha*, which together form the word *hatha* after which the well-known school of yoga is named.

Yin Tissues and Yang Tissues

Yin and yang are relative terms and need a context to be appropriately applied. They can be used as adjectives, although they are often used as nouns. Within our bodies, if we use the context of position or density, the yang tissues could be said to be our muscles, blood, and skin compared to the yin tissues of ligaments, bones, and joints. The contexts of flexibility or heat could also be used; muscles are elastic, bones are plastic.[5] Muscles love to get hot while ligaments generally remain cool. However, we are not making an absolute definition here. In the context of water content, the muscles are yin and the ligaments are yang. Muscles love to get juicy, thus, they have lots of water in them, which is a yin quality; ligaments have less water content, which means they are relatively yang.

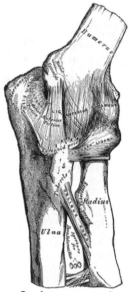

In the context of elasticity, our bones and their ligaments can be considered yin-like compared to our more yang-like muscles. ᴀ

Despite the context of water, there are more ways in which the muscles are yang-like relative to the ligaments than they are yin-like. This is one reason this particular style of yoga is called Yin Yoga. Yang styles of yoga generally target the muscles and employ rhythmic, repetitive movements to stress the fibers of the muscles. Being elastic and moist, the muscles appreciate this form of exercise and respond well to it. Yin tissues, however, being dryer and much less elastic, could be damaged if they were stressed in this way. Instead, the more plastic tissues appreciate and require gentler pressures, applied for longer periods of time, in order to be stimulated to grow stronger. This is why orthodontic braces must be worn for a long time, with a reasonable (and not always comfortable) amount of pressure, in order to reshape the bones of the jaw.

---

[5] Elastic materials return to their original shape once the stress upon them ends. Plastic materials retain the new shape.

Our joints can be seen simply as spaces between the bones where movement is possible. Stabilizing the joint are ligaments, muscles, and tendons, which bind the bones together. The tendons and muscles also provide a force to move the bones relative to each other. Generally one of the muscles' jobs is to protect the joint; if there is too much strain on the joint, the muscle will tear first, then the ligament, and then finally the joint itself may become damaged. In this regard, yang yoga is designed to *not* stress the joint. This is why there is so much care taken to align the body and engage the muscles correctly before coming into asanas in the yang practice. However, Yin Yoga is specifically designed to exercise the ligaments and to create space and strength in the joints. The topic of tissues is discussed more fully in the Chapter Three: Our Bodies and Yoga's Benefits.

An example can help explain the different roles of the muscles and ligaments. Take your right index finger in your left hand. Tighten the muscles of the right finger and try to pull it away from the knuckle. Notice that there is no movement there. The muscles' job is to bind the bones together and limit the range of motion allowed in the joint. Now relax the finger completely. Shake it out for a moment. Now, keeping the muscles passive again, try to pull the finger away from the knuckle. Notice the slight dimpling there? Perhaps you can feel only the slight pulling away. When the muscles are relaxed the stress is moved to the ligaments binding the joint. The joint can open a little now and the ligaments can receive some of the stress. The first exercise was yang-like, whereas the second exercise was yin-like.

The Theory of Exercise

All forms of exercise share two features in common:

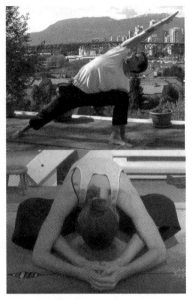

- first we must stress the tissues,
- then we must let the tissues rest.

Yang tissues do better when stressed in a yang manner and yin tissues do better when stressed in a yin way. Stress has many negative connotations in our culture because we forget the "rest" part of this equation. But to have no, or little, stress in our life is just as damaging as having too much stress. We need to stress the body, and we need to rest it. There is a yin/yang balance here that leads to health. Too much of anything is not healthy.

Yang exercise targets the yang tissues: the muscles. Muscles love to be rhythmically and repetitively moved. Any static holds are brief. The muscles are elastic and can take this type of exercise. However, to apply yang exercise to yin tissues could damage them. Yin tissues, being more plastic, require gentle but long-held stresses. Imagine bending a credit card back and forth one hundred and eight times every morning. It wouldn't take many mornings of this for it to snap in half. The credit card is plastic, just as our ligaments are. To rhythmically bend ligaments over and over again, as some students do when doing drop back from standing into the wheel, can, over time, damage the ligaments, just like the credit card was damaged. The warning here is … **do not apply yang exercise techniques to yin tissues!**

Applying a yin exercise to yang tissues could also be damaging! Holding a muscle in a contracted state for a long period of time is called "tetany"[6] and may damage the muscle.

---

[6] Tetany is an involuntary cramping of a muscle.

Is it better to tighten muscles (yang) or relax them (yin)? That depends on your intention. We tighten our muscles to protect our joints. We relax our muscles so we can exercise our joints. What is your intention in the pose you are doing?

Many health care professionals shudder at the thought of exercising joints; they have the mistaken view that all exercise is yang exercise. Despite this concern it is possible to exercise ligaments, bones, and joints. In fact, it is necessary. However, being yin tissues means we must exercise them in a yin way. And then, please remember the important second part of this equation – we must let them rest![7]

There is a lot of research proving the importance of stress and rest beyond just developing strength physically, but it is beyond the scope of this journey to go into it further.[8]

---

[7] As an aside, the theory of exercise applies beyond the tissues of our body. We need to have stress, and then rest, in all areas of our life in order to be healthy. This can include our relationships, our mental abilities, and even our immune system. For example, cancer patients rarely get colds before getting their cancer. Their immune systems were not exercised by colds and thus were weaker than the immune system of people who did get colds regularly. We need to stress our immune systems, appropriately, in order for them to be strong. But we also need rest. Migraine sufferers rarely have heart attacks because their migraines force them to slow down and adopt a yin lifestyle for the few days that their migraines occur. Like our tissues, our lives require periods of stress and rest.

[8] If you are curious about the above examples, feel free to start a discussion in the www.YinYoga.com Kula discussion board.

Chapter Two: The History of Yin Yoga

Yin Yoga has been described as new, yet ancient. While Paul Grilley has done much to publicize and popularize this form of yoga,[9] he did not invent it. Paul combined three lines of inquiry in a unique way. This is the hallmark of genius. In his own book, *Yin Yoga*, Paul dedicated his work to three teachers who guided his three lines of inquiry:

- Dr. Garry Parker ... who taught him anatomy
- Paulie Zink ... who taught him Daoist Yoga
- Dr. Hiroshi Motoyama ... who reminded Paul of yoga's greater purpose

While Paul has done more than any other individual to spread the teachings about Yin Yoga in the West, its practice goes back thousands of years. In this section we will discover the distant roots of Yin Yoga. We will also hear Paul's own story, the stories of Dr. Motoyama, Paulie Zink, and the other great teacher of Yin Yoga, Sarah Powers, whose style of teaching is very different from Paul's.

Original Yin

There are many documents describing yoga; some were written hundreds and even thousands of years ago: the Hatha Yoga Pradipika, the Gheranda Samhita, the Yoga Sutra, and many more.

---

[9] It was actually Sarah Powers who coined the term "Yin Yoga" that is commonly used today.

However, none of these ancient texts were meant to be read alone. They all required the guidance of a guru, to ensure understanding. The books were used more like notes – shorthand reminders of the real teaching. Much of the real knowledge was deliberately kept hidden; only when the teacher felt the student was ready was the knowledge revealed. We cannot tell simply from reading these old texts how the physical practice of yoga was performed. What we can say, with some certainty, is that the purpose of the physical practice was to prepare the student for the deeper practices of meditation.

In the earliest spiritual books of India, the Vedas, yoga is not described as a path to liberation, and asana practice is not described at all. Rather, yoga, among its many other meanings, meant discipline, and the closest word to asana was *asundi*, which described a block upon which one sat in order to meditate. By the time the Yoga Sutra was compiled,[10] yoga was defined as a psycho-spiritual practice aimed at ultimate liberation. Asana, however, was still a very minor aspect of the practice. The Yoga Sutra mentions asana only twice[11] in all one hundred and ninety-six aphorisms. And all that is said about asana is that it should be *sthira* and *sukham*: steady and comfortable. These are very much yin qualities, compared to the style of asana we see performed today in yoga classes. When we are still and the mind undistracted by bodily sensation, meditation can arise.

The point of yoga practices is to enter into a meditative state from which realization or liberation may arise. Different schools of yoga have different techniques for achieving this. Some even claim that one cannot become liberated while in the body. The goal in these dualistic schools is to get out of the body as fast as possible, but this must be done in the right way. Other schools rejected that approach and suggested, since we can meditate and practice yoga only while in the body, we must treat the body well. The body must be healthy. The focus of the Hatha Yoga schools was to build a strong, healthy body that would allow the yogi to meditate for many hours each day. In Hatha Yoga, the practice of asana began to take on a new, broader importance. However, the ultimate goal was still to be able to sit comfortably and steadily for hours.

---

[10] Arguably around 200 C.E. and mythically attributed to the sage Patanjali.
[11] Yoga Sutra, II-29 and II-46.

The Hatha Yoga Pradipika was written around 1350 C.E. by Swami Swatmarama. It is almost twice as long as the Yoga Sutra and has generated a lot of commentary since its writing. It is one of the oldest extant documents we have describing Hatha Yoga. Compared to today's practices, however, it too has very little asana practice in it. There are only sixteen postures described, and of these, half are seated postures. These are quite yin-like in their nature; however, many of the other postures are very definitely yang-like. The peacock (*mayurasana*) is prescribed, and if you have seen this posture performed, there is nothing relaxing or yin-like about it. We are told that one of the sixteen postures is supreme; once one has mastered *siddhasana*, all the other postures are useless.[12] Siddhasana is a simple, yin-like seated posture.

The Hatha Yoga Pradipika claims that Lord Shiva taught the Hatha Yoga sage Matsyendra eighty-four asanas.[13] Other myths claim there are eighty-four thousand or even eight hundred and forty thousand asanas. Regardless, only sixteen are listed in the Pradipika. And of asanas it is said that these should be practiced to gain steady posture, health, and lightness of the body.[14] Not mentioned in any of the Hatha texts is how long one should hold the pose. This is where the guru's guidance is necessary. However, one can

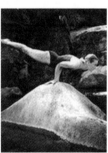

Sarah Powers in Mayurasana

assume that the seated postures were meant to be held a long time while the more vigorous poses like the peacock were held for briefer periods. It is in the seated postures that the *vayus* (the winds or the breath) become trained through *pranayama*.[15] The Lotus Pose (*padmasana*) is the prescribed pose for conducting pranayama.[16]

As time went on, later texts expanded the number of asanas explained. The Gheranda Samhita, written perhaps in the late 1600s, a few hundred years after the Pradipika, describes thirty-two asanas,

---

[12] Hatha Yoga Pradipika, I-43.

[13] Ibid, I-35.

[14] Ibid, I-19.

[15] Pranayama is one way to harness the inner energies we work with in yoga. This is described in more detail in Chapter Five: The Energy Body.

[16] Ibid, II-7 and 8.

of which one-third could be said to be yin-like and the others more yang-like. A trend had begun: more yang asanas compared to yin asanas. A few decades later, the Shiva Samhita listed eighty-four asanas. By the time of the British Raj, when England began to colonize Indian culture and change the school system, asanas were beginning to become blended with forms from the gymnasiums. Wrestling, gymnastics, and other exercises were cross-fertilizing the asana practice. By the end of the nineteenth century there were thousands of asanas. Krishnamacharya[17] said he knew around three thousand postures but that his guru, Ramamohan Brahmachari, knew eight thousand. The era of yang yoga was upon us.

This gradual, and then sudden, evolution of asana practice moved the practice away from the original yin style of holding seated poses for a long time as a preparation for the deeper practice of meditation to the more active yang style of building strength and health. One is not better than the other; they are simply different. To sit for long periods of time in deep, undisturbed meditation requires a body that is open and strong. This opening, especially in the hips and lower back, is developed through a dedicated yin practice. However, if one is in ill health or weak, it is very difficult to sit with focus. A yang practice helps to build a "diamond" body, readying the student for the rigors of advanced yoga practice.

The original styles of physical yoga were very yin-like in nature. Over the past two hundred years the style has changed to be more yang-like. As in all things in life, harmony comes through balance. By combining both styles, progress in practice is more assured.

---

[17] Whose students included BKS Iyengar, Pattabhi Jois and TKV Desikachar.

Paul Grilley's Discovery of Yin Yoga[18]

In the spring of 1979 Paul Grilley was inspired to study yoga after reading *Autobiography of a Yogi* by Paramahansa Yogananda. After two years' study of anatomy with Dr. Garry Parker, he relocated from his home in Columbia Falls, Montana, to Los Angeles to continue his studies at UCLA. While in

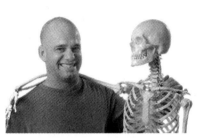

Paul Grilley and Friend

L.A., Paul furthered his study of yoga and began to teach.

Paul's personal yoga practice took him into Ashtanga, where he experienced the joys (and consequent dangers) of doing too many drop backs into *urdhva dhanurasana* (the Wheel). He also ran a Bikram's studio and studied that form of practice. One day, Paul stumbled across a locally televised martial arts interview that featured Paulie Zink. While Paulie's martial arts demonstration was impressive, what really caught Paul's attention was his flexibility. Paulie kept stressing the importance of yoga practice to do martial arts effectively and without injury. Paul contacted Paulie through the TV station. Paulie invited him to attend an ongoing class, which included two hours of long holds of simple postures, and Paul was hooked. Paul became Paulie's student.

In 1990 Paul met Dr. Hiroshi Motoyama. Through Dr. Motoyama's teachings Paul began to see the connection between the asana practices he had been doing and Dr. Motoyama's theory of the meridians. Paul went to Japan to learn more about the way our body's physical and energetic structures are connected through the chakra system. Paul continues to study with Dr. Motoyama as well as host seminars with him.

Paul combined the knowledge he had been given on anatomy, Daoist Yoga, and the meridian theory into the core of his Yin Yoga teachings. His teachings resonated with many people who recognized the benefits of the practice and related to the model of the body/mind/soul Paul offered. One student, who found this practice

---

[18] Adapted from *Yin Yoga* by Paul Grilley.

compelling and highly beneficial to her meditation practice, was Sarah Powers.

From 1998 to 2000 Paul took a sabbatical and relocated to Santa Fe where he earned a master's degree from St. John's College in the study of the Great Books of the Western World. In 2005 he received an honorary PhD from the California Institute of Human Science, founded by Dr. Motoyama. He currently teaches yoga and anatomy worldwide and lives in Ashland, Oregon, with his wife Suzee.[19]

Paulie Zink

Paulie Zink is the fifth-generation master of the art of Ta Sheng Men, or Monkey Kung Fu. He is also a seventh-generation master of the art of Pek Kwar (Ax Fist) Kung Fu. Three times he has been grand champion, with and without weapons, at the Long Beach International Karate Championships. He has been studying kung fu since 1977 and has written many articles and books. He has also 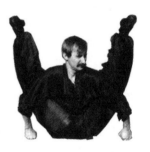 created many videos on Daoist Yoga. For the last few years Paulie has been living near Billings, Montana, and teaching Daoist Yoga throughout the USA and Canada.

The following more detailed biography is from Paulie's own Web site (www.PaulieZink.com).

Paulie Zink began studying yoga and martial arts as a teenager. While he was in college he met a Kung Fu master from Hong Kong named Cho Chat Ling. Master Cho had been imparted with secret martial arts knowledge by his uncle and was obligated to pass on the legacy. He wanted to choose a proficient, worthy practitioner who could show the art to the Western world. He found in Paulie the potential and the tenacity of spirit necessary to meet this aim.

---

[19] You can learn more about Paul at his own Web site: www.PaulGrilley.com.

After some time Master Cho chose Paulie to become his sole protégé. Master Cho came to Paulie's home and instructed him privately every day for six to eight hours. About three hours of his daily practice were devoted to Taoist Yoga and Chi Kung. Paulie was taught Taoist Yoga and Chi Kung as a foundation for his martial arts training. Master Cho taught Paulie three distinct Kung Fu styles combined into a discipline that demanded tremendous mental concentration, harsh physical exercise, and esoteric spiritual practices.

With this intensive level of study it took Paulie seven years to master the art of Taoist Yoga. At this time Master Cho began to taper the frequency of his visits, although Paulie continued to train just as vigorously. By the tenth year Master Cho declared Paulie to be his own master and his training ended. He told Paulie he had transmitted to him in ten years time what would usually require twenty years or more to learn. Paulie is the only Westerner to be traditionally trained in these Kung Fu styles in a direct Chinese lineage from the arts' originators. Master Cho never charged Paulie for his tutelage.

Master Cho insisted Paulie compete in the martial arts arena. Paulie entered in the "Empty Hands" and "Weapons" divisions of approximately one hundred martial arts tournaments from local to regional to national levels. He won the Grand Championship in all of them, often in both divisions. Master Zink's tournament career culminated with him winning the Grand Championship at the Long Beach International Karate Championships three consecutive years.

Master Zink has been inducted into four Martial Arts Halls of Fame. His personal effects are on display at The Martial Arts History Museum in Los Angeles, California. Master Zink has co-authored two books on Monkey Kung Fu. He has starred in numerous martial arts and Taoist Yoga training videos. Dozens of articles about Master Zink and his art have been published in several major martial arts magazines. And he has been featured on many magazine covers. For more information on Master Zink's martial arts background, go to www.monkeykungfu.com.

Master Zink continues to evolve his art of Taoist Yoga. Through many years of study, practice, and teaching he has further developed this ancient tradition into his own distinctive and dynamic style.[20]

Dr. Hiroshi Motoyama

Dr. Motoyama was the inspiration for Paul Grilley, and later Sarah Powers, to delve deeper into the mysterious connection of the physical movements in yoga and the movement of energy through the subtle body. Sarah has described Dr. Motoyama as a yoga adept. He was born of a mother who was an accomplished yogini with advanced psychic abilities. Early in his life Motoyama was also taken under the wing of his mother's teacher who adopted the young Motoyama. Her name was Kinue Motoyama[21] and she was the founder of the Tamamistsu Jinja religious organization.

Tidbits of Dr. Motoyama's life are sprinkled throughout his books. Curious readers can find more details in the book *Awakening of the Chakras and Emancipation*. Here we learn about the rigor of Motoyama's early training and the awakening of his many *vibhutis*, or powers: his ability to see the energy fields, his ability to influence and correct faulty energy, to heal both those close to him and those in need far away.

Dr. Motoyama's brilliance is not limited to his psychic abilities. He holds two PhD degrees. He is also a Shinto priest, one highly respected in Japan. His ability to move freely between the worlds of the spirit and of the physical allowed him to investigate his own abilities using the rigors of Western science and medicine. With the aim of making the subtle measurable, he created instruments that he and others have learned to use to verify the flow of energy through the subtle body.

To further his research and spread his findings, Dr. Motoyama created institutes both in Japan and in the USA. It was during his travels that Paul Grilley came across him. Paul, as noted earlier, was inspired by what Dr. Motoyama revealed and went back with him to

---

[20] To order Paulie's Daoist Yoga videos, or to see his teaching schedule, you can go to his Web site at www.PaulieZink.com.
[21] She was also called Myoko no Kamisama.

Japan. Later Paul introduced Sarah and others to Motoyama and they too embraced the teacher.

Even though he is in his eighties, Dr. Motoyama still travels and teaches. He often comes to Encinitas, California, where he established the California Institute of Human Science (CIHS). His formal biography is available from this Web site.[22]

Sarah Powers

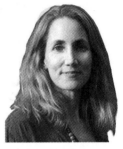

Sarah Powers' journey into the world of Yoga was unplanned. Her initial goal was to learn how her mind worked. She was working on a master's degree in psychology when the detour that was to consume her occurred: she chose to study a topic based upon a book that had been lying around her home for many years. It was a book on yoga; Sarah fell in love.

Fortunately, Sarah was already married at the time this new direction appeared in her life. Supported by her husband Ty, she was able to delve deeply into the practice of yoga. She took teacher training courses and began teaching in Malibu. Her practice gravitated to the yang styles, but at that time she had no awareness that yoga could be yin or yang.

One day, after a lovely and sweaty Ashtanga class, Sarah tried a class Paul Grilley was teaching. That was her first taste of yin; it was delicious. Sarah loved sinking deeply into the poses. However, at that time Paul's classes were mostly conducted in silence; he didn't explain the various and deep benefits that Yin Yoga has for the body. Eventually life's changes took both Sarah and Paul along separate paths. Sarah did not see Paul again for many years.

After several years of building her physical yoga practice, Sarah decided it was time to face her mind. Ty had been studying the mind and consciousness for many years already, and Sarah felt like she was still just catching up to him. She decided to do a ten-day vipassana retreat in Asia. Despite the very flexible muscles and wide range of motion that her yang practice gave her, Sarah found sitting for an

---

[22] www.cihs.edu.

hour several times in a day to be excruciating. She was amazed how poorly prepared she was physically for the practice of meditation. It is hard to face your mind when all you can hear is your body screaming.

Fortunately Sarah's path again crossed Paul's. She returned to the yin practice she had dropped a few years before. This time, Paul explained the benefits of the practice. This understanding convinced Sarah she needed to stick with both the yin-style and the yang-style of asana practice. Her next vipassana retreat was a completely different experience: she was able to sit calmly and go deeper into mindfulness without the distractions she suffered earlier.

Ty and Sarah had been investigating Buddhist mindfulness: Sarah began combining this aspect of the practice with the physical and energetic work of yoga. Their Tibetan teacher, Tsoknyi Rinpoche, influenced them greatly as did their Zen teacher, Toni Packer.

Today Sarah interweaves the insights and practices of yoga and Buddhism into an integral practice to enliven the body, heart, and mind. Her yoga style blends both a yin sequence of long-held poses to enhance the meridian and organ systems, combined with a flow or yang practice, influenced by Viniyoga, Ashtanga, and Iyengar teachers.

Sarah feels that enlivening the physical and pranic bodies, as well as learning to open up to our emotional blockages, is paramount for preparing us to deepen and nourish insights into our essential nature – a natural state of awareness. She draws from her studies in transpersonal psychology, as well as her in-depth training in the vipassana, Tantric and Dzogchen practices of Buddhism. She now teaches trainings and silent retreats internationally with Ty. They live with their teenage daughter Imani Jade in Marin, California. [23]

---

[23] For more information, please visit Sarah's Web site at www.SarahPowers.com. Here you can find her DVDs *Yin and Vinyasa Yoga* and *Insight Yoga.*

Chapter Three:
Our Bodies and Yoga's Benefits

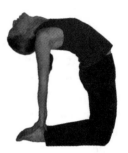

The benefits of a yoga or meditation practice have been known for millennia in the East. In the West, the claims were not believed until very recently. Fortunately these benefits have become accepted in the West through the efforts of many broadminded scientists and medical researchers. Benefits can be found in virtually every aspect of human health: physically, emotionally, and mentally as well as, oftentimes underappreciated, spiritually.

To understand the benefits of yoga we need to first understand ourselves. Yinsights into the way the body works, how energy flows and even how our minds operate, provide a baseline upon which we can observe how a dedicated yoga practice influences us. This requires us to first investigate ourselves, before observing the changes yoga can have upon us.

Models

The way we study reality is by creating a model to explain what we observe and to predict behavior. The way to study ourselves also requires us to create models. The problem is, most people forget that their knowledge is conceptual and the model is not the reality. We can never know reality; our perceptions are too limited, and our methods of describing reality are self-limiting. What we can do is create conceptual constructs that are useful for predicting and explaining behaviors. Whether we are creating scientific models using

Western methodologies or creating models based on metaphors using Eastern experiences, these are all still models. Please do not confuse the model with reality.

Understanding the model nature of our knowledge is important. Too often people dismiss a perfectly valid model because they believe it is not "real." A model is never meant to be real – it is meant to be useful. And there are many different ways to model the same thing. For example, a map is simply a model of a territory. A map of the city of Vancouver is never mistaken for Vancouver itself. One map (one model) may show all the roads and traffic lights, which is very useful for navigating around the city. Another map (a different model) may show all the parks and trees. This is also useful if you are trying to figure out where to buy a home or where to walk your cat. These are two very different models of the same underlying reality.

The same dichotomy occurs even in the scientific domains. Physicists use one model to describe the nature of light when they are observing light as a wave; they use a completely different model when they are observing light as a particle. Reality has not changed but we require more than one model to be able to explain reality's behavior. We need more than one map to completely describe the city of Vancouver too. This does not mean the models are wrong; it is just an admission that models are not reality, and it is useful to have competing models or views of reality.

A scientific model is considered valid when it can predict all the observed behaviors and make forecasts of as yet unobserved behaviors that can be verified through well-designed experiments. To be considered well designed these experiments must be reproducible by anyone using the same techniques under the same circumstances, and the results must be consistent. If this is so, we consider the model to be valid. But scientists never believe the model to be reality. It is simply one possible description of how reality works.

Generally in the scientific world, we strive to unify competing or smaller models into one large, more comprehensive view. This is not always possible and the grand unified theory is still being sought by physicists as a way to combine the models for the forces of electromagnetism, the strong and weak nuclear forces, and the force of gravity. In the research of yogis throughout the centuries, many different psycho-spiritual models have been developed. This leads to confusion because so many of these models sound similar on the surface. There is a danger for a student who is not being taught by a teacher intimately familiar with the chosen model. The student may attempt to combine (or her teacher may present) pieces of different models without understanding the risk in doing so. Cobbling together elements of different models does not lead to a new coherent model. Be cautious of teachers who blithely recite bits of teaching from different schools, implying that all these techniques will yield the desired results if practiced diligently. It is useful to understand many models, but the unification of different models requires a lot of testing to make sure the new model is valid.

In our school system we expect our post-secondary teachers to be very experienced. Professors should teach from their own base of knowledge. Also, when we are beginning to seriously study advanced yoga practice, we need to seek a teacher who has experience with a complete and coherent model, and teaches from what she knows through her experience. In the earlier school levels, we can gain value from teachers who haven't had the direct experience of the highest teaching. The same benefits apply in our earlier yoga studies. We can learn the basics from many people. But once you start to study at a deeper level, you will need to find the teacher who really knows. Yoga, in the end, is experiential not theoretical; you will need an experienced teacher.

As we have just discussed, models are found in the psycho-spiritual investigations of yoga. As one example, we will look at a model called "the Chakra Theory." This is not an attempt to state definitively that we all have chakras and they all operate exactly as the models describe. Rather, like all models, the chakra model is an attempt to explain observed behaviors and predict what would happen if certain conditions arise. The challenge in psycho-spiritual investigations is – not all participants are capable of reproducing the same results, because their skills vary considerably. Science attempts to minimize (but rarely eliminates) the skill of the observer. This is not possible in the subjective sciences that we will be dealing with.

Do not mistake the map for the territory. If you remember this, then your mind may stay open longer when it is faced with things outside your normal experience.

The Kosha Model

To begin our investigations into ourselves, and the way Yin Yoga affects us, we will adopt a very old but still useful model: the *koshas*. In the Taittiriya Upanishad[24] a model of our self is given. Each layer of our being is described as a sheath, or a bag, called a "kosha." Five such sheaths exist, each one being more subtle than the previous. They are like layers of an onion, or a child's toy of nested dolls stacked one inside the other.

The layers are

1. The *annamaya* kosha
   … the physical sheath
2. The *pranamaya* kosha
   … the energy sheath
3. The *manomaya* kosha
   … the lower mind sheath
4. The *vijnanamaya* kosha
   … the higher mind sheath
5. The *anandamaya* kosha … the bliss sheath

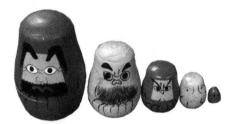

Russian dolls are a good metaphor for our koshas. [B]

Inside the final sheath is our true being, which cannot be described in words, only experienced.

While the kosha model is a rather primitive and early attempt to describe ourselves, it is a nice, simple way to investigate how our bodies work, and how yoga affects us. Following this simple model we will investigate our first three sheaths and see how Eastern and Western views compare.

---

[24] The Upanishads are Hindu sacred texts compiled after the Vedas. Some are over twenty-eight hundred years old while others were written only two hundred years ago. The Taittiriya Upanishad is just one of the hundreds of Upanishads, but it is one of the earliest.

The Physical Body
The Annamaya Kosha

There are three things that we physically do to our bodies in yoga asana practice: we compress tissues, we stretch tissues, and we twist tissues. Technically these three movements are called compression, tension, and shear. The drawings show each of these movements. For example, in back bends we compress the facets of the vertebrae into each other (which, as we will see, is very healthy for the bones); in forward bends we stretch the fascia, muscles, and ligaments along the back of the spine; and in twists we provide a shearing force between the vertebrae and the ribs, which both compresses and stretches the tissues between each pair of ribs.

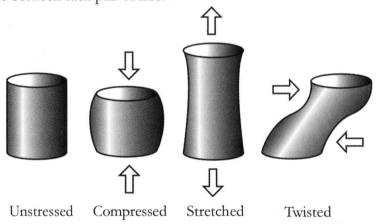

Unstressed   Compressed   Stretched   Twisted

These three forces affect the body on many levels. Through twisting, elongating, and compressing of tissues, our bodies become rejuvenated in the same way an old sponge can be resurrected, by soaking it in warm water and twisting, squeezing, and stretching it – the old grungy particles trapped in the tissues of the sponge are released and carried away by the warm water. Similarly our tissues are massaged by asana practice, releasing toxins and waste products. Even old scar tissue can be broken down and removed.

Yoga promotes the flow of energy in the body through both stimulating energy release (especially in the active yang practices) and through removing deep blockages to the energy flow (especially in the more passive yin practices). Our blood and lymphatic systems serve the same function as the warm water in the example of cleaning a sponge. Another analogy is a garden hose that has been left unused for years, lying in the grass of an overgrown back yard. Insects and mud (toxins) eventually clog the hose (which could be called a *"meridian"* or *"nadi"*). When the water (which could be called our energy or *"prana"*) is turned on, it can't flow. These clogs have to be removed, and we do so by turning on the water and bending and stretching the hose. Once the flow of energy has been freed or increased, information and nourishment flow throughout the body. Chapter Five: The Energy Body, describes this in more detail.

Our physical bodies are made up of many types of tissues and these tissues respond differently to exercise. Yang yoga is excellent at working the muscle tissues. Yin Yoga is especially effective at working the deeper connective tissues of the body. To fully understand the benefits of yoga, we need to understand the nature of these tissues. The next several sections take us further along our journey of exploration by investigating the:

- Tissues (and their flexibility)
- Muscles
- Fascia
- Connective tissues

When we have finished this segment of our journey we will take a closer look at our joints.

Tissues

Tissues are simply aggregations of cells in our body that have a similar purpose and arrangement. Obviously tissues are found everywhere throughout the body and have many functions. Generally though there are four main kinds of tissues. These are:

- Epithelia tissue (skin, linings of our organs, etc.)
- Nervous tissue
- Muscle tissue
- Connective tissue (CT)

Yoga most obviously affects these last two, although it actually affects the whole body. Every time we move we are engaging muscle to create the movement, and each movement stretches, twists, or compresses all the tissues in the area affected by the movement as well as areas farther away. For our investigation of how yoga affects and benefits the physical body we will look more closely at these last two types of tissues:

- Muscle tissue – including its fascia
- Connective tissues – including collagen (the principal component of CT) and ground substance (the fluid component)

Before we head into a closer examination of our muscles and connective tissues, it is helpful to understand one more facet of our physical body. Let's spend a moment understanding what stops us from being more flexible. What limits our flexibility?

Limits of Flexibility

As we discussed earlier, all of our physical yoga practice does one of three things to our tissues: we stretch the tissues, compress them, or apply a shear to them. This simple fact dictates what stops us from going deeper into any posture. The resistance to stretching, or said another way, the limitation on our flexibility, is due either to tension along the tissues, which resist further movement, or compression, where two parts of the body come into contact and prevent further movement.

If tension is stopping the movement, it is felt in the direction away from the movement. For example ... stand up and fold one leg backward, moving your heel toward your buttock. If the heel stops before the calf presses into the back of the leg it may be due to tension in the quadriceps. This tension in the quadriceps is in the opposite direction from the movement of the lower leg. If compression is stopping the movement, it is felt in the direction of the movement. In this example, compression may occur when the calf is squeezed into the back of the thigh or when the heel pushes into the buttock.

In some cases whether tension or compression is limiting movement is not easy to determine, and part of our practice is to pay attention to what is happening in the body when we move. A useful mantra to repeat during asana practice is "What is stopping me from going further?" The answer to that question may influence your practice considerably.[25]

The range of motion (ROM) we have in our joints, if it is limited by tension, can be increased through asana practice, breathing, and even diet. When the limit to the ROM has been reached and compression is stopping further movement, no amount of yoga will increase it; you have reached the limit of flexibility that asana practice will provide you. However, diet, injury, surgery, and other interventions may reduce the point of compression thus increasing the ROM. For example, a woman nine months pregnant may not be able to touch her toes due to compression of her belly and her legs. Yoga will not help her now! Once she has delivered her baby, the point of compression has changed, and her range of motion in that direction will increase again.

When tissue's resistance limits the ROM, the resistance has been found to come in four main areas: the skin, the tendon of the muscle, the muscle itself and its fascia, and the joint capsule – all provide

---

[25] A more general mantra useful at any time in life is a similar question, "What is stopping me?" The answer to that question is also extremely illuminating, although often very difficult to find.

tensile resistance to movement. The following table shows how the resistance is distributed relatively in these four areas:[26]

Muscle (and its fascia)	41%
Tendon	10%
Skin	2%
Connective Tissues (the joint capsule)	47%

As shown, the biggest single limit to flexibility, when it is caused by tension, is the joints' rigidity, followed by the muscle and its fascia. Yang yoga is excellent for opening us to the limits of flexibility of our muscle tissue, its fascia, and our skin. Yin Yoga is required to safely open the joints to their healthy limits. [27] As we continue to investigate the muscles and connective tissues, we will learn how we can open them more deeply. The exercises to open connective tissues will be examined in the second part of our journey down the Yin River – The Practice of Yin Yoga. For now, let's look closer at the muscles.

Muscles

Muscular tissue has three main jobs: create motion, maintain posture and balance, and create heat. There are three basic kinds of muscular tissues:

- Skeletal muscles … which move our limbs
- Cardiac muscles … which make our hearts pump
- Smooth muscles … which line our blood vessels and other tubes

---

[26] Johns and Wright, 1962.

[27] It is not recommended to deliberately try to lengthen the tendons; these tissues need to remain at their normal length to help maintain fine control of our movements. Since tendons are directly connected to muscles, it is very difficult to target a Yin Yoga exercise strictly at a tendon. However, since the material in a tendon is closer in makeup to a ligament, the tendon, being more yin-like, will not respond well to yang-type exercise. Thus the muscle protects the tendon by taking up the stretch.

The active, yang, styles of yoga specifically target the skeletal and the cardiac muscles. But again, the whole body does benefit from an active yoga practice. However, the major benefits of a yang style of asana practice are the strengthening and lengthening of our muscle tissues.

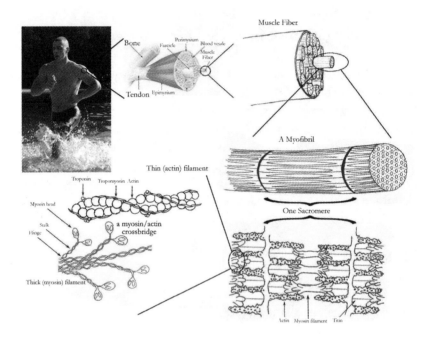

Muscles illustrate the "tubes within tubes" model of our body. C

The Make-up of Muscles

Muscles are connected to the bones via tendons. That is a simplification; in reality there is continuum of tissues from the muscles that turn into tendons, which in turn gradually become bone. The body is not made up of discontinuous pieces. Everything is connected and a part of everything else. But it does help us to understand the body if we employ simplifying models. So let's go with this simplification of bones, tendons, and muscles for now.

If we look closer at the muscle itself, we find it is composed of tubes nested within tubes within tubes. This is a common feature of the body. Most of the body can be considered a system of tubes; the muscles are just one example. If we zoom in, we eventually find a single fiber of muscle tissue, which is called a "myofibril." Again, this tube of myofibril is made up of smaller fibers. One unit of the fibers, called a "sarcomere," contains interconnected filaments of actin, myosin, and titin. The actin fibers are thin filaments; the myosin fibers are thick filaments. The titin fibers connect the myosin fibers to the wall of the sarcomere (called the "Z-line," which is not named in the diagram).

Around the myofibril, the single contracting fiber, but still within the muscle itself, are connective tissues or fascia. Connective tissue can make up as much as thirty percent of the mass of the muscle. It contributes to the muscle's ability to stretch and allows the neighboring fibers to slide along each other. Any program of exercise trying to lengthen the muscles will also affect the muscle's fascia.

Contracting Muscles

The function of the muscle is to create tension, which is called contraction. Usually this contraction creates movement or maintains posture. One theory on how this works is that the sliding of the actin between the myosin filaments draws the walls of the sarcomere closer together. If the actin filaments get too close to each other they may overlap. Maximum contraction is reached when the myosin filaments hit the walls. When maximal compression happens the sarcomere may be shorter by twenty to fifty percent. This can vary depending upon the type of muscle and where it is in the body. Contraction requires the consumption of energy[28] in the muscle's cells, but now we are getting too technical.[29]

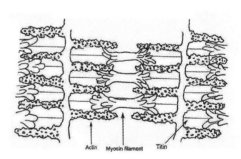

Actin   Myosin filament   Titin

The sliding nature of the muscle fibers is evident in this illustration. D

---

[28] This is provided by the conversion of adenosine triphosphate (ATP) into adenosine diphosphate (ADP) and phosphate (P).

[29] For more information on this topic you may want to read *The Science of Flexibility* by Michael Alter.

Stretching Muscles

When a force from outside the muscle is applied that moves the walls of the sarcomere apart, stretching occurs. The muscle cannot stretch itself. Studies[30] have shown that a muscle can normally stretch up to fifty percent or in some cases sixty-seven percent longer than its resting length, before rupturing occurs.

Again, in the sliding theory, stretching occurs when the filaments simply slide along each other, until the titin filaments can't be extended any farther. Neither the actin nor the myosin filaments (in this theory) change lengths, but the titin filaments can and do lengthen. The theory postulates that the titin fibers are folded up like an accordion, with many V's adjoining each other. Once pulled to its maximum length, the V's get shallow and become straight. Once they are straight, the maximum length of the sarcomere is reached.[31]

The lengths of the resting sarcomeres are generally constant. A prominent theory holds that increased strength and range of motion in a muscle is caused by a large increase in the number of sarcomeres along the length of the fibers. Several studies have shown that the adding (or subtracting) of sarcomeres is not regulated by neuronal control (i.e., this is not directed by the brain), but by responses within the muscle itself.

Changes in Our Muscles as We Age

The normal aging process and injury can result in a loss of strength and range of motion of the muscles. This is termed atrophy, and can be caused by both a reduction of the number of sarcomeres in a muscle as well as a shortening of the remaining sarcomeres. The

---

[30] Again, see Alter's book.

[31] At the scale of the whole body, when we stretch a muscle we want to feel the stretch in the middle of the muscle not at the attachment. This is true for the full muscle (do not stretch so much that you feel strain in the tendon, which is where the muscle attaches to the bone) as well as within the individual sarcomeres. During the first stage of stretching, the myosin and actin filaments move apart. Eventually the titin starts to unfold. Since the titin anchors the myosin filaments to the wall, too much stretching here can cause damage and tear the filaments.

number of nerve cells in the muscles also decreases, and the muscle fibers are replaced by fatty and fibrous tissues (known as "collagen"). Collagen does not stretch nearly as well as the sarcomeres. As we age, the collagen content in our muscles continues to increase, further weakening the muscle and reducing its range of motion. This effect can also be caused prematurely by immobility of the muscle, the classic – use it or lose it – syndrome. Yoga, obviously, counteracts this tendency, by using the muscles.

As muscles shorten due to age or immobility, they also become less flexible. The size change is due to fewer sarcomeres. The rigidity is caused by an increasing number of collagen molecules. This is the worst of all worlds ... we lose strength, size, and flexibility in muscles that grow older or are not used.

Yoga's Effect on Muscles

Yoga can strengthen and lengthen the muscles: this is unique. Most forms of exercise that strengthen muscles also tend to shorten them. If a muscle is habitually held in a shortened position for long periods of time, due to strongly contracting the muscle, the body removes sarcomeres along the length of the fibers while adding them in parallel to the remaining sarcomeres.

As shown earlier, shorter muscles tend to become stiffer due to the increase in collagen. Yoga, however, lengthens the muscles, while they are being strengthened, stimulating sarcomeres to be added in both the horizontal and vertical directions. Yoga also prevents the increase of collagen.

The myofibrils and their sarcomeres are not the only component of a muscle. What is not seen in the image shown earlier is the material that surrounds and supports the myofibrils. This is the fascia of the muscle, and it plays an important role in the strength and elasticity of the muscle. Our journey continues with a visit to our fascia.

Fascia

The term fascia is a Latin word that means "band" or "bandage." It is used when we are discussing fibrous connective structures that don't have a more specific definition. You would be safe to think of fascia as any connective tissue that doesn't have a more specific name.[32]

Fascia can vary in thickness and density depending upon where it is, and what it is being used for. Often it is found in sheets. There is a type of fascia located just beneath the surface of the skin (called the "superficial fascia" or "hypodermis") and another type directly beneath this (called the "deep fascia"), which is usually tougher and tighter than the superficial fascia. Embedded inside this deep fascia are the tissues of the muscles, the blood vessels, and all the other tubes that wind through the body. A third kind of fascia lines the body's cavities. For our purposes we are mostly interested in the deep fascia and how it contributes to the flexibility of the muscles.

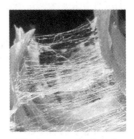

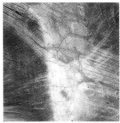

The fascia exposed. [E]

As seen in these three images, muscle fibers are embedded inside the deep fascia. In the first image the fascia has been teased so that it is easy to see.[33] The second image again shows muscles and fascia, the fascia being the streaks of white. The third image shows the pervasiveness of the fascia. Normal anatomy drawings don't show the fascia and concentrate only on the muscles, leading to a misguided impression that the muscles (and the bones, etc.) are distinct, separate systems within our body. Distinct they are – separate they are not.

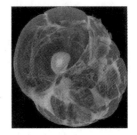

The facia is deeply embedded in all our tissues. [F]

---

[32] Later we will have a more general description of connective tissues.

[33] The thick fibers are muscle fibers; the thin white streaks strung between the muscle fibers are strands of fascia.

In reality, as shown here, everything is interconnected, and all the tissues work together. The deep fascia merges with all the other tissues embedded within it. Even the organs cannot be completely separated from the bed of deep fascia. The organs are continuous with the fascia. The muscles are the same. We can make only an arbitrary definition as to what is muscle tissue and what is deep fascia. They are actually one continuum. What we do to one, we do to all. For this reason some modern texts and body workers prefer to use the term "myofascial" to refer to the muscle and fascia together. After all, it is impossible to contract or stretch our muscles without also compressing or stretching our fascia.

The fascia can make up thirty percent of the tissue in the muscle. There are probably three functions of the intramuscular fascia (or the connective tissue, as it is also called):

1. It binds the muscle together, while ensuring proper alignment of the muscle fibers, the blood vessels flowing through the muscles, the nerves and other components of the muscle.
2. It transmits the forces applied to the muscle evenly to all parts of the muscle.
3. It lubricates the various surfaces that need to move or slide along each other.

These are important functions. It is the fascia that allows the muscle to change shape and lengthen. When we work to increase the range of motion of a muscle, it is not only the muscle fibers (the sarcomeres) that need to be freed up or lengthened; the fascia provides a great deal of the tensile resistance found in a muscle and needs to be released as well.

The fascia is not only continuous with the muscles, organs, and all tissues found within it, the fascia is connected together throughout the body. In one model of our body, it is the fascia that holds us together. It is fascia that keeps the bones connected and upright … without fascia the bones would collapse to the floor, like a medical school skeleton without its wires.

This continuity within the fascia means a small movement in one area of the body pulls on the whole web of fascia connected throughout the body. If you are paying close attention, the slightest movement at one end of the body can be felt at the other end. This is what makes it possible to feel the movement of the breath everywhere in the body – all it requires is attention and practice.

As briefly mentioned above, fascia is sometimes called connective tissue. In fact, fascia can be considered to be a particular type of connective tissue but CT is even more pervasive than fascia and has a big impact as well on our flexibility and health. To really understand why yoga is so beneficial for us, we need to also understand our connective tissues.

Connective Tissues

Normally it is thought that our connective tissues provide support to the structure of the body, giving it the shape we have, and provide binding or rigidity to the whole system. However, this view misses many other important functions of our connective tissue and fascial network. Beyond meeting the needs of the body for stability and flexibility, the connective tissue is important for our ability to respond to demands. For example, the CT plays a role in healing the body following certain traumas, such as a broken bone.

Connective tissue is a broad term that refers to biological tissues that are used to bind, support, and protect other tissues. CT is extra-cellular, which simply means the tissues are not cells in themselves, but are the materials surrounding and in between cells. Because they are not cellular, many people feel CT is not alive. However, as we will see, CT is very much alive. It responds to stimuli and reacts to keep the body healthy. It is CT that creates and maintains the matrix of the body.

Fascia and connective tissues can be confusing terms. There are many and various cells found inside the body, as shown in the image on the next page. These include nerve cells, fat cells (adipose), blood cells (macrophages, plasma cells, mast cells, and lymphocytes), and blood vessels (capillaries). Weaving their way through all this are fibers, such as collagen and elastin, which are connecting the tissues together. As the name implies, elastin is elastic and lends flexibility while binding the structure.[34] Collagen is relatively inelastic and

---

[34] Within the context of flexibility, elastin is yang-like.

provides rigidity to the structure.[35] The collection of elastin and collagen can be considered the fascia for this area of the body. Not so obvious, at first, is the ground substance that flows around all the cells. This ground substance is worth studying, as it affects us in many ways, but we will look at this later.

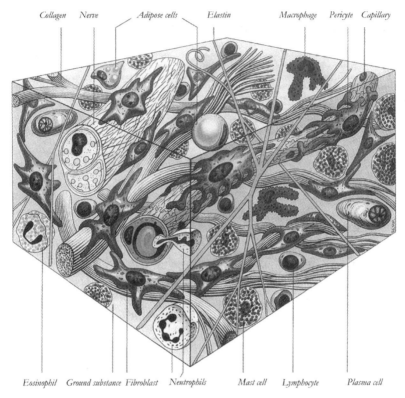

Collagen   Nerve   Adipose cells   Elastin   Macrophage   Pericyte Capillary

Eosinophil Ground substance Fibroblast   Neutrophils   Mast cell   Lymphocyte   Plasma cell

Extracellular materials include many connective tissues. G

Connective tissues are considered to be of four types. These are:

- Bone
- Blood
- Cartilage
- And all the others

---

[35] Collagen is yin-like.

Under "others" we can include, for example, dense CT that includes our tendons and ligaments. When we have no other name to give the CT, fascia is often the term used.

Our connective tissue is what gives us shape and helps to restrain our movements. Bones are the most resistant to movement; cartilage is softer than bone and restrains our activities less strongly. Ligaments, which bind bones together, also act to restrain movement depending upon their location or arrangement surrounding a joint. And then, even less constricting than any of the above but still contributing to restriction of our activities (sometimes more than we would prefer!), there is the fascia (loose connective tissues) that binds and stabilizes the body.

Bones and Cartilage

Our bones are not at all like the bones you may have seen in labs, on a skeleton, or even after a non-vegetarian meal. Usually people see or notice only the "hard" parts of a bone. This is the mineralized bone, which is generally made up of calcium salts that are deposited between the collagen fibers of the bone. What is missing is the mesh of collagen, which is much more leather-like than hard. In living bone there is a significant portion of both collagen and calcium salts. The mineral salts help us tolerate compression of the bone while the collagen helps us resist tension that would bend or break the bone.

If the bone was made only of mineral salt and was subjected to extreme pressure, it would snap the way an old tree branch breaks: cleanly. However, healthy, especially young bone, with a high degree of collagen meshing, breaks more like a living branch of a tree. If you have ever tried to snap off a living branch you know that is just bends, crumpling one side while fraying the side away from the pressure.[36]

Examined closely, the inside of our bones appears porous. This sponge-like scaffolding allows the bones to be light and yet incredibly strong. The spongy-looking part is called "trabecular" bone and it is

---

[36] If this is hard to imagine, go find a green branch and try to break it cleanly. It can't be done. Only old, dried-out branches snap in half. The same difference is found in young and old bones.

more elastic than the harder outer skin of the bone, which is called "cortical" bone. Trabecular bone is more active, more subject to bone turnover, to remodeling. The ratio of trabecular to cortical bone varies throughout the body depending upon the need. For example, the bones of the rib are not weight bearing and so they have much higher trabecular content. Our leg bones have much more cortical bone.

Cartilage is similar in makeup to bone but has a different ratio of collagen to mineral salts and other components. The cartilage in our nose, for example, has much more hydration[37] than our bones. The cartilage in our ears is even more flexible thanks to the presence of more elastin fibers. In our intervertebral disks we have fibrocartilage with a higher proportion of collagen to chondroitin. This allows the cartilage in our spines to have greater weight-bearing support than we would find in the cartilage in our ears.

Cartilage supports tissues and provides a degree of structure and firmness. Bones do exactly the same thing, but to a different degree. Of significant interest to the student of yoga are the three kinds of the "other" connective tissues: tendons, ligaments, and the fasciae. Each of these has different degrees of flexibility, caused by their different makeup. We have already looked at fasciae, so now let's look at tendons and ligaments.

Tendons and Ligaments

Tendons are connective tissues that join muscles to the bones. Gradually the tissues of the muscle become the tissues of the tendon, which in turn gradually evolve into bone tissue. Once again we see that the body is not segregated, as many medical models imply. Such separation of parts of the body is just a convenience for learning, not reality.

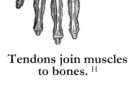

Tendons join muscles to bones. [H]

---

[37] Thanks to chondroitin-sulfate.

It is the muscles' job to provide the varying degrees of tension that allows precise movements to occur. The tendon does not change its shape when the muscle does. If the tendon were to change shape or stretch, it would affect the precise control the body has over desired movements. We rely upon the nervous system to control the muscular contraction to create movement. The only nervous system interaction with the tendon comes from sensors in the tendon that tell us when a stretch has become too strong. When this happens, cells, called the "Golgi tendon organs," embedded in the tendon, signal the nervous system to quickly and suddenly relax the muscle.[38] A stretch of four percent in a tendon is considered the limit to its elasticity. Forces that would stretch the tendon farther than four percent could permanently damage the tendon.

Ligaments

Ligaments are similar in construction to tendons but their function is to bind bones together, usually supporting a joint. Unlike tendons, ligaments come in a variety of shapes: they can be chords, sheets, or bands. Where tendons are generally white in appearance, ligaments can be darker due to their mixture of elastic and finer fibers. Ligaments can be pliant and flexible in the directions where they are not binding the body.[39] These qualities make ligaments ideal for protecting joints, which may move in a variety of ways. Ligaments are tough, strong, pliable, and yet inelastic. The illiotibial band running down the outside of your thigh, for example, is strong enough to support the weight of a car without snapping!

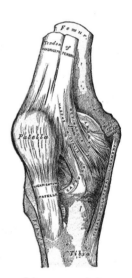

Ligaments join bones to bones. [H]

---

[38] This is noticeable at the end of an arm wrestling match when the losing competitor collapses suddenly … his body is reacting to a stretch signal that is telling him he is close to damaging himself and thus the effort ceases.
[39] Imagine a credit card … it is pliant and flexible, yet it will resist being stretched longer or wider.

Not all ligaments are rigid along their lengths; some ligaments have a higher proportion of elastic fibers (elastin) than collagen. Elastin[40] gives us an ability to stretch tissues just like muscles do. They distribute stress instead of maintaining it in one place. The ligaments in the vertebral column of our lumbar spine and in our necks are especially elastic in this way. In fact, the ligaments in the lumbar spine are the most flexible ligaments in our body. When elastin fibers age they become mineralized and cross-linked with other fibers – they become stiffer.

The tendons and ligaments are quite dry compared to the muscle or other tissues of the body. They generally contain only one to three percent "glycosaminoglycans," the molecules that hydrate our tissues.[41]

Plastic Versus Elastic

Like tendons, ligaments that are stretched suddenly and farther than about four percent will be damaged and tear or remain stretched.[42] In this regard ligaments and tendons are said to be plastic rather than elastic. Elastic materials, like our muscles or an elastic band, can be stretched considerably, and once stretched they will still revert back to their original shape. Plastic materials, like our ligaments or plasticine, if stretched will remain in the new shape. Once a ligament or tendon is stretched, it will not recover its original shape or size on its own. However, the body may repair it over time. For these reasons, the way in which we exercise plastic tissues must be different from the way we exercise elastic tissues.

This does not mean we should not exercise our ligaments or tendons; we just have to take care when we do so that we don't exceed their limits. We do not have to worry about our tendons normally … the muscles will do the stretching for us. However, even here we do have to be careful that we don't overdo the effort. Damage to tendons can happen and generally pain is present as a

---

[40] Which is produced by our fibroblasts, as explained in our next section.
[41] See the section Ground Substances for more details on glycosaminoglycans.
[42] There are exceptions, such as the ligaments in our spine, as noted earlier.

signal that something is wrong. Listening for these warning signals is the best way to prevent tearing anything.

Now that we know what connective tissue is, we look at what it is made of. Mostly what it is made of is collagen.

Collagen

The reason tendons and ligaments do not stretch (very much) is that they are made up predominantly of collagen. Collagen is a ubiquitous and amazing substance found throughout our bodies. It is made up of a protein, the most abundant one in our body. What makes this protein so useful are its

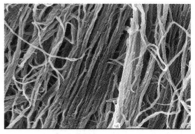

One example of collagen fibers. [1]

strength and resistance to stretching. Unlike most proteins, which form clumps when gathered together, collagen is fibrous and can form mats, sheets, or chord-like structures.

Collagen is what makes our teeth strong, yet it gives our skin its elasticity and strength. When it degrades it creates wrinkles. The word itself comes from the Greek language and means "glue producer." That gives us a sense of what it does for us … it helps hold us together.

Of the twenty-seven of types of collagen, it is the Type 1 collagen that is of the most interest for this exploration. Type 1 collagen is found in our skin, bones, ligaments, and tendons. It is found in the scar tissue that is present after healing. It was collagen that plastic surgeons used to use to enhance the lips of women looking for something better than what Mother Nature provided.

Like the general structure of all tissues in our body, connective tissue has substructures that follow the tubes-within-tubes model. For example, a tendon has bundles within it called "fascicles," and within these are found fibrils. Within fibrils are subfibrils, and then microfibrils. These in turn are made up of collagen molecules that are composed of chains and cross-links. These cross-links are one of the reasons that collagen is so strong. The more cross-links there are, the stronger the net is. These cross-links are like welds joining together the individual strands in a rope, making them stronger. Of course, the stronger the rope, the less flexible it will be.

Collagen is continually being laid down and absorbed by the body. Cells called "fibroblasts"[43] produce collagen. If the rate of production of collagen is faster than the rate of absorption, then more cross-links are created and the fibers are more resistant to stretching, but are stronger. If the opposite occurs, and the rate of absorption is faster than the rate of production, then fewer cross-links are produced and the fiber is more elastic. Researchers[44] speculated that exercise or mobilization can restrict the number of cross-links, thus increasing flexibility while reducing rigidity. Thus we can see how the practice of yoga can make collagen fibers more flexible.

Collagen in the Bones

Fibroblasts create the collagen fibers found in our connective tissues, but they are not the only cells that create fibers. Other cells also create the connective tissue fibers found in our bones. In this case, instead of fibroblasts, osteoblasts are laying down new bone fibers. Over ninety percent of the bone is made from Type I collagen. Other cells, called "osteoclasts" do the opposite; osteoclasts reabsorb collagen, cleaning up old bones by degrading the collagen and releasing its components into the bloodstream.

Directional Stress on Connective Tissues

The direction of growth of the collagen fibers is key. When the osteoblasts or fibroblasts create collagen fibers, they are randomly laid down in all directions. When a stress is applied along a predominant direction, electrical fields are generated by the fibers that experience the stress.[45] This electric field prevents the osteoclasts from reabsorbing those fibers, but fibers that are not being stressed, and thus have not created an electric field, are reabsorbed. Over time,

---

[43] Fibroblasts produce a wide variety of other substances found in the extracellular matrix, such as elastin.

[44] W.M. Bryant, 1977; Shephard, 1982.

[45] See Chapter Five: The Energy Body, for more about how this happens.

the body absorbs all fibers that are not supporting stress, leaving behind the fibers that are meant to do the work.

Astronauts in orbit, who are thus weightless, have no stress upon the collagen fibers in their bones. Their osteoclasts are free to reabsorb their bones everywhere. Studies of cosmonauts and astronauts who spent many months on space station Mir revealed that space travelers will lose, on average, one to two percent of bone mass each month. In some astronauts the lack of stress has resulted in a much greater loss of bone density – up to twenty percent over a six-month stay in space! This loss of bone density generally occurred in the lower body and the lumbar vertebrae (the lower back).

Connective tissues respond to demands, to stresses upon them. Stressing the body is essential in order to keep it healthy. Bones need stress to remain strong: so too do ligaments and tendons. Simply walking is a great way to stress the bones of the legs, pelvis, and spine. Yin Yoga is another way to provide this stress, in an intelligent and safe way, to targeted areas of the body. Specifically, Yin Yoga targets those areas where the astronauts suffered the most bone loss – the legs and lower back.

Aging or Damage of Connective Tissues

When the collagen fibers within the connective tissues are healthy they generally line up quite straight, and along the direction of the predominant stress. The top image here indicates this in a simple graphical way. Shown are the major parallel lines of collagen fibers in a tendon.

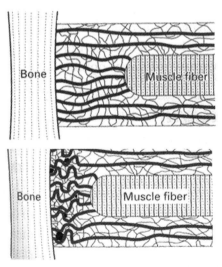

As the body ages or is damaged, these relatively straight fibers become tangled or bent and as a result they are shorter, drawing the muscle and the bone closer

Collagen fibers change as we age ┘

together and decreasing the range of movement possible. The bottom image shows how this shortening occurs. Notice also that within the tangled area of the fibers, particles can become trapped. When the fibers are long and straight there is less likelihood of particles being trapped inside the fiber. What is trapped can be toxic to the body – waste products from the metabolism of nearby cells or particles of pollution from outside the body, like smoke or pesticides.

Once these particles are trapped they can remain in the body for a long time, even forever. Massage and yoga, which move the tissues of the body, can loosen up the bonds that trap these particles. Once freed, the particles can be swept into the blood system or lymphatic system and carried away, eventually eliminated from the body. It has long been known in the East that yoga is a detoxifying practice; understanding how the body works helps us to understand why this is so. Yoga stretches and compresses the collagen network of the body, which lengthens fibers and frees toxic particles – just like we do to that old, gnarly sponge we all have hiding under our kitchen sink.

One final topic will round out our investigation into how muscles, fascia, and other connective tissues create stability, strength, and elasticity in our body. This next topic involves the ground substances, the fluids that fill the spaces between the fibers and cells in our tissues.

Ground Substances

Imagine the inner tube of your bicycle wheel is deflated. Imagine holding it in your hands; notice how limp and flexible it feels. You can bend it and twist it any direction you like. Now imagine the same inner tube filled with water. Try to flex it now and feel the rigidity that has suddenly appeared. Water, which normally seems to be quite yielding, is very difficult to compress. When contained, water provides a tremendous resistance to being squeezed. This is the basis of hydraulic systems – fluids, such as water, when they have been contained or constrained, resist compression and transfer forces placed upon them into areas of lesser resistance.

As was mentioned when we looked at our connective tissues, our tissues are filled with a variety of extracellular substances such as collagen fibers, elastin, etc. What weren't described were the fluids that flow around everything. These fluids are called our "ground substances." Sometimes these are called "cement substances" and they are found widely distributed throughout our connective tissues and supporting tissues. Ground substances act very much like the water in the inner tube analogy; they provide strength and support to the tissues. But they do so much more than just that.

Ground substances are the non-fibrous portion of our extracellular matrix (the stuff outside the cells of our bodies) in which the other components are held in place. They are made up of various proteins, water, and glycosaminoglycans.[46] Water can make up sixty to seventy percent of the ground substances, and it is attracted there because of the GAGs. One of the most important GAGs is hyaluronic acid (HA[47]). Various researchers have estimated that HA can attract and bind one thousand to eight thousand times its volume of water. Another estimate suggests each HA protein in the extracellular matrix has fifteen thousand molecules of water associated with it! Another important kind of GAG is chondroitin-sulfate.

When GAGs combine with proteins they are called "proteoglycans" and it is in this form that they attach to water molecules and hydrate our tissues. The proteoglycans are very malleable and move about freely. However, being made of water they also resist compression tremendously.

With water as a principal component of our ground substances, we can see why the ground substances are an excellent lubricant between fibrils, allowing them to move freely past each other. Water gives our tissues a spring-like ability, allowing them to return to their original shapes once pressure has ceased. This is crucial to our tissues' ability to withstand stresses; however, a cyclic loading and unloading of the tissue is important to maintaining health. One study

---

[46] That's a mouthful, which is easy to gag upon when trying to pronounce. So let's just call these GAGs for short.

[47] To be more current, we could call this hyaluronan.

found that the alteration of loading and unloading of pressure on the tissue, as long as it is not excessive, maintains cartilage health.

The fluid in our joints (called "synovial fluid") is also a lubricant and it too is made up substantially of GAGs. HA and two kinds of chondroitin-sulfates are essential to keeping our joints working properly.

When the extracellular matrix is well hydrated, cells, nutrients, and other components of the matrix can move about freely. Toxins and waste products can migrate out of the matrix into the blood or lymphatic system to be removed from the body. The ground substances, which are also formed by the fibroblasts (remember, fibroblasts also produce collagen), are also helpful in resisting the spread of infection and are a part of our immune system barrier.

Unfortunately, as we age, the ability of the body to create HA and other GAGs diminishes. We have fewer fibroblasts available to us, and those we do have produce less HA. As a consequence, the extracellular matrix becomes filled more and more with fibers. As these fibers come closer together, they generate cross-links that bind them to each other. As a result of that, our tissues become stiffer, less elastic, and less open to the flow of the other components in our matrix. Toxins and waste products[48] become trapped in the matrix and cannot get out, but harmful bacteria can migrate around more easily.

Fortunately exercise like yoga and massage, which stress the extracellular matrix, can help us maintain the number of fibroblasts and keep them functioning properly. This helps to keep the matrix hydrated, open, and strong.

We need these fluids everywhere in the body. The fluid of the eye is made up mostly of ground substances. Our skin needs HA to remain soft. Recently cosmetic surgeons have been using HA injections, instead of collagen, as a soft tissue filler to increase the size of lips or remove skin wrinkles. The effects, however, last only six to twelve months. Chondroitin is an often-used supplement to help increase lubrication of joints. However, injections and supplements

---

[48] Called "ama" in yoga.

are very inefficient ways to hydrate the body.[49] More effective is to coax the body to increase its own production.

Ground substances can be fluidic or gel-like, and under certain conditions they change from one to the other. When they are gel-like they provide more stability, but they are less open for the passage of materials of the matrix. When they are fluid they have less rigidity, but more openness to the flow of materials. Compression of the tissues, via yoga and other means, can temporarily transform the ground substance from gel to fluid. During the fluid state, toxins and wastes can be transported out of the matrix. Once again, yoga is an excellent way to detoxify the body.

---

[49] One study showed that oral ingestion of chondroitin-sulfate resulted in only a five percent absorption rate, which meant that large doses were required to have any effect.

Chapter Four: Our Joints

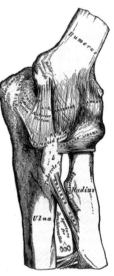

The elbow joint K

A joint is simply the joining of two or more bones. Normally a joint allows movement of the body to occur. Joints also provide support to the body. Muscles attaching to the bones via tendons provide the force or leverage to move one bone relative to another. Wrapping around the joint itself are ligaments that support and protect the joint. Inside the joints may be found synovial fluids or cartilage, or both, depending upon the type of joint and its function.

Not all joints are meant to provide large ranges of motions. Some joints do not allow any movement at all, but they are still the joining of two bones together. There are three basic kinds of joints:

- Fibrous joints, where the bones are held together by connective tissues. An example of this kind of joint is the joining of the plates of our skull. No movement is desired here so the joints are fibrous, held tightly together.
- Cartilaginous joints, where the bones are held together by cartilage and allow slight movement. Examples of these kinds of joints are the pubic symphysis (where the two ends of the pubic bones are connected by cartilage), between the ribs and their connection to the sternum, and in the spine in the region between adjoining vertebrae. Slight movement is

allowed in all these areas but large ranges of movement are not desirable.

- Synovial joints, where there is a space (the synovial cavity) between the bones. This type of joint provides the greatest degree of movement in a variety of ways.

Yoga does not try to increase the range of movement in all three kinds of joints; however, for a cartilaginous joint that has grown too tight, Yin Yoga can help to restore the normal range of movement. For the synovial joints, Yin Yoga definitely helps rebuild and even extend the current range of movement, depending upon the type of synovial joint we are targeting.

Synovial Joints

As shown in the drawings on the right, there are several kinds of synovial joints in our bodies:

1. Ball and socket joints, such as the hip joint. These allow a wide range of movements.

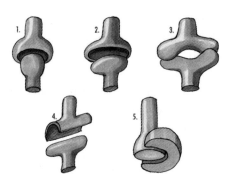

2. Condyloid (or ellipsoid) joints, such as the knee. When the knee is extended, there is no rotation; when it is flexed, some rotation is possible. A condyloid

Five of the six kinds of joints [L]

joint is where two bones fit together with an odd shape (e.g., an ellipse), and one bone is concave, the other convex. Some classifications make a distinction between condyloid and ellipsoid joints.

3. Saddle joints, such as at the thumb (between the metacarpal and carpal). Saddle joints, which resemble a saddle, permit the same movements as the condyloid joints.

4. Hinge joints, such as the elbow (between the humerus and the ulna). These joints act like a door hinge, allowing flexion and extension in just one plane.

5. Pivot joints, such as the elbow (between the radius and the ulna). This is where one bone rotates around another.

6. Gliding joints, such as in the carpals of the wrist. These joints allow a wide variety of movement, but not much distance (not shown).

The Joint Capsule

The ends of the bones are coated in cartilage of varying and sometimes uneven thickness. Cartilage is softer and more pliable than the bone itself due to a higher proportion of proteoglycans to collagen. In some joints, even with the cartilage lining of the ends of the bones, the bones do not fit together snugly. In these cases, multiple folds of fibro-cartilage are employed, such as in the meniscus of the knee, to allow the bones to slide smoothly.

Around all the synovial joints is the synovium, a membrane that covers all the surfaces in the joint. The synovium forms the capsule of the joint and secretes synovial fluid into it, to keep the articulating surfaces lubricated. As we age, the synovial fluid begins to dry up. Like a leaf in autumn, we grow dryer and smaller, more yin-like. This fluid (as was discussed in the section on Ground Substances) is made up of water-attracting molecules like hyaluronic acid and chondroitin-sulfates. We will discuss this drying up more in the next section.

A Demonstration

As we pointed out earlier, the job of our muscles is to protect the joints. The muscles do this by tightly closing the joint. There is an easy way to see this, which we described at the beginning of our journey. Take your right forefinger in your left hand. Relax the right hand and finger and apply a gentle pull with your left hand. Observe the base of the right finger … you may notice a slight dimpling or extension across the knuckle. Even if you can't see any movement, you will definitely feel an opening there. Now contract the muscles of the right finger tightly and try to pull the finger. Notice the difference? There is no movement at all. The muscles have actively bound the joint so that no movement is possible.

The reason so much time and care is given to aligning the body and engaging our muscles properly in our active, yang-styles of yoga is to make sure the joints are not damaged by our yang movements. This is wise. As the above demonstration showed, the muscles act to protect the joint and do not allow the joint to open.

As we will soon see, however, a chronically closed area of the body, whether it is in our muscles, our fascia, or in our joints, becomes permanently closed. If we only close our joints and never allow them to resume their full range of movement, we will lose the original range of motion. Yang yoga is not designed to open the joints. Yin Yoga is. In fact, Yin Yoga has four major benefits for our joints. We will examine these next.

Yin Yoga and Our Joints

If you are aiming to strengthen or maintain the health of your joints, there are four reasons to add Yin Yoga to your practice. The reasons are to:

- Prevent contracture
- Prevent degeneration
- Reduce fixation
- Provide hydration

Let's investigate each one in more detail.

Contracture

Contracture is a loss of mobility in a joint. There are many possible causes of contracture of a joint: illness, nerve damage, muscle atrophy, or problems with the cartilage or ligaments of the joint. We are going to investigate the case where problems in our ligaments cause contracture.

Everyday life can create microscopic tears in our ligaments. These small wounds are healed by the insertion of ligament tissue in between the torn edges. This function has been known for a long time; however, what was mysterious was … if the body naturally lengthens ligaments due to their constant tearing and rebuilding, why then aren't our ligaments extremely long? As Paul Grilley likes to ask, "Why don't our knuckles drag on the ground when we walk?"

A researcher at the University of North Carolina, Professor Laurence Dahners, was investigating this question. What he discovered was a mechanism in which the body shrink-wraps our joints by removing materials from our ligaments. There are similar functions in many areas of our body; one part of the body creates materials (like the osteoblasts in our bones, which create bone tissue) and another part consumes or removes materials (like the osteoclasts, which dissolve bone). Health is usually the balance of these two functions.

An example of shrink-wrapping contracture is the classic "frozen shoulder syndrome." Grandpa falls and breaks his arm, the bone is reset, and the arm rests in a sling for several weeks. When the time comes, the sling is removed, the bone has healed, but the shoulder is frozen. Movement there is not possible. What happened? While there are multiple causes of frozen shoulder syndrome, such as inflammation, this cause was the lack of use of the shoulder joint. The body took away materials no longer needed[50] so that when the time came to use the shoulder again, it couldn't respond.

The treatment for contracture is not surprising for any student of yoga: mobilization. You can do this yourself through Yin Yoga techniques and stretches, or through mechanical means. In the latter case, devices such as the Continuous Passive Motion machine move the limb through the patient's tolerable ranges of motion. This is exactly what we do in Yin Yoga … we gently but persistently move the body through its tolerable ranges of motions and hold the body there. Eventually we regain or even expand the original range of motion of the joint and combat contracture.

---

[50] Again we see the "use-it-or-lose-it" syndrome.

Degeneration

As we have, seen the body continually creates bone and absorbs bone. If this gets out of balance we can start to gain bone mass, causing strengthening of the bone, or we can start to lose bone density and the bone degenerates. Up until our mid-twenties to mid-thirties we generally gain bone mass. If we exercise conscientiously, we can continue to maintain or even add bone mass past these early years of life. However, eventually the balance is tilted more and more in the opposite direction and we start to lose bone density. This condition is known as osteopenia or, in more severe cases, osteoporosis. This condition is more common in women than men, especially as women approach menopause.

One estimate suggests that ten million Americans suffer from osteoporosis and another thirty-four million suffer from osteopenia, or low bone mass, which leads to osteoporosis. This weakening results in almost one and a half million bone fractures each year, with the majority of them occurring in the lower back.[51] Other common sites for breakage are the wrists and hips, all areas with higher trabecular bone, as compared to cortical bone. Generally, it is a continual weakening of the trabecular bone that develops into osteoporosis.

Eventually fifty percent of all women and twenty-five percent of all men in North America will develop osteoporosis. Starting just before menopause, and over a four- to eight-year period thereafter, women begin to lose bone density. Eventually twenty to thirty per-cent of their trabecular bone mass is gone, and they also lose five to ten percent of their cortical bone mass.

For a variety of reasons, osteoblast (bone-creating) activity may diminish or osteoclast (bone-absorption) activity may increase, causing osteoporosis. A lack of vitamin D or calcium can cause bone degeneration. Certain hormonal deficiencies such as testosterone, estrogen, or parathyroid hormones can also contribute to bone loss. So too can immobilization or lack of use.

Fortunately physical activity can cause bones to grow stronger, and actually change size and shape. It is well known that active

---

[51] Specifically in the lumbar spine.

people are less likely to develop osteoporosis. Autopsies have shown that attachment sites, where muscles join to the bone, grow bigger through continued use. One example is the lesser trochanter.[52] In runners this site is highly developed. Too much stress, however, can be dangerous; marathon runners have been known to develop osteoporosis late in life.[53] As in everything, balance is needed.

The bones need to be stressed to remain healthy. And the stress needs to be appropriate. Yin Yoga provides compressive stress on the bones, especially the lumbar spine. Other forms of yoga also stress the bones; most standing postures will do this. In Yin Yoga the stresses are held longer, allowing the bones more time to be stressed. This generates a larger recovery response – the bones having been stressed longer will grow stronger. Very few active yoga postures will stress the lumbar bones like Yin Yoga does.

Fixation

Ever wonder what causes all those pops and cracks you hear as you move your body? There are lots of urban myths about the cause of these, but usually there are only three causes: fixation, friction, or a release of gas. Most people are aware of only the last two.

Sometimes bubbles of nitrogen form in the synovial fluids of our joints. When these bubbles release they make a popping sound. Once the bubble is gone you won't be able to pop the joint again for a while. Friction, on the other hand, can be repeated again and again without any waiting. Friction occurs when two surfaces rub against each other. Friction is the noise made when we snap our fingers. Try it now … just before the two fingers release there is pressure building up between them. Once the pressure becomes greater than the friction between the fingers, they release. As finger strikes the base of the thumb, a sound is created. The same thing can happen in a joint; two ligaments, tendons, or pieces of cartilage may get temporarily stuck or rub against another piece of the body. If the pressure builds up enough to overcome the friction, the pieces release, usually with a snapping sound.

---

[52] An attachment site on the inner femur.
[53] See www.arthritis.org for more on the risks of running.

Cracking knuckles is a good example of friction-generated noise. With friction you don't have to wait to recreate a noise; it can be done over and over again quickly. Often people do this as a nervous habit. Many myths, promoted by mothers who can't stand the sound of their sons cracking their knuckles (yes, it is usually boys who do this), promise that continued cracking of the joints will lead to arthritis. However, no scientific studies have verified this. At worst, continued cracking may loosen the joints minimally. Even snapping your fingers over and over again could be harmful to the tissues in your thumb. But, it would take a lot of snapping for that to happen.

On the other hand, sometimes torn flaps of cartilage or ligaments getting caught in the joint cause the friction. This kind of cracking is not healthy. The key is the presence or absence of pain. Noises accompanied by pain are not good and should be avoided or investigated.

The third cause of joint popping is "fixation." This is the cause we are really interested in. Fixation is a temporary sticking together of two surfaces. The cracking sound is generated when the surfaces are released. That nice pop you might get in your ribs or lower back when you go into a twist or some other pose is probably caused by releasing fixation. Usually it feels good … pressure has been released.

There are three conditions for fixation to occur: first, the two surfaces that are getting stuck together must be smooth; second, there must be some liquid lubricant between the surfaces; finally, the surfaces must be under some pressure that pushes them together.

A good example of fixation is familiar to most readers who aren't yogis. A frosty glass of beer creates condensation (the liquid lubricant) all over the glass, including the bottom. The bottom of the glass is smooth, just like the surface of the coaster the glass is resting on. The weight of the beer in the mug provides enough weight to press the glass onto the coaster. When we pick up the glass (strictly for experimental purposes mind you … yogis don't drink, right?) the coaster comes along with it.

This is fixation. When you pull the coaster off the bottom of the mug a sound may be audible. When you break the fixation between two bones in the body a sound may be even more noticeable. Even without the sound you will definitely feel the release.

Why do we care about breaking fixation? Well, it feels good for one thing; generally the release is enjoyable. But the main reason to break fixation is to prevent fusion of a joint. Often in older patients who suffer a broken bone, the doctor will fix the two pieces together with a pin to keep the edges in contact. This kind of fixation allows the bones to fuse back into one piece; this use of fixation is good. However, in a joint, if two ends of a bone are held together for a long period of time, they too will fuse together. This use of fixation is not good. The joint becomes useless when the bones are fused.

Fusion can happen to anyone. The joint between our hips (ilium) and our tailbone (sacrum), called the "sacroiliac joint," can become fused together. A 2006 study in Israel showed that 34.2% of men examined by computer tomography had a bridge formed between their sacrum and ilium. The rate for women was far lower, 4.6%. This incidence of fusion, via the bridge, was age related; the older subjects had a higher incidence of bridging. For some older people the joints of the lumbar spine also start to fuse.[54] Loss of flexibility here is very noticeable and a big problem.

Fusion begins with fixation; fixation is cured by mobility; and mobility of the joints is one of the big benefits of Yin Yoga.

Hydration

An inevitable fact of life is that we get older. That's not a bad thing or a good thing; it is just the way the world works. Part of getting older is, hopefully, gaining experience and wisdom. Another part of getting older is becoming more yin-like … we dry up like a brittle leaf in autumn. As we dry up, we also tend to curl up and get smaller. One of the benefits of practicing yoga is to delay this inevitable trend.

The gradual, inevitable decay at the end of life can take many years, even decades. Many people linger in ill health for a substantial portion of life before the cycle is completed. Dedicated yogis, however, have a much quicker demise. A yogini may not have a

---

[54] Sometimes with degenerative joints, a procedure called arthrodesis is used to deliberately fix joints, to allow them to fuse together.

longer life span than others[55] but what is noticeable is that the level of health remains high for a much longer proportion of her life. When the final days approach, the decline is quite sudden. That may not sound so appetizing but which would you really prefer?

Yoga helps the body remain hydrated, fluid, and flexible long into the later years. This is one of the contributing factors to a longer period of good health late in life. Hydration applies to all our tissues. This was explored in detail in the section on Ground Substances. With respect to our joints, hydration is essential to their proper functioning.

We have seen that fibroblasts produce the molecules that attract and hold water in our tissues. There are four main molecules that do this for us, but hyaluronic acid (HA) is the biggest contributor to hydration. HA and the other hydrating molecules make up the synovial fluids that are key to keeping our joints lubricated. And the key to this is the number and productivity of the fibroblasts.

As we age we lose fibroblasts; the body just doesn't produce as many. And those that the body does produce lose their productivity – they produce less HA. This is a double whammy that reduces the level of hydration in our tissues. This is why we dry up, curl up, and get stiffer as we age.

The treatment for this condition is not just replacing the lost HA, although there are many companies promoting supplements and injections just for this purpose. We cannot stop the age-related drying-out process, but we can delay it. The best approach is to not replace the missing HA and other water-attracting molecules, but to stimulate the growth of more fibroblasts and increase their production of these water-loving substances.

Fibroblasts are stimulated through stress. Squeezing, compressing, and stretching the connective tissues where fibroblasts reside stimulates them to produce more HA. The body also creates more fibroblasts under such conditions. With more fibroblasts, and more production from each one, the body rehydrates our tissues and joints more.

We have to make sure we are providing the stresses the tissues need and in an appropriate way. That is what yoga does. Yin Yoga

---

[55] There are no known studies available yet.

specifically does this for the joints and the deeper connective tissues, but all yoga will do this for the more superficial and myofascial tissues as well.

We have just looked at four key reasons why we should add Yin Yoga to our yoga practice to protect and enhance our bones and our joints. There is another major reason relating to our joints and that is the benefits our spine gets from Yin Yoga. We will take a quick look at this next.

Spinal Curves

The ancient Romans employed a wonderful invention in their architecture – it was called the arch. Arches allowed stresses built up from the weight of the Roman building materials (stones) to be distributed, which meant fewer stones were needed to support walls and domes.

Arches distribute stress. The same principle applies in our bodies. When you look at the body you never see a straight line. Everything is curved to a greater or lesser degree. Even the longest bone, the femur, has a curve to it. Curves are everywhere but probably the most noticeable curve is the spine.[56]

The spine has four curves. It forms a double S, with the curves in the neck and lumbar moving in opposite directions to the curves in the thorax and sacrum. The forward curve of the lumbar and cervical spine is termed "lordosis." The backward curve of the thoracic spine is called "kyphosis." These four curves are immensely important for an animal that walks upright; these four curves distribute the stress of keeping the torso vertical.

The spine, when healthy and possessing all its normal curves, acts like a spring. Every time we increase the pressure on our body – for example, by walking or running – the spine flexes. The curves deepen and then they release. If our spine were a straight rod, the stresses would fall in between the vertebrae, and the disks cushioning the vertebrae would wear out quite quickly. Of course, the ligaments

---

[56] Okay, we are deliberately ignoring a woman's more obvious curves, which to men are far more noticeable. But even these curves are due partially to the spine's shape.

wrapping the spine also take some of the strain, but these are more responsible for taking the strain of passive activities, such as sitting or standing. Our muscles support the dynamic movement of the spine.

For many people the curves in the spine become exaggerated in one direction or the other. Of most concern are changes in the lumbar and cervical spine. If the lumbar spine curves too far forward, hyperlordosis occurs. If the lumbar spine curves too far backward, hypolordosis occurs. These two conditions are arbitrary diagnoses; there is no standard that health care professionals apply to determine if an individual is hyper- or hypolordotic. The therapist has to decide, based on her own experience.

A study in 2002 at the University of Waterloo in Canada[57] noted, "Tissue failure can result from excessive strain." The study measured the position of least strain for the spine and noted how people varied from that optimal position while walking, standing, and sitting. The authors noted, "Research supports the proposition that individuals with hypolordotic or hyperlordotic lumbar spine posture have more tissue strain and a smaller prefailure tissue safety margin when performing various … tasks such as sitting, standing, and walking." This simply means that if you have too little curve or too much curve in your lower back, you are at risk of lower back pain and more severe problems later in life.

The study also asked if the conditions of hyper or hypolordosis could be changed by exercise. The result of the study was a qualified yes. The authors also noted, "As this is the first study documenting whether lordosis should be and is trainable, no literature exists for comparison. People with hypolordosis appear to have greater posterior tissue strain when seated than do people with hyperlordosis … The results indicate that a person with hypolordosis could be at greater risk for strain-related tissue failure when sitting than a person with hyperlordosis."

This makes intuitive sense. If the normal ranges of motion for your back are reduced or exceeded significantly, you will have problems. A person who already has a significant forward curve in her lower back can cause hyperlordosis by standing for long periods, as this causes greater extension of the lumbar. On the other hand,

---

[57] *Lumber posture – should it, and can it, be modified?*

someone who sits for long periods of time leaning against the back of a chair (the familiar slouch position) will tend to decrease lordosis leading to hypolordosis.

Sitting, it turns out, is one of the worst things we do to our spines, especially if we are already slightly hypolordotic.

The *American Family Physician* in its April 1998 publication stated, "Up to 90 percent of the U.S. population may have significant low back pain at some point. In 1984, it was estimated that over 5 million persons were incapacitated as a result of lower back pain. The financial impact in terms of health care dollars and lost work hours reaches billions of dollars each year in this country."

That is a lot of people with lower back problems … but when you watch virtually everybody who sits in a chair today, you can see one possible source of the problem. When people slouch in their couches, they rotate the top of their pelvis backward, flexing the spine and reducing the normal lordosis in the lumbar. Imagine doing this for many hours every day for decades (and for most of us, this is not hard to imagine!) Eventually the spine will lose that nice normal shape it had when we were young, and the damage from the constant strain upon the lower back will add up. Another problem from this posture is the weakening of the muscles of the back. If you rely upon the chair back to support your upper body, you rob your muscles of the chance to remain strong or grow stronger.

It is no wonder that all fitness coaches will advise you to bend your knees when you try to pick something up. Your back has gotten so weak from years of sitting that you had better baby your back or you will break it! Farm workers who spend hours every day working in the fields do not need to bend their knees.[58] They just simply bend over. But their backs are strong. Most Western backs aren't.

One remedy – stop sitting in chairs! If you love your back, if you want to strengthen your spine and open your hips (another problem area for most Westerners), start sitting on the floor every chance you get. Give your chairs away. Live as close to the ground as you can get. Eat at your coffee table, read with books on the floor. Watch television while lying on the floor in seal pose.[59]

---

[58] Which is a very inefficient way to pick something up, after all.
[59] See the Asana section for details.

All forms of yoga can help strengthen the back. Yin Yoga can help reestablish the normal range of motion of the lumbar ligaments as well. But remember, there is no agreed-upon definition for when someone is hyper-this or hypo-that; everybody's bones are different. When you practice moving your spine through its full and natural ranges of motion, be aware of going too far. Be aware of pain or its precursors, small tweaks. Don't stay in a pose when the sensations of the poses are too great. The essence of the yin practice is to maintain a gentle, but persistent, pressure for a long period of time.

Our exploration of the physical body, the first kosha, has revealed many benefits of the Yin Yoga practice. The compression, twisting, and stretching of our body works deep into our connective tissues, and this frees up toxins and other materials that have become trapped. Yin Yoga helps to detoxify the deep tissues of our body. Additionally, Yin Yoga has many benefits for our joints: fighting contracture, fixation, and degeneration of the bones, while assisting in rehydrating the synovial fluids and moistening the ligaments. Understanding these physical benefits is useful. It is time now to look at the second kosha, the energy body, and discover what benefits Yin Yoga brings to us energetically.

Chapter Five: The Energy Body
The Pranamaya Kosha

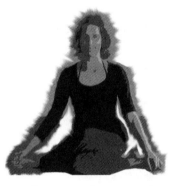

Man does not live by bread alone and our food sheath, the annamaya kosha, is not all there is. Beneath the outermost sheath is the pranamaya kosha: the energy body. Our journey now takes us beneath our physical manifestation so we can investigate the vital energies of the body and learn how yoga affects these energies.

In the East we find many metaphors and concepts concerning energy. Many yoga texts teach us about prana in its various forms. Many scholars believe that the knowledge of yoga and prana filtered into China over 2,500 years ago. Once there, the Chinese built upon the spiritual uses of these sciences and developed a more complete physiological understanding. In the Daoist explorations, prana became known as Chi[60] and it has many different manifestations. In the West, scientists and doctors had little time for the metaphysical aspects of Eastern energy. But even in the West, there are various interpretations of the word "energy." There is the energy of our nervous system that is electrical in form. There is chemical energy transported by our blood system. And, as we will see, there are many other forms of energy now being investigated by Western scientists.

We will look more closely at the three major ways of exploring energy beginning with the most ancient philosophy of India, then the

---

[60] Chi is often spelled Qi. In Japan it is also called Ki.

Daoist view, and then the evolving Western understanding. Finally, we will look at how we can measure this energy flow using modern instruments. In the second half of our journey, when we visit The Practice of Yin Yoga, we will come back to this investigation and discover various ways to stimulate the flow of energy.

The Yogic View of Energy

In India a psycho-spiritual science (called "pranayama") developed around the concept of energy (called "prana"), the little rivers the energy flowing within our bodies (called "*nadis*"), and the major energy plexuses (called "chakras"). We can call this a science because it meets the classic requirements of any scientific investigation; a model is posited that predicts certain testable behaviors, which can be verified by anyone who duplicates the conditions of the inquiry. The challenge is – very few people are equipped with, or can develop, the abilities to meet these conditions of inquiry.

A Western definition of energy is the ability to do work. An Eastern explanation is not so different; energy allows us to be, to live, and act in the world. Just as we use the term "energy" to denote all the various kinds of energies that exist, so too in the yogic models one term is used to encapsulate all of the various kinds of energies. This one word is prana.

An understanding of prana is important for the yogi. The control of our energies, our prana, allows us to maintain or improve our health, to provide the energy needed to delve deeper into the mysteries of our existence, and to calm the inner winds that blow our minds from one thought to another. Yin Yoga helps us to manage our pranic energies in several ways. But before we learn how to release or restrain these energies, it is valuable to understand a bit more about prana, the channels along which it flows, and the major plexuses that bridge our various bodies.

Prana

Life is possible only because of prana. Prana is the universal energy of existence. The word literally means "breathing forth." It is usually synonymous with the breath or with air (vayu). In the Rig Veda, the oldest Hindu text, prana is claimed to be the breath of the cosmic purusha.[61] But prana itself is an overarching term with many subcategories. Learning how prana works and how to free this energy is part of the psycho-spiritual practice known as pranayama.

Vayu, meaning air, is another synonym for prana. Inside the body there are five major kinds of prana, or vayus, and five minor ones. The major vayus are:

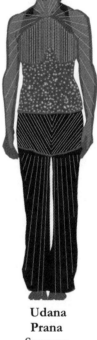

Udana
Prana
Samana
Apana
Vyana

1. *Prana* … the upward lifting energy. This can be confusing; the vayu prana is a subset of the overall term for all energies, also called prana. The vayu prana is responsible for the energy of the heart and the breath. When we see a tree's branches reaching upward to the sun, that is prana energy being expressed. When we feel our inhalations lift our spirit, along with our shoulders, that too is prana.

2. *Apana* … the downward, rooting energy. Apana is responsible for elimination, both through the lungs (eliminating carbon dioxide) and the digestive tracts. The roots of a tree searching downward for stability are expressing apana. The rooting downward of our exhalations tap into the same energy.

---

[61] Purusha is the cosmic man or the original Self from which all comes.

3. *Udana* … the "up breath" or upward moving energy. Udana is responsible for producing sounds and is the energy of the five senses. Some texts place this only in the throat but other texts say that it circulates in all the limbs and in the joints.
4. *Samana* … the balancing energy. Samana is responsible for digestion and the metabolism of our cells.
5. *Vyana* … the outward moving energy. Vyana is responsible for the movement of our muscles and for balancing the energy flow throughout our body.

None of these energies exist in isolation. One of the challenges in our yoga practice is to detect the presence of all these energies when one of them is most obvious. For example – take a deep breath. The energy of prana is obvious, but can you detect at the same time the subtle rooting energy of apana? More simply put, can you feel the apana in the prana? Try this on the exhalation too. Can you feel the prana in the apana? It may be useful to follow the movement of your diaphragm as you try this. On inhalations, despite the obvious lifting upward of the chest and shoulders, the diaphragm is descending. Following this movement may help you find the apana in the prana and vice versa. Once you can do this for the breath while sitting, try following these energies while you do your asana practice.

Sensing the flow of energy is a meditation practice all on its own. Just sitting for a few minutes watching the apana in the prana and the prana in the apana requires attention. Any time we follow our energies, we are meditating.

The five minor pranas are not important unless the student is going into advanced practices. This is fortunate as different sages describe different and conflicting effects of these minor energies. A generalization of these energies is compiled below, but the reader is warned that some teachers have very different observations:

- *Naga* … causes salivation and hiccups
- *Kurma* … causes opening of the eyes and blinking
- *Krikara* … causes sneezing and sensation of hunger
- *Devadatta* … causes yawning and sleep
- *Dhanamjaya* … pervades the entire body; causes hair growth and lingers even after death

Energy does not just simply exist; it flows. Just as our nerves channel electrical energy and our blood vessels channel chemical energy, so too prana is channeled in our bodies. These channels are known as nadis.

The Nadis

Just as water requires banks before it can become a river, prana requires a path along which to travel. These pathways are the nadis. This Sanskrit word means "little river." It is hard to pin down just how many of these channels exist in our body. Some ancient texts, such as the Shiva-Samhita, claim there are three hundred and fifty thousand nadis. Many texts claim there are seventy-two thousand. The Tri-Shikhi-Brahamana Upanishad tells us that the number is

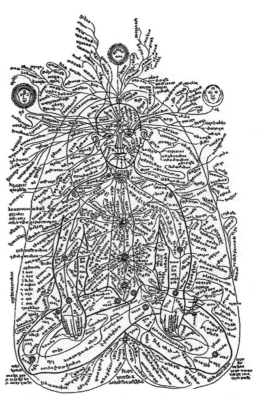

This depiction of our nadis is attributed to the 19th century Tibetan sage Ratnasara. [M]

countless. That is probably the best way to interpret any large number given in the ancient texts. Whether the number is seventy-two thousand or three hundred and fifty thousand, the sage was most likely advising us that the number was beyond counting.

Despite the large number of nadis detected by the yogic sages, usually only eleven or twelve are named, and of these only three are really discussed. However, even here the texts vary considerably in the descriptions of each nadi. Dr. Hiroshi Motoyama has researched various texts' views of these channels and has published his findings in his book *Theories of the Chakras*. We recommend that the dedicated student acquire this book. It will be referred to again.

The three nadis of most importance are:

- The *sushumna* nadi
- The *ida* nadi
- The *pingala* nadi

We will look at the main central channel first.

The Sushumna Nadi

The most important nadi is the sushumna nadi. Most texts agree that this channel begins in the muladhara chakra[62] at the base of the spine. The channel corresponds to the Governor Vessel meridian in the Daoist view of energy flow. The sushumna flows inside the core of the spine, but it is not the spine; it is subtler than that. The perceived function of the sushumna depends upon the school of yoga one is studying. Dr. Motoyama claims that the sushumna governs the six yang meridian lines, but here he is combining his unique experience of both yoga and Daoism to explain the way our body works.

In Tantra and Kundalini Yoga, and in many Hatha Yoga schools, the sushumna is the key channel within which *shakti* energy[63] flows. Kundalini is said to be a special form of energy or the highest form of prana. The term refers to the power of the snake, which is envisioned to lie curled in three and a half coils at the base of the spine, dormant and awaiting wakening.[64]

Georg Feuerstein in the *Shambhala Encyclopedia of Yoga* explains that prana may be considered like the energy in an atomic bomb, while kundalini energy is like that of a hydrogen bomb. An apt

---

[62] See the Chakra section for details.

[63] Sometimes called the *kundalini* energy.

[64] Sometimes we find shakti written with a capital S and sometimes without. When the word is capitalized, it generally refers to the goddess Shakti. When it is not capitalized, it is referring to the energy of the goddess but not the goddess herself. But don't be alarmed if this is not universally done.

metaphor as the release of this energy is quite dramatic. Shakti energy is directed upward from its home just below the *muladhara* chakra toward the *ajna* chakra (according to Dr. Motoyama) or the *sahasrara* (according to Georg Feuerstein).[65] The intention is to bring kundalini up the sushumna to the top of the head where Shiva awaits reunion with Shakti. [66]

Once the kundalini has been awakened and raised up the sushumna to the top of the head, many psychic phenomena may occur. Inner sounds, special sight, and insights can be perceived. *Vibhutis*[67] may be manifested such as clairvoyance, telekinesis, telepresence, and telepathy. Living liberation is achieved in this manner – that is, liberation while still residing in the body.

The Ida and Pingala

Running alongside the sushumna nadi, on either side of the spine, are the ida and pingala nadis. Ida refers to the *chandra* (yin) energies of the moon while pingala refers to the *surya* (yang) energies of the sun.[68]

---

[65] The chakras mentioned above will be defined a little later in our journey.

[66] Again here we find very different models taught by different sages. Many schools claim the kundalini energy is supreme and must be stimulated to rise up the central channel. These teachers make a distinction between the kundalini awakening and the activation of ordinary prana. Others, such as the sage who wrote the Yoga Yajnavalkya, claim the kundalini snake at the base of our spine is an impediment, a blockage, which must be burned away before prana can rise. The snake is a guardian of the gate to the sushumna and must be woken up so it can be moved away. In this model, it is just prana that needs to be concentrated in the body and directed up the sushumna nadi. And yet another school claims that Shakti's energy actually descends downward to meet Shiva, who is awaiting her at the base of the spine. This is represented in the *Shri Yantra* where the downward-facing triangles are said to be Shakti and the upward-facing triangles are Shiva, pointing in the same direction his symbolic lingam is always pointing. We can avoid being confused if we consider the different teachings as simply different models; do not try to use one model to explain the symbolism of another model.

[67] Vibhutis are special powers.

[68] The two words that make up the word "Hatha" in Hatha Yoga are *ha* and *tha*. Most teachers interpret ha to mean the sun and tha to mean the moon.

The flow of these two channels is disputed. Modern teachers generally teach that the ida begins in the muladhara at the base of the spine and rises up the left side of the spine until it reaches a chakra. It switches sides at each chakra until it reaches the back of the head. Climbing over the head, it comes down the forehead until it ends in the left nostril. The pingala runs similarly but begins on the right side and ends in the right nostril. Together they form a caduceus, two snakes spiraling their way around the sushumna nadi.[69]

Dr. Motoyama's research reveals that none of the yogic texts actually describe in detail the paths of the ida and pingala. There is certainly no discussion of the nadis crossing at the chakras. Implied is that the nadis flow up alongside the spine much like the Urinary Bladder lines in Chinese medicine. His experience shows that these channels pass through the nostrils on their way to their termination in the ajna chakra (at the point between the eyebrows.)

An interesting thing happens to the flow of energy in our ida and pingala channels: about once every ninety minutes or so, our breath switches sides. See if you can tell which nostril is more open right now. Generally if you close one nostril while you breathe, and then the other, you can tell which one is more open. When we are healthy, the breath switches nostrils regularly, every ninety minutes or so. When we are ill, the time between switching is longer, maybe every few hours. It has been said that when death is near, the breath does not switch nostrils at all; we will all get to test out that theory one day.

When the breath is flowing out of the surya (the solar or right) nostril, we are in a yang, energized state. When the breath is flowing out of the chandra (the moon or left) nostril, we are in a yin, passive state. There are several forms of pranayama that help to balance the

---

Thus the right nostril, being the solar channel, is the ha channel and the left nostril, being the lunar channel, is the tha channel. However, as usual in the world of yoga, even here there is no unanimity. T.K.V. Desikachar in his book *The Heart of Yoga* defines ha to be the moon and tha to be the sun. But even he admits the left nostril is the lunar channel.

[69] Which, curiously enough, looks a lot like the old logo of the American Medical Association, which the AMA borrowed from the caduceus of the Greek god Hermes.

surya and chandra energies such as *nadi shodana* (an exercise designed to cleanse the nadis).[70]

According to many teachers, there are certain activities that must be abstained from if the wrong nostril is open. For example, Pattabhi Jois, in the book *Yoga Mala,* warns that one must not make love when the sun is shining, or when the right nostril is open. When the right nostril is open, it is the same as the sun shining. Most students do not think to check their breath before commencing lovemaking; however, if you do decide to check and you notice that conditions are not optimal, don't despair. There is a way to change the flow of the breath so you won't have to tell your anxious lover to wait for a couple of hours. A sinus reflex can be stimulated, allowing the breath to switch sides within a few minutes. There are a couple of ways to tap into this reflex. One way is to lie on your side that is already open with that arm extended over your head and used as a pillow. Another approach is to sit and shift your weight to the buttock of the open nostril. However if neither intervention works, please do not blame yoga for your lover's frustration.

Warning

As with all forms of pranayama, or controlling of energy, caution is advised. Many students who have managed to raise their kundalini energy without properly cleansing and preparing their bodies have suffered severe physical and psychological damage. These techniques should be practiced only under the guidance of a teacher who has been there before and knows the way.

---

[70] These pranayamas will be described in Chapter 15: Moving Energy.

Chakras

Within the human body there are almost one hundred plexuses. A plexus is a joining together (as opposed to a branching apart) of nerves forming a nerve net. The best known is the solar plexus, which is an autonomous cluster of nerve cells behind the stomach and below the diaphragm. Some scientists call the solar plexus our second brain. Other channels can form plexuses too. Blood vessels can form plexuses, such as the choroid plexus in the brain. And yogic sages tell us that nadis also form a network creating plexuses, which they call "chakras". A chakra is literally a wheel or circle.[71]

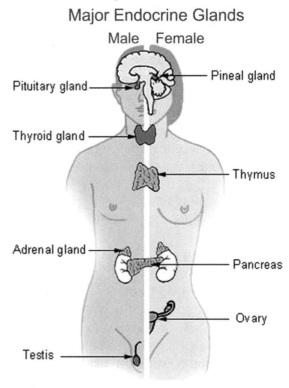

Major Endocrine Glands

Male   Female

Pituitary gland
Pineal gland
Thyroid gland
Thymus
Adrenal gland
Pancreas
Ovary
Testis

The endocrine glands are not along the spine.

Chakras are models of the way the subtle energy in our bodies can be networked into gathering points, in the same way nervous energy may be networked in our solar plexus. Once again the student of yoga is cautioned not to believe that the models used to explain observed behavior are reality. A model is just a model; if it is useful, it is a good model.

---

[71] Often it is spelled "cakra." In fact, usually when you find a Sanskrit word translated into English with the letter "c" by itself, you can visualize a "ch" instead; the pronunciation of "c" is "ch" as in "church."

Buddhist yogis developed one of the earliest models of the chakras fifteen hundred years ago. They helped develop the Tantra school of yoga. Being Buddhist, their model posited five chakras, one for each of the meditation Buddhas. In the Tantra school of yoga, as practiced in India by Hindu yogis, seven major plexuses were detected, one for each heavenly plane of existence (or *lokahs*), ranging from the earth to the highest heaven.[72]

The theories of chakras are varied and diverse. There is no consensus on the number of chakras we have (some texts describe twelve or more), their location, the description of each chakra, or even the purpose or function of chakras. Often chakras are depicted in diagrams as having a certain number of lotus petals, a particular color, sound, and symbol. But here too there is a wide diversity. What is commonly agreed is that the chakras are energy centers of the subtle body.

Chakras is not another term for the nerve plexuses or endocrine glands found in the physical body, such as the solar plexus or the ovaries, even though they may reside in the same physical location (as shown in the image on the facing page). Similarly, chakras are not to be considered physical organs of the body. Much has been made of the close proximity and similar functions of the chakras and the endocrine organs. However, the yogic texts do not make such claims, and it has been only in the last few decades that some teachers have made this association. These glands and plexuses are found outside the spine, whereas chakras are always described as being anchored in the spinal column.[73]

There are many books available today that describe chakras in detail. *Tantra, the Path of Ecstasy* by Georg Feuerstein has a good introduction to this topic. It is difficult to find a definitive explanation of what chakras are supposed to do, but it is safe to say that a chakra is a center of subtle energy (prana or kundalini) that needs to be manipulated in order to achieve complete physical and spiritual health, and eventually enlightenment. In ordinary individuals,

---

[72] It is from this hierarchy that we derive the saying "being in seventh heaven" to signify our greatest joy.

[73] Dr. Motoyama's personal investigations lead to a different understanding and a different model of the chakras. We will look at his findings a little later.

the chakras are undeveloped or even dormant. The practice of yoga helps to awaken the chakras, allowing prana to flow through them. Eventually, when all six of the lowest chakras have been opened, energy is free (*ayama*) to reach the highest chakra, and liberation is possible.

It is time to look at each of the seven chakras individually.

The Seven Chakras

The Muladhara Chakra

Each chakra has an associated home and function. The lowest chakra is the muladhara, located at the base of the spine. Mula means root. The coiled serpent, the kundalini, lies just beneath this chakra, making the muladhara key to awakening the shakti, which must rise up the sushumna nadi. Being the lowest chakra, this center is the most base and is associated with the element *prithivi*, or earth.

Joseph Campbell, in his book *Transformation of Myth through Time*, has a metaphor for the muladhara chakra that is quite delightful – the dragon. This chakra is a dragon. Dragons don't do anything of value, but they guard that which is valuable. Dragons hoard jewels and they kidnap beautiful women, but have no idea what to do with either one. They are only concerned with existing.

Purananda, in the Shat-chakra-nirupana text he wrote in 1577, tells us that meditation on this chakra can make a man "an adept in all kinds of learning. He becomes free from all disease and his inmost spirit becomes full of great gladness."

The Svadhisthana Chakra

The next chakra is called the "*svadhisthana*." Campbell liked to interpret this to mean "her favorite resort." The svadhisthana is associated with the element *apas*, or water, and thus the many bodily functions that are fluid in nature are controlled here. Sexuality blossoms here, with all the joy and suffering that accompanies it. Often the svadhisthana is said to be located at the genitals.

Purananda tells us that meditation on this chakra frees a man "from all his enemies such as lust, anger, greed and so forth." When this chakra is undeveloped, a man (or woman) is at the mercy of sexual impulses. Campbell reminds us that at the purely physical level, sex is the aim of life. Everything sexual is exciting, but the frustrations of sex are also here. When the frustration is high, these sexual energies are often sublimated into other avenues. Campbell believes civilization is a result of such sublimation.

The Manipura Chakra

Manipura translates as the "city of the shining jewel." This chakra is located at the navel, although some sages claim it is located at the solar plexus. The energy here is aggressive, concerned with power. Meditation here gains one the "power to destroy or create (the world)," according to Purananda. The associated element is *agni*, or fire.

Campbell points out that people living at the levels of these first three chakras are mostly concerned with the lowest forms of religious awareness. They seek health, wealth, and progeny. They have no interest in higher spiritual attainment. Their prayers are requests of, or rather bargains with, a god for the fulfillment of the base desires of life. The true yogi, however, seeks to quickly purify these lowest three chakras so energy can flow up to the heart.

The Anahata Chakra

This is the heart chakra. The name *anahata* is the sound that is *not* made by having two things hit each other. It is the un-struck sound of *Om*. This is the level of transformation – of turning away from the material and sensual, to the spiritual. Purananda tells us that he who meditates here "is pre-eminently wise and full of noble deeds. His senses are completely under control." The associated element is *vata*, or air.

Once all six chakras are open and functioning, and Shakti has reached Shiva at the seventh chakra, the yogi who wishes to return to life while residing in the body, returns and dwells in the heart. The heart is the balancing point between the first and seventh, the second and sixth, and the third and fifth chakras.

The Visuddha Chakra

Visuddha means pure. What is pure is not exactly clear from reading the texts; many suggestions are offered. Apparently, if you have to ask, you don't know. This chakra is located at the throat and is associated with the element *akasha* or space, the subtlest of the five elements. It is also associated with the sense of listening. Richard Freeman, in his audio book *The Yoga Matrix,* explains that, when we listen, we create space. The two are intimately connected. For Freeman, yoga begins with listening, with creating space.[74]

Purananda tells us that this chakra is the doorway to becoming "a great sage, eloquent and wise and (one who) enjoys uninterrupted peace of mind."

The Ajna Chakra

Ajna can mean command, power, or authority. This is the highest chakra that is actually a part of our body. It is located right between the eyebrows, a location often referred to as the third eye. Indian women commonly wear a dot, called a *"bindu,"* here. Georg Feuerstein claims that this is the site of the organ of clairvoyance and other paranormal powers.

The subtle mind, known as *manas*, resides here, according to Purananda. He also says that meditation here allows those accomplished in yoga to become "all knowing and all seeing. He becomes the benefactor of all … long lived … the creator, destroyer and preserver of the three worlds."

The Sahasrara Chakra

This is the highest of the chakras. Sahasrara means one thousand lotus petals, which is the symbol for this chakra. The chakra is located just above the crown of the head. Campbell reports that between the sixth and seventh chakras, the soul beholds God. Here

---

[74] This can be understood by recalling a time when you really listened to a friend. Normally when we listen, we are busy thinking about what we are going to say when our friend gives us a chance. But when we really listen, we create space for her to be whatever she needs to be in that moment.

at the seventh chakra, the soul merges with God. Shakti and Shiva have come together, and the sage is liberated.

For unenlightened yogis, the sahasrara is responsible for the mental functions higher than manas (the lower mind). Discernment here may be manifested as a mystical experience or even illumination.

Let's leave the final word on the final chakra to Purananda. "That most excellent of men who has controlled his mind … is never born again … as there is nothing in the three worlds which binds him. He possesses complete power to do all which he wishes and to prevent that which is contrary to his will. He ever moves towards (God) …"

Dr. Motoyama's View

The practice of yoga is the gradual cleansing and opening of each chakra. Once these energies' vortexes are open, the flow of kundalini, or shakti energy, can rise up the central channel and consciousness merges with God. The impression is easily gained that these chakras must be opened sequentially, beginning with the lowest and moving upward. This is not actually stated in any of the ancient texts on yoga. Many people may have one or two chakras already open but have lower ones blocked.

In Dr. Motoyama's experience the chakras should be opened in a specific sequence but not starting from the muladhara. He strongly advises the student begin with the ajna, and says, "… if the ajna is awakened first, the overpowering and potentially dangerous karmic forces hidden in the lower chakras may be safely controlled." After awakening the ajna, the yogi moves on to opening the muladhara and then the svadhisthana chakras.

Through his clairvoyant visions, Dr. Motoyama reports that chakras are less like wheels and more like cones, with the root of the cone in the spine and the top, open end of the cone on the front surface of the body. He calls the front of the chakra the receptor. The following table summarizes some of the attributes of each of the seven chakras, mostly from Dr. Motoyama's *Theories of the Chakras*.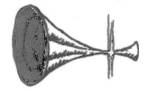

Chakra	Receptor	Root	Element	Sense	Petals	Bija Mantra
Muladhara	Perineum (pelvic floor)	Coccyx	Earth	Smell	4	Lam
Svadhisthana	1~2inches below navel	2nd/3rd sacral vertebra	Water	Taste	6	Vam
Manipura	Around the navel	2nd lumbar	Fire	Sight	10	Ram
Anahata	Halfway between nipples	8th thoracic	Air	Touch	12	Yam
Visuddha	In the throat	1st thoracic/ C7	Space	Hearing	16	Ham
Ajna	Between eyebrows	Medulla oblongata	-	-	2	Om
Sahasrara	Top of head	-	-	-	1000	-

There is one major difference between Dr. Motoyama's view of the function of the chakras and those of most authors on yoga: Dr. Motoyama has determined that the chakras are bridges between the three bodies we each possess. These three bodies are:

- The physical body and its mind: the consciousness associated with the physical.
- The astral or subtle body and its mind: the consciousness associated with emotion. This is the home of prana or Chi. It is interesting to note that Chi obeys physical laws. It weakens over space and time.

- The causal body and its mind: the consciousness associated with wisdom and intellect. This is the home of a higher psychic energy known as "Psi." It is also interesting to note that physical laws do not bind Psi. It does not weaken over space and time, but like a laser stays powerfully focused wherever it is directed.

Dr. Motoyama tells us that the physical body is yang compared to the yin nature of the astral and causal bodies. It is the chakras that link these bodies together and allow information and energy to flow between them. It is due to this linkage that yogis throughout the ages have been able to perform normally impossible feats. For example, a master buried alive for weeks with no air, food, or water survives because of her ability to transform astral energies into physical energy.

Now that we have models of energy (prana), its pathways (nadis), and the main energy centers (chakras), all that is left to explore is the practice of moving the energy. This practice is pranayama.

Pranayama

Prana is life. It is the energy of the universe. Prana is also often considered to be our breath. In Latin, the word "spiritus" also means breath. When our breath leaves us, it is the same as our spirit departing. Pranayama is a freeing of the breath, of the spirit.

The word pranayama is really two Sanskrit words: prana and ayama. This is often misunderstood, and many students think the two words are prana and *yama*. Yama means to restrain or control, ayama is to not do that. Thus in a pranayama practice we are trying to free up the energy of prana, not restrain it. This can be confusing as many teachers and authors prefer to interpret pranayama as controlling the breath. Perhaps a better way to think of pranayama is to consider it regulating the breath, but in such a way that the prana is actually freed or extended in a controlled way.

Why would we want to regulate the breath? Consider this analogy: the mind and the breath are like two fish in a school; when one fish moves the other moves with it. If you have ever attempted to meditate and still the turnings of your mind, you know how difficult this is. Zen is one discipline that attempts to still the mind through sheer willpower. This is a most difficult way and it is not surprising that Zen was a practice of the samurai; it is a hard practice and not for everyone. Yoga sought an easier route to the same goal, through regulating the breath. If the breath is quiet, the mind is still. If you really pay attention, you may discover that the moments between breaths are the moments between thoughts.

Almost two thousand years ago an important book was written: the Yoga Sutra. Myths abound about the author of this sutra, and a thousand years after its compilation people began to say that the author was a sage named Patanjali. We may never know who wrote the sutra, but that doesn't stop it from being an excellent source of knowledge on Classical Yoga. Like all ancient texts, it was never meant to be used as a standalone teaching. A guru's knowledge is required to really understand the sutra. Perhaps we should consider the Yoga Sutra a sort of "Coles Notes" condensation of a guru's teaching.[75]

In the Yoga Sutra, the aim of Classical Yoga was given in the second line: *Yogas-citta-vritti-nirodhah*; Yoga is the stilling of the fluctuations of the mind-stuff. Within the sutra are given many methods for accomplishing this rather daunting task. Pranayama is the fourth stage of an eight-limbed method offered in this sutra.[76]

According to the Yoga Sutra,[77] the practice of pranayama should be *dirgha* (extended) and *sukshma* (subtle). This means the practice should allow the breath to become long without being forced. The sutra then describes the four components of the breath and the three phases of pranayama. The four components are:

1. Placement ... where are you putting the breath?
2. Time ... how long is your breath?
3. Number ... how many repetitions are you doing?
4. Intensity ... how much force are you exerting?

---

[75] For our American readers, consider the Yoga Sutra as the "Cliffs Notes" of Classical Yoga.

[76] People have taken to calling these eight limbs the *ashtanga*; however, the author of the Yoga Sutra never used this term.

[77] Yoga Sutra, II-50.

The three phases of the breath are:

1. Inhalation … *puraka*
2. Exhalation … *rechaka*
3. Retention … *kumbhaka* or holding of the breath, either between the inhalation and exhalation (*antara kumbhaka*), or between the exhalation and inhalation (*bahya kumbhaka*).

When the breath is extended and the practice is mature, then a fourth phase of the breath arises: *kevala*. Kevala means isolated. In this state the breath naturally suspends itself, without any effort or force. Later sages explained that in this stage, the kundalini awakens and thus the prana is freed.

Almost every sage from Patanjali onward noted that pranayama was more valuable than the practice of asana. Asana is a preparatory stage, allowing the body to be strong and healthy enough to engage in pranayama. In the same way, pranayama can be considered just one step on the path toward the practices of meditation. When the breath is regulated, the mind can be approached; insight becomes possible.

All yoga involves the breath; how can it not? All life involves breathing. And so, even in our asana practice, the breath is present, providing us the opportunity to regulate it. Yin Yoga is no different. We are given the opportunity to free and extend the breath. Regulating the breath, however, is not the only way to stimulate the flow of prana. Pranayama is just one method. Other methods include massaging the body, directing our awareness, being in the presence of others, and … yes … even the performance of asanas. How we can stimulate prana to flow as part of our Yin Yoga practice is discussed in Chapter 15: Moving Energy.

Chapter Six: The Daoist View of Energy

Five thousand years ago, and earlier, throughout all cultures, shamans blazed the spiritual paths. In India the shamanic traditions evolved into the yogic practices and philosophies we have been investigating. But this evolution was not confined to the valleys of the Indus, Saraswati (now gone), and Ganges rivers. In Europe (mostly in Greece), the Middle East, and in China, the same discoveries were being made. Over centuries, despite the distances and difficulty of travel, knowledge filtered out and was shared among the cultures. It is not surprising that we find sim-

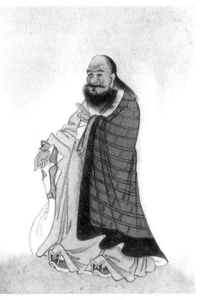

Lao-tzu °

ilar concepts being discussed in the spiritual practices and philosophies of each region. However, the models and metaphors were modified to fit the local cultural landscape.

The concept of spirit (breath) in the European world had its counterpart in prana (breath) in India. In China the same energy was known as Chi. Chi is just one of several concepts central to Chinese medical practices. These concepts evolved out of native spiritual practices grouped together under the name Daoism.[78]

There are many forms of Daoism and many ways to practice the teachings. The Dao is sometimes personalized as a god, but most often it is impersonalized as a benevolent but disinterested power: the way of the universe. Live in harmony with the way and you will benefit. Struggle against the way things are and you will suffer.

Most Westerners know of the Dao only through the book by Lao-tzu called the Dao De Ching: the Way of Virtue.[79] In the Dao De Ching we learn that the Dao is the source of everything. It is nameless because whenever you try to capture the essence of the universe in a concept, you miss the totality of what you are trying to name. The Dao is infinite and inexhaustible. Only the Dao is unchanging and unchangeable.

Since everything is part of the Dao, it follows that the earth, sky, rivers, mountains, stars, and humans are also part of the Dao. Man is not outside of all this, man is a part of all this. In the Dao De Ching the message is: Get involved! Help, but help in a non-intrusive way. When finished, retire. Yang is acting. Yin is retiring. The Dao is the balance between the two.

In the Daoism of Lao-tzu, the sage is one who cultivates life. The sage learns physical techniques to do this: he regulates his breath, he hones his body, he garners health, and he manages his internal energies including the important sexual energy. Along with the physical techniques, the sage also follows ethical principles and regulates his own mind through meditation. Diet is also an important part of building and maintaining health. Through all these practices, the sage seeks to change his body and mind to recover youth and vitality and live in peace.

There are actually five main systems in Daoism. Let's look at each one briefly.

---

[78] Daoism is often spelled "Taoism" but since it is pronounced more with a "D" than a "T" we are adopting the former spelling.
[79] *Dao* is the way; *de* means "virtue", however, it is often translated as power; *Ching* is a book or story.

The Five Major Systems

The five major systems of Daoism are sometimes contradictory and confusing, especially to people of different cultures. Many of the practices of one system are used in the other systems. Thus the lines between these systems are not fixed and final. The five systems are:

1. **Magical Daoism** – the oldest form of Daoism still practiced today. In this practice, the powers of the elements of nature and spirits are invoked and channeled through the practitioner to gain health, wealth, and progeny.
2. **Divinational Daoism** – based on understanding the way of the universe and seeing the great patterns of life. Knowing how the universe works allows us to live in harmony with those universal forces. As in heaven, so on earth. Divinational Daoism utilizes the study of the stars and patterns found on earth to help us live harmoniously. The I-Ching (the book of changes) is a divinational book.
3. **Ceremonial Daoism** – Originally Daoism was a spiritual practice. Unlike yoga, which remained a personal spiritual practice, one branch of Daoism evolved into a religion.[80]
4. **Action and Karma Daoism** – Proper action leads to accumulating merit. Following the introduction of Buddhism into China, ethics took on a greater role in spiritual practice. But it did not start there; Confucius also taught the value of

---

[80] Religion is the spectator sport of spirituality. In religion we give up our authority to another who will perform sacred rituals on our behalf. In a spiritual practice, responsibility remains with us. When a spiritual practice becomes a religion, ceremony is required. Ceremonies, rituals, and sacrifice bind the powers of heaven to the needs of man. Because we are separate from the powers, we require an intermediary, or priest, to conduct the rituals for us. As in all religions, a hierarchy develops between the person who needs help and the powers that can render it. Only if the rituals are correctly performed will help be given. Monks defer to abbots who are more experienced and who, in turn, defer to even more senior members of their faith.

proper behavior and morality. Good deeds result in rewards, both in this life and the next.

5. **Internal Alchemy Daoism** – Immortality is the goal of this practice. The seeker works to change her mind and body to achieve health and longevity. It was in this practice that Chi became recognized as the key to health and long life. Chi is gathered, nurtured, and circulated through very strict practices. Incorrect practice is dangerous, and this path of Daoism absolutely required an expert teacher. It is mostly from this system that Chinese medicine evolved.

An investigation of all these forms of Daoism is beyond the scope of this journey but if you would like to further study this fascinating field, you could start with the book *Taoism* by Eva Wong.[81] From there you will be led to many other texts by Eva Wong and others. For our part, we will journey through the way of alchemy and transformation. The next step in our journey involves understanding the forms of energy, beginning with Chi.

Chi and Daoist Energy

In Chinese medicine, a model of the body is used that is based upon energy and the passages along which energy flows to nourish the organs. Just as prana has many forms, there are three major energies in the Chinese model: Chi (Qi), *Ching* (*Jing*) and *Shen*. The passages, similar to the yogic nadis, are called "meridians." And where the yogic models include psycho-energetic centers called "chakras," in the Chinese models the organs are the important centers for energy storage and distribution. In the Chinese model, the organs are actually functions residing, not just within the physical location of the organs as we know them in the West, but within every cell of the body.

Chi is derived from the word "breath," just like prana or spirit, and also denotes this essential life force. Chi is the mystical, subtle force that moves the universe. One meaning for the word is

---

[81] We are using Eva Wong's definitions for the five systems of Daoism.

"weather." Another is "heaven's breath." Chi is the pulsation of the universe itself. It is found everywhere, in all things. It is not quite energy or matter; rather, it can be considered energy on the verge of becoming matter, or matter on the verge of becoming energy. Chi is becoming and being. Chi doesn't cause things to happen, as Chi is always present before, during, and after any change or event.[82] Whether Chi is real or merely a metaphor is debated. In the next chapter, The Western View of Energy, we will look closer at these subtle energies and join that debate.

When we looked at the Yogic view of energy, we noticed that there were five main kinds of prana within the body. In a similar manner, the Daoist yogis and doctors discerned five kinds of Chi, called "the fundamental textures," including the three major kinds we just saw. These are:

- Chi
- Blood
- Ching
- Shen
- Fluids

Blood is what we would normally think of as blood in the West but with a bit more to it. Blood moves constantly throughout the body, flowing in both the blood vessels we are familiar with in the West, and also through the meridians. Blood nurtures, nourishes, and moistens. Blood is a yin complement to the yang Chi. Where Chi excites, Blood calms. Where Chi advances, Blood remains.

Ching (Jing) is essence. That definition is not overly helpful and there are many interpretations on what exactly Ching is and does. Ching can be considered the material basis of our body that nourishes and fuels our cells. Ching also cools the body and thus is yin in nature. One definition of Ching claims it is a form of Chi found in sexual fluids. Another possible consideration has Ching being the carrier of our original physical nature. It is in the DNA that our cells build upon – the gift from our parents. Ching is stored in

---

[82] A more complete introduction to Chi can be found in Ted Kaptchuk's book *The Web That Has No Weaver*.

the kidneys and is carried in the semen and menstrual fluids. There are two kinds of Ching: "before heaven" – the Ching that is allocated or given to us before our birth; and "after heaven" – the Ching that we gain from living, eating, and exercising. Unfortunately our store of the prenatal Ching is fixed and cannot be replenished. Once it is used up, life is over. Ching is consumed constantly by just being alive; however, some activities consume Ching too quickly: stress, illness, too much sex or improper sex, or abuse of substances. Some activities restore Ching, but only the postnatal Ching. The secret to longevity is to use up as little before-heaven Ching as possible while building up a store of after-heaven Ching through Daoist practices, such as Chi-gong, Tai Chi, or Yin Yoga.

Shen is a broad term. Sometimes Shen is used as the word for God by Chinese Christians. It is the opposite density from Ching; Shen is the most refined and subtle form of Chi. Shen is the inner strength underlying Chi and Ching, and is closely associated with consciousness. Shen is awareness. It is also associated with creativity. If Shen is weakened, a person will suffer in many ways; forgetfulness and foggy thinking, insomnia or erratic behaviors may arise.[83]

Fluids are all the other liquids we have not yet discussed. These include saliva, urine, perspiration, and all the digestive liquids. Some Fluids are dark and heavy, while others are light and clear. Fluids lubricate and nourish. Fluids feed the skin, the hair, muscles, joints, the brain and all the organs, our bones, and our marrow. While related to Blood, these other Fluids are not as deep or as important as Blood.

---

[83] To be complete we would need to investigate the five subcategories of Shen: *Yi*, which means consciousness of potential; *Hun*, our non-corporeal souls; *Zhi*, or our will; *Shen* again, but this time as our spirit; and *Po*, which is our animal soul that dies when the body dies. Unfortunately this level of investigation is beyond our scope. The reader is once more directed to *The Web That Has No Weaver* to learn more.

Other Forms of Chi

The above categorization of Chi is not the only model used. Some Chinese practitioners break Chi into many kinds. Just as the yogis in India discovered ten kinds of prana, some Daoist scholars have found thirty-two different types of Chi. Chi has been described as:

- Yuan Chi – Original Chi given before birth, which governs our zang/fu organs.[84]
- Gu Chi – Chi from food, also called Grain Chi.
- Kong Chi – Chi from air.
- Zong Chi – Gathering Chi created by combining Gu Chi and Kong Chi. Zong Chi circulates the blood.
- Zheng Chi – True Chi created from Zong Chi when it is acted on by Yuan Chi. This is the Chi most often referred to in texts.
- Ying Chi – Nourishing Chi, which nourishes the organs and produces blood.
- Wei Chi – Defensive Chi, which protects and warms the body.

Like Ching, a certain amount of Chi is given to us before our birth but we can also gain more Chi through our diet, breath, exercise, and meditation.

Function of Chi

One very important purpose of Chi is to support the function of the organs. Chi helps to digest food and transform it into blood and energy. Chi defends the body against infection and pathogens. Chi also maintains the body's temperature and circulation; it keeps the organs in place, keeps the blood in its vessels, and governs

---

[84] See the section The Organs coming up for details.

elimination of excess materials. Chi makes all movement and growth possible When Chi is out of balance it can become deficient or stagnant; these are opportunities for disease and illness to arise.

From these functions it is clear how important Chi is to our health. From a purely pragmatic perspective, learning to acquire and utilize Chi properly, to keep it strong and mobile, will assist in extending a person's lifespan. The quality of that life depends upon other aspects of Chi as well: the strength of the Shen (spirit) energy and the health of the organs.

Energy, as we have described before, can be considered the ability to do work. Work requires something physical to be acted upon. When a force is applied against a substance, energy is expended, and work is achieved. We have just seen what energy is in the Daoist models, but what is substance? Let's take a brief journey into the Daoist view of the nature of matter before continuing on to look at the organs and meridians.

The Five Daoist Elements

The Greeks developed a model of the universe that posited four elements underlying all physical existence: earth, fire, water, and air. In their model, the yogis of India, following the Samkhya philosophy, included space as a fifth element. The yogis, however, extended the model to all experience, not just physical forms. In China, the pragmatic Daoist also saw five base elements; however, they noted a couple of key differences. The five elements in their model are earth, fire, water, metal, and wood. They developed this model from the patterns of the universe easily observable to anyone who watches.

The Elemental Cycle

Rain (water) causes plants (wood) to grow. These plants and trees are scorched in summer and feed the flames when fire comes. From the fire the plants turn to ash, which become earth. Within the earth are formed metal ores. Metals, when cold, cause water to condense, forming the rain that begins the creative cycle all over again.

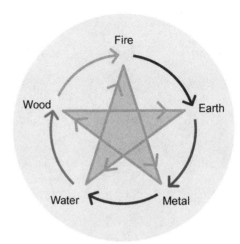

Each element nourishes another element and controls a different element but in turn is controlled by a different element.

Here we find a universal method of checks and balances. Water promotes the existence of wood, which promotes fire, which burns things to the earth. In the earth we find metals, which through condensation promote the formation of water.[85] However, water douses or controls fire, which melts or controls metal, which cuts or controls wood, which plows or controls earth, which soaks up or controls water.[86] Harmony requires checks and balances. If any one element becomes too strong or too weak, imbalance occurs, illness sets in, and harmony is lost.

While these observations were noticed in the external world, the Daoist, like the yogis of India, associated these elements with everything experienced in life. Harmony in our internal world requires checks and balances as well. Physically we suffer if there is too much fire in our body or too little water. Health requires the five elements to be balanced.

---

[85] Follow the outer circle of the diagram clockwise to see how one element nourishes its neighbor.

[86] In the diagram, looking inward follow the left-hand line to the opposite element to see how one element controls another. Following the right-hand line shows how each element is controlled by another.

The five elements became associated with the five directions, the five colors, five bodily tissues, five fluids, five solid organs, and five hollow organs.

Wood	Fire	Earth	Metal	Water
East	South	Center	West	North
Green	Red	Yellow	White	Black (or dark blue)
Tendons	Blood Vessels	Muscles	Skin	Bones
Tears	Sweat	Saliva	Mucus	Urine
Liver	Heart	Spleen	Lung	Kidney
Gall Bladder	Small Intestines	Stomach	Large Intestines	Urinary Bladder
Anger	Joy/Fright	Worry	Sadness/Grief	Fear

As seen above, the elements are also associated with emotions. There are seven emotions in the Daoist models: joy, fright (a sudden panicky feeling), worry, sadness, grief (or shock), fear, and anger. Any excess in these emotions can be harmful. This may seem strange to our Western sensibilities; how can we have too much joy? But in the Daoist model, an excess of joy can be just as harmful to our spirit as an excess of anger. The excess joy referred to here may best be seen in the youthful exuberance of a gang of revelers whooping it up in the streets late at night. Their joy creates disturbance all around them and within themselves too. Joy as defined here is not the deep bliss, our true nature, sought after by seekers of spiritual truth.

Strong emotional states are often triggered by imbalance in, or dysfunction of, our organs. When the checks and balances are not working, illness will arise. If the water function of the kidneys is impaired, the fire in the heart will be out of control, allowing fire to attack the metal of the lungs. Asthma and grief can result. A Chinese doctor may not look to a respiratory remedy for the asthma, but may rather prescribe tonics for the kidneys to cure the condition.

This is a very simplistic view of the Daoist model. We have only just scratched the surface. There are many excellent texts that describe the model more fully. The interested reader may wish to begin with *The Web That Has No Weaver* by Ted Kaptchuk to learn more about this topic. For now our journey takes us to visit the organs.

The Organs

In Chinese medicine the organs are not merely physical entities, they are functions. These functions reside throughout the body, not in one place. Just as the body overall needs these functions to maintain health, each cell also requires the same functions. We cannot say that just the body needs oxygen and needs to eliminate wastes. The function of respirations (via the Lungs) and elimination (via the Kidneys) are pervasive: every part of the body needs to be fed, nourished, and its wastes taken away.

These organ functions were discovered through observation, not dissection.[87] Because of this different approach, Chinese medical models often refer to the organs with a capital letter to differentiate their model from the Western view of organs, which are denoted by a small letter. When you see the word Heart with a capital "H" you will know you are dealing with the function of the Heart organ, rather than the physical heart organ, as we know it in the West.

The functions of the body are based upon the five solid organs, referred to as the *zang* organs. These are the Heart, Spleen, Lungs, Kidneys, and Liver. Everything in life requires yin and yang for balance; thus these solid, yin-like zang organs have their yang counterparts in the hollow *fu* organs of the Urinary Bladder, Gall Bladder, Small Intestines, Stomach, and Large Intestines. Each pair of organs is connected via meridian channels. Each of the zang organs is also associated with one of the five elements of Daoist cosmology and, through these elements, the emotions. This is somewhat comparable, in the yogic view, to the connection of the five lower chakras to the five elements.

---

[87] Chinese physicians never dissected bodies and thus had to develop keen observational skills.

Organ	Type	Paired	Emotion	Element	Function
Stomach	Fu	Spleen	Worry	Earth	Reservoir for food and water
Spleen	Zang	Stomach		Earth	Controls digestion, stores intention or determination
Liver	Zang	Gall Bladder	Anger	Wood	Stores blood, regulates Chi flow, controls tendons, seat of soul
Kidney	Zang	Urinary Bladder	Fear	Water	Regulates water volume, coordinates respiration, stores Ching
Urinary Bladder	Fu	Kidney		Water	Storing and discharging
Gall Bladder	Fu	Liver		Wood	Reservoir for bile (Liver Chi): Gung ho! Decisiveness/dithering
Heart	Zang	Small Intestine	Joy/Fright	Fire	Blood circulation, mental functions
Lungs	Zang	Large Intestine	Sadness/Grief	Metal	Controls Chi and respiration, regulates water flow
Small Intestines	Fu	Heart		Fire	Receives and contains food and water
Large Intestines	Fu	Lungs		Metal	Involved with transport and transformation
San Jiao	Fu				Digestion
Pericardium					Circulation

The Zang Organs

These are the viscera of the body, the solid organs. These organs store our energies and fluids: Ching, Chi, and Shen as well as Blood and other bodily fluids that are created and stored within each organ. These organs can be considered yin relative to their partner fu organs. The zang organs regulate. The five organs are the Heart, Spleen, Lungs, Kidneys, and Liver.

- **The Heart** (and pericardium)

The Heart is the ruler of all the zang organs. The Heart controls our mental activities and the circulation of blood. Problems with the Heart are often seen in the face and in the complexion. Curiously, in this model, it is not the brain that controls our thoughts. The brain is simply the place where thoughts are received and stored. Our mental health, our ability to think, and the vigor of our blood are directly related to the strength of the Chi in our Heart. Weak Chi here can result in insomnia, disturbing dreams, poor sleep, dullness, and heart palpitations. Due to the Heart's meridian passing by the tongue, problems with the Heart can often be seen in the tongue.

- **The Spleen**

Most people in the West don't really know what the spleen is or does. This is a vague organ. In Chinese medicine, however, the Spleen is very important. The Spleen is essential to the process of digestion and distribution of nourishment. If the Spleen's Chi is strong, the food's essence is spread throughout the body. If Chi here is weak, the body becomes undernourished and weak. This same distribution function occurs for water too; the Spleen ensures proper hydration of our cells and the elimination of water through the kidneys. Because our blood is mostly water, the Spleen directly affects the quality of our blood. The Spleen also controls the proper functioning of our limbs and maintenance of our skeletal muscles. The Spleen affects our mental function; especially our intention, determination or willpower, and the awareness of possibilities for changes we could make. Weakness in the Spleen can often be seen in the lips and mouth. If things taste good, the Spleen is working well. If the Spleen Chi is weak, worry may be a constant companion.

• The Lungs

The Lungs control Chi (breath), and since this is the first contact with the external winds, the Lungs have to be vigilant. They are associated with Defensive Chi to ensure nothing harmful enters the body. The Lungs send Defensive Chi to the body's skin to assist in this protection. Due to Lung Chi flowing downward, the Lungs help to control water and fluids. Edema (water retention) may be caused by a weakness in the Lungs. Since air passes through the nose, the Lungs are associated with the nostrils and our sense of smell. The quality of Lung Chi is often seen in the skin and body hair. Sadness that won't go away may be a sign of weakness in the Lungs.

• The Kidneys

The Kidneys store Ching. Here this essence of our body can be converted into Kidney Chi, which is used to help the Kidneys control water. This is a function shared with the Lungs. The Kidneys send clear healthy water upward to circulate in the body and send used, turbid waters downward for elimination. It is not just the distribution of water that the Kidneys govern but also the utilization of it. Because blood and bones are so intimately connected to water, the Kidneys are also responsible for their proper functioning. Determination is also said to be stored in the Kidneys. The Kidneys are also directly connected to reproductive health and function. Problems with the Kidneys can be seen in the ears and genitals. Problems may also result in anxiety or emotions of fear arising at inappropriate times.

- **The Liver**

The Liver is the home of Shen, the soul. This may seem strange to us in the West; we are used to thinking that the heart is the seat of the soul. In Daoist belief, the Heart is the home of thinking. When our Shen is calm, the Liver is functioning well and we can watch the world unfold dispassionately. The Liver also has many physiological functions but mostly it regulates the amount of blood in the circulation. While the Heart may govern the flow of blood, it is the Liver that stores and releases it. Because of this, Liver Chi is important for the vitality of all parts of the body. In fact, acupuncture treatments often focus on releasing Liver Chi, to dispel stagnation throughout the body. Weakness in the Liver can be seen in the eyes and in our tendons. Aching knees are one indicator of weakness, yellow eyes are another. When the Liver Chi is weak, we may suffer from too much anger or irritation or be unable to express anger at all.

The Fu Organs

The fu organs are the receptor organs. These hollow organs receive the fluids and energies from their zang counterparts. They receive, digest, absorb, and transmit nutrients and excrete wastes. They are considered yang relative to their paired zang organ. We can generalize and say that the fu organs transform and transmit. There are six fu organs: they are the Small Intestines, Stomach, Large Intestines, Urinary Bladder, Gall Bladder, and an interesting one called the "San Jiao," also known as the Triple Burner.

- **The Small Intestines**

Paired with the Heart, the Small Intestines receive and store water and food. Just as we understand in the West, the Small Intestines are believed to digest food, convert it into nutrition, and send the unusable bits downward for excretion. A Chinese doctor would call the bits for excretion "turbid" and the nutritious bits "clear." If we are suffering from too much heat or too much dampness, problems may arise in our urinary system and turbidity will increase.

• The Stomach

Paired with the Spleen, the Stomach receives and digests food. It also stores food and water. If Stomach Chi is weak, food stagnates and all manner of digestive problems arise.

• The Large Intestine

Paired with the Lungs, the Large Intestines compact our solid wastes. Just as the Lungs' Chi energy controls water, the Large Intestines also affect water through the ability to absorb it. Too little absorption and we suffer loose bowels, too much and we become constipated.

• The Urinary Bladder

Paired with the Kidneys, the Urinary Bladder stores and excretes urine. If there are problems with Kidney Chi, this may show up in urinary problems such as frequent micturition or the need to get up at night many times to urinate.

• The Gall Bladder

Paired with the Liver, the Gall Bladder stores and excretes bile. In Chinese medicine, bile is considered to be Liver Chi, not the byproduct of the liver's digestion of fats, as we believe in the West. Together with the Liver, the Gall Bladder builds and controls the blood and our overall Chi levels. When weak, the Gall Bladder may cause us to be indecisive or hesitant. When strong, the Gall Bladder allows us to be decisive and bold.

- **The San Jiao**

This organ has no Western counterpart. Sometimes referred to as the Triple Burner, this organ's function relates to digestion and elimination overall. There are many different views of what the San Jiao is exactly and what it does. It is often considered to have three separable functions:

- the Upper Jiao, located above the diaphragm, distributes water in a mist form throughout the body, assisting the Heart and Lungs
- the Middle Jiao, located between the diaphragm and the navel, assists the Stomach and Spleen with digestion and the transportation of nutrients
- the Lower Jiao, located below the navel, assists the Kidneys and Urinary Bladder in their roles of elimination

Sometimes the San Jiao is believed to be paired with the Pericardium, which in some models is considered to be a zang organ separate from the Heart.

A more detailed online summary of these organs and the zang/fu theory can be found at a Web site called TCM[88] Basics.[89] Beyond these five (or six) zang and six fu organs are six other miscellaneous organs in the Chinese models. These are organs of consciousness, and are associated with Ching energy. They include the Brain, Bone Marrow, Blood Vessels, Uterus, Gall Bladder (again!), and the Meridians.

---

[88] TCM stands for Traditional Chinese Medicine.
[89] www.tcmbasics.com.

The Meridians

In Chinese medicine the channels that conduct energy throughout the body are called "meridians." These conduits form a network. If the network is disrupted, if blockages occur, the body will not function properly – Chi, Ching, and Shen do not flow as required, the organs will not perform their function, and imbalance arises. When the meridians are clear and open, energy flows freely and all is well once more.

When we looked at the highways within our subtle body from the yogic perspective, we discovered the ancient yogis sensed thousands upon thousands of individual passageways, which they called the nadis. Some text suggested there were seventy-two thousand nadis while other texts claimed there were three hundred thousand. The use of large numbers is not meant to give an exact tally of how many lines of energy there actually are in the body. Large numbers simply signify that there are too many to count. The learning to be taken here is that our bodies are full of conduits for the subtle energies that flow within us.[90]

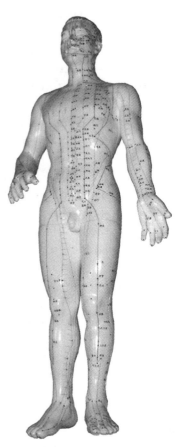

The Meridian Man

As in India, the Chinese mystics realized that not all channels are equally important. The Indian yogis described eleven nadis by name

---

[90] In Thailand a similar model of energy movement evolved through a cross-fertilization of Indian and Chinese influences. The lines of energy manipulated in Thai Yoga massage are called sens. Thai massage can be considered a form of acupressure which stimulates the flow of energy along the sen lines.

and further claimed that only three were really important for spiritual practice. In China, with a greater concern over physical well-being and longevity, seventy-one meridians were named and of these, fourteen were most important. Each of the ten major organs has its associated meridian, and the meridian may be yin or yang, depending upon the zang or fu nature of the organ it pertains to. Additionally, the pericardium and the San Jiao also have their associated meridians, which, along with the others, make up twelve major meridians, known as a group as *Jing Mai*. We can consider these twelve to be major channels.

Each of the major channels has one or more collateral channels, side roads leading to destinations other than the pertaining organ. Along the meridians are found special points that can be stimulated, through acupuncture, to mobilize energy or remove blockages. On the major meridians, there are three hundred and sixty-one regular points, although during an examination a Chinese doctor may discover even more. In more recent times, a branch of acupuncture focusing just on the ear has discovered fifty-four additional points on each ear.

In all there over two thousand acupuncture points used to help maintain or rebuild health. That is far too many for us to investigate in this journey. The interested reader can take up the trail by studying one of the many textbooks used in Traditional Chinese Medicine[91]

---

[91] It should be noted that the Traditional Chinese Medicine is not the original Chinese Medicine! Mark Seem, a former president of the Council of Colleges of Acupuncture and Oriental Medicine, writes in his book *Acupuncture Imaging*:

> The label [TCM] is inappropriate for two reasons. First it obscures the fact that there has never been one traditional medicine in China. Second … this very modern reformulation of Chinese medicine is … a recent invention.

In the forward to this book, Bob Flows writes:

> …[TCM] … refers to a specific style of Chinese medicine developed and taught in the People's Republic of China over the last forty years…TCM is a style of Chinese medicine rather than its totality…

training such as the newly compiled *Chinese Acupuncture and Moxibustion,* published by the Shanghai University. Even more highly recommended, and easier to follow, is Ted Kaptchuk's book *The Web That Has No Weaver.*

We will limit our investigation to the fourteen most-discussed meridians. There are six meridians that begin or end in the feet. Relative to their position in the body these meridians can be considered yin meridians, compared to another six that begin or end in the hands, which can be considered yang meridians. Being yin meridians, these lower ones are more strongly affected during a Yin Yoga practice than the higher yang meridians. We will begin our investigation with these six lower lines. Note that we will describe each meridian as a single line but usually there are two meridians; one for each side of the body.

Flows notes that TCM focuses mostly on the fourteen key meridians but ignores "the other fifty-seven of the seventy-one channels and collaterals described in classical Chinese acupuncture."

The Lower Body Meridians

The six meridians that begin or end in the lower body are of most interest to Yin Yoga practitioners. These are the lines affected the most by the yin asanas. They are the Liver, Gall Bladder, Kidney, Urinary Bladder, Spleen, and Stomach meridians.

The Liver Meridian

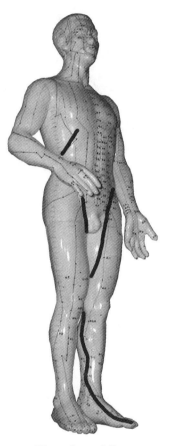

The Liver meridian begins at the inside of the nail of the big toe and runs along the top of the foot. It climbs the front of the ankle and then runs up the inside (medial) part of the leg (running just beneath the Spleen meridian) until it reaches the pubic area. From here it curves around the external genitalia and goes into the lower abdomen[92] where it enters into the liver and the gall bladder. Rising higher, it branches in several directions, with one branch connecting to the Lung meridian. Rising still higher, the Liver meridian follows the throat and connects with the eyes before branching again. One branch reaches down across the cheeks and circles the lips, while a higher branch goes across the forehead to the crown where it links with the Governor Vessel meridian.

Lower back pain, abdominal pain, or mental disturbances may be a sign of disharmony of the Liver. Frequent or unreasonable anger or irritation may also be a sign of dysfunction here.

---

[92] Unfortunately, we can't see the inside lines on Mr. Meridian Man.

The Gall Bladder Meridian

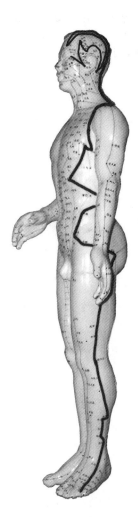

The Gall Bladder meridian begins at the outer corner of the eye (close to the Liver meridian, which passes through the center of the eye) and immediately branches into two lines. A main branch remains on the surface and winds back and forth across the side of the head and above the ear, before turning downward along the side of the neck. After following the top of the shoulder, it passes under the arm and zigzags along the side of the ribs to the hips. The other branch goes inside the cheek and descends to the liver and gall bladder. From there it descends farther and emerges in time to rejoin the first branch at the front of the hip. The single line then descends, running along the outside (lateral) thigh and knee until it reaches the ankle. It runs across the top of the foot until it reaches the fourth toe; however, another branch leaves at the ankle to run across the top of the foot and join the Liver meridian at the big toe.

Headache, blurred vision, and pains along the side of the body including the eyes, ears, and throat may be an indication of problems with the Gall Bladder meridian.

The Kidney Meridian

The Kidney meridian begins at the outside of the little toe and immediately goes under the sole of the foot. It follows the arch, makes a circle around the inner ankle and then it runs through the heel, and comes up the inmost (medial) side of the leg (just beneath the Liver meridian) and into the tailbone. It follows the spine to the kidney and then branches. One branch heads to the Urinary Bladder, where it comes back to the surface of the abdomen and up the chest, ending at the clavicle. The other branch touches the liver and diaphragm and moves up through the lungs and throat until it ends beside the root of the tongue.

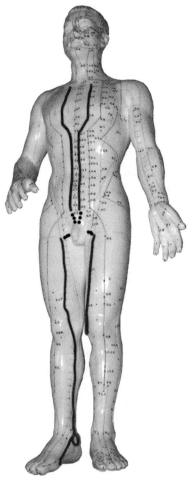

Disharmony of the Kidney meridian is suggested by gynecological problems, genital disorders, and problems in the kidneys, lungs, and throat. Examples may include impotence, frequent urination, and weakness in the lower limbs. Emotional problems may also occur related to anxiety and fear.

The Urinary Bladder Meridian

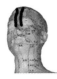 Like the Gall Bladder meridian, the Urinary Bladder meridian also begins at the eye. The Urinary Bladder line starts at the inner eye and then goes up, across the forehead, to the crown. One branch splits here, enters the brain, and then reemerges at the scapula and runs just inside the line of the scapula down the spine to the buttocks, where it reenters the body and runs to the urinary bladder and the kidney. The second branch from the crown flows down the back of the neck and shoulder and runs just outside and parallel to the first branch. This branch continues down the back of the buttocks and legs, circles the outer ankle, runs along the outer edge of the foot, and ends in the small toe where the Kidney meridian begins. Dr. Motoyama believes that the ida and pingala nadis correspond to the Urinary Bladder meridians, because they run along either side of the spine.

Signs of disharmony in the Urinary Bladder may include backaches, headaches, an inability to urinate, mental problems, and disease of the lower limbs.

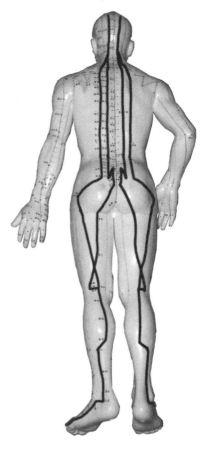

The Spleen Meridian

Starting at the inside of the big toe, the Spleen meridian runs along the inside of the foot, then turns and runs up the inside of the ankle and the shin. It runs just in front of the Liver meridian and enters the abdominal cavity, just above the pubic bone. It connects to the spleen and then the stomach, where it branches. The main branch comes to the surface and runs up the chest to the throat where it again enters the body, going to the root of the tongue, where it spreads out. The second branch remains internal and reaches the heart, connecting to the Heart meridian.

Indications of Spleen disharmony include stomach problems, flatulence, vomiting, and bloating. Unreasonable worry may also arise.

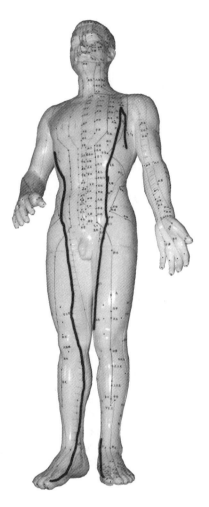

The Stomach

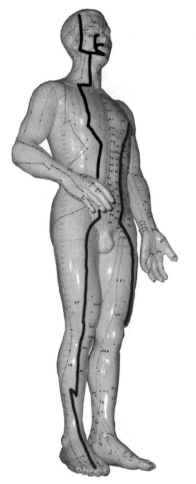

Beginning at the side of the nose, the Stomach meridian rises to the corner of the eye (where it connects to the Urinary Bladder meridian) before descending along the side of the nose, to enter the upper gum, and follow the outer lips to the lower jaw, toward the joint of the jaw. It branches here with one branch ascending along the front of the ear to the forehead. The other branch descends through the body to the diaphragm, and runs to the stomach and spleen. A third branch emerges from the lower jaw and runs across the outside of the body, crossing the chest and belly, until it terminates in the groin.

The line that runs through the stomach reconnects with this third branch and runs downward along the front of the leg, reaching the top of the foot. Here it splits again, with the main branch ending in the outside (lateral) tip of the second toe. The other branch reaches the inner (medial) side of the big toe where it meets the Spleen meridian. Just below the knee an additional branch splits off and runs to the lateral side of the third toe.

Like the Spleen meridian, problems with the Stomach meridian may be indicated by abdominal problems such as bloating, vomiting, pain in any of the areas the meridian passes through (mouth, nose, teeth, etc.), as well as mental problems.

The Upper Body Meridians

There are six meridians that begin or end in the fingers of the hands. They all pass through the shoulder or armpit. The Yin Yoga practice does not often target these lines.[93] The six upper body meridians are the Heart, Small Intestine, Large Intestine, Lung, Pericardium, and San Jiao.

The Heart Meridian

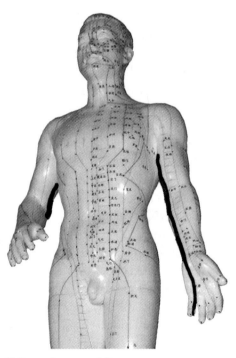

The three branches of the Heart meridian begin in the heart. One branch flows downward through the diaphragm to meet the small intestines. Another rises up alongside the throat and ends in the lower eye. The third runs across the chest, through the lungs, and comes out through the armpit. It flows along the midline of the inside upper arm, through the inner elbow, along the midline of the inner lower arm, until it crosses the wrist and palm, before ending in the inside tip of the little finger where it connects to the Small Intestine meridian.

---

[93] Sometimes, when in a reclining pose, the student may choose to bring her arm or arms over her head and this will stimulate one or more of these upper bodylines. However, for many students, having the arms raised over the head cuts off the flow of blood and energy to the hands. This results in a pins-and-needles feeling, which is not desirable. In those cases the arm should be brought lower.

Disorders of the heart and chest such as palpitations, pain, insomnia, night sweats, and mental problems may signal problems with the Heart meridian.

The Small Intestine Meridian

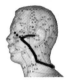 Starting where the Heart meridian ends, the Small Intestine meridian begins at the outer tip of the little finger. It runs along the back edge of the hand, through the wrist, upward along the outer forearm and upper arm, to the shoulder. After circling the back of the shoulder, it meets the Governor Vessel meridian. Here it branches, with one branch going inside the body and descending through the heart, diaphragm, and stomach before ending in the small intestine. Another branch ascends along the side of the neck to the cheek and outer corner of the eye from where it then goes to the ear. Another small branch leaves the cheek to run to the inner eye where it meets the Urinary Bladder meridian.

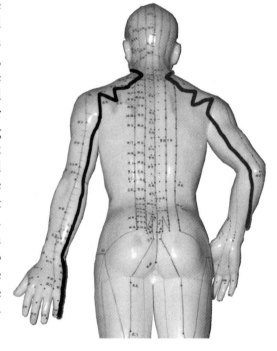

Disharmony in the Small Intestine meridian may be indicated by ear, eye, or stomach problems such as deafness, pain in the lower abdomen, or pain in the shoulders or neck.

The Lung Meridian

The Lung meridian begins inside the belly just above the navel, and drops down to the large intestines. From here it comes back up through the diaphragm and connects to the stomach. It ascends through the lungs and follows the throat before coming to the front surface of the shoulder from under the clavicle. From here it runs along the outer, thumb side (medial/radial) of the upper arm and the front (anterior) of the lower arm. It crosses the wrist and ends at the outer tip of the thumb. A small branch goes from the wrist to the tip of the index finger, where it connects to the Large Intestine meridian.

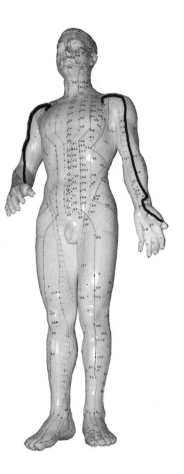

Respiratory problems like coughs, asthma, and chest pains may signify Lung meridian dysfunction. Extreme and persistent sadness and grief may also indicate problems here.

The Large Intestine Meridian

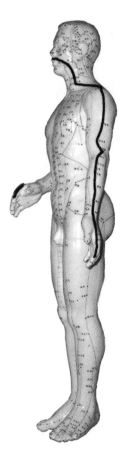

Beginning at the tip of the index finger, the Large Intestine meridian runs between the thumb and forefinger and along the outside (lateral side) of the arm. It comes over the outside top of the shoulder and along the back of the shoulder blades to the spine. Here it branches, with one branch descending through the lungs, diaphragm, and the large intestines. The second branch ascends along the neck and the lower cheek, and enters the lower gum, circling the lower teeth. On the outside, this line also circles the upper lips, crosses under the nose and rises up to join the Stomach meridian.

Problems in the mouth, teeth, nose, and throat such as toothaches and sore throats, as well as problems with the neck and shoulders, may indicate disharmony of the Large Intestine meridian.

The Pericardium Meridian

The pericardium covers the heart and is considered in Chinese medicine to be an organ function of its own. The Pericardium meridian begins in the chest and connects to the pericardium. From here it moves down the chest, connecting the three sections of the San Jiao meridian. Another branch moves horizontally across the chest, coming to the surface of the ribs, moves up and around the armpit and down the front of the bicep and forearm to the palm, and ends at the tip

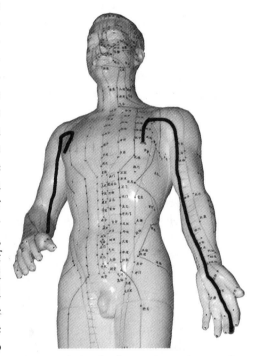

of the middle finger. A small branch leads from the palm to the tip of the ring finger where it connects to the San Jiao meridian.

Pain in the heart area, poor circulation, some stomach problems, and mental problems may indicate disharmony of the Pericardium meridian.

The San Jiao Meridian

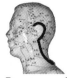

The San Jiao meridian is often called the "Triple Burner" or "Triple Energizer." It begins in the ring finger where the Pericardium meridian ends. It runs over the back of the hand, the wrist, and lower arm. It passes the outer point of the elbow and the back (lateral) of the upper arm to the back (posterior) shoulder. From here it comes over the shoulder to the front of the body and enters the chest beneath the sternum. Here it branches, with the main branch running to the pericardium and continuing down through the diaphragm to the three burners: upper, middle and lower. The second branch ascends along the side of the neck, circles the back of the ear and then circles the side of the face. Another small

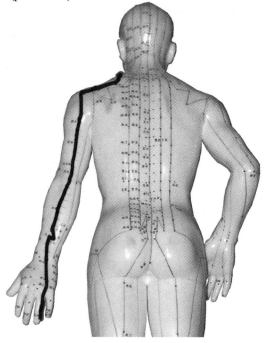

branch emerges from the back of the ear and connects to the Gall Bladder meridian at the outer corner of the eye.

Problems associated with the San Jiao meridian may occur in the side of the face, neck, or throat, or in the abdomen. Examples could include deafness, ringing in the ears, bloating, and urinary difficulties.

The Extra Meridians

As we have just seen, the meridian system is made up of the lines connecting the five yin and six yang organs plus the pericardium. Beyond these twelve, there are eight additional meridians that a Chinese doctor must know. These remaining eight are beyond our scope; however, we will visit the two most important: the Governor Vessel and the Conception Vessel meridians. These two are considered important because they have acupuncture points separate from those on any of the other twelve main meridians. All the other extra meridians share points with the main meridians.

The Governor Vessel

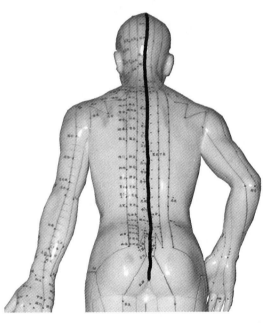

Dr. Motoyama associates the Governor Vessel with the sushumna nadi. It begins within the lower belly and splits in three. Two smaller branches ascend to connect to each kidney. The third, and main branch descends to the perineum where it enters the tip of the spinal chord and then rises up the spine to the brain. This branch comes over the top of the skull, down the middle of the forehead and nose, and terminates in the upper gum. Dr. Motoyama recommends the practice of nadi shodana to purify this meridian.[94]

---

[94] See the section on pranayama.

The Conception Vessel

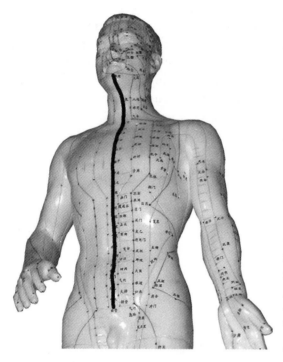

This meridian also begins in the lower abdomen next to the Governor Vessel. It has only one branch and it too descends to the perineum. Emerging from the muladhara (halfway between the anus and the "vegetables"), it ascends along the front midline of the body through the neck and chin to the mouth. At the mouth it splits and goes around the lips before sending branches to the lower eyes.

The Governor Vessel and Conception Vessel run along the front and back of the torso. These lines also contain the front and back of each chakra. When we breathe and draw energy up the Governor Vessel and down the Conception Vessel, we are completing the Microcosmic Orbit, which will be discussed in detail in Chapter 15: Moving Energy.

Eastern Energy/Western Energy

As we have seen, in the East energy has several aspects or forms. There are the ten forms of prana and the thirty-two forms of Chi. Each form of energy has a particular purpose or function. But what do the doctors and scientists in the West think about these models? Can these models really be accurate descriptions of the underlying reality? Our journey takes us westward...

Chapter Seven:
The Western View of Energy

In India, the yogic sages observed ten forms of prana through subjective experience. In China, the Daoists observed thirty-two forms of Chi. Some seers have intuited even more than this number. To our Western scientific minds, these claims seem fanciful and unsubstantiated by objective study. Within our bodies we

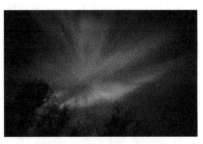

The energy of the sun is displayed via an aurora. P

have two main kinds of energy: chemical and electrical. That's it ... at least, according to the predominant Western models in vogue currently.

Chemical energy is transmitted via the blood system. Electrical energy is transmitted via the nervous system. These are the two great communication systems we are aware of and can prove exist. Due to their proven existence, many Eastern sages and Western new age pundits have tried to link the blood and nervous systems to the nadis or meridians. Efforts are made to show how the nadis are just another way to describe the nervous system, and the meridians are just another way to describe the blood system. These efforts are not very satisfactory and fail on many counts. Probably the biggest reason they fail is because what we are modeling in the prana/nadi models or the Chi/meridian models are different communication structures entirely.

Our chemical and electrical systems are not the only ways for information to be transmitted within the body!

Recent research has resurrected many nineteenth century theories about electro-magnetic fields, and how they are an integral part of the body's operation. As we shall discover, there are many other forms of energy being employed by the body to maintain its healthy, normal functioning. Why these forms of communication are just now being given credence is an interesting aside and may help to explain some of the difficulties the Eastern models have faced over the years.

A History of Energy Research

James Oschman, in his book *Energy Medicine: the Scientific Basis*, notes that the earliest known use of electricity in medicine was around 2750 B.C.E., when electric eels were used to shock ill people back into health. It was the Greek Thales who discovered static electricity around 400 B.C.E. The use of magnets in healing may be even older than electrical treatments. The ancient Egyptians and Chinese used magnetite (also known as lodestone) to heal the sick. In 1773 Anton Messer tried magnets to heal his patients; scientists of his day ridiculed his claims. The nineteenth century witnessed an explosion of electrical healing devices.

In the nineteenth century popular awareness of electricity was new. Like the computer in the late twentieth century, there was a fascination with this latest technology. Many people thought electricity could solve or explain most problems. Doctors and scientists experimented with electric fields and applied to them to the human condition. Oschman says that by 1884, ten thousand American physicians were using

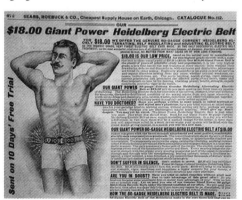

Sears, Roebuck advertised the healing power of electricity in the early 1900s.

electricity daily in their practice. Intriguing discoveries were made, but this was the time of unregulated medicine.

Fraud was commonplace and, as with any new fad, there were many entrepreneurs eager to cash in on the public's interest. Serious science was swamped by bogus claims of miraculous cures. More people were harmed than cured by this unregulated, Wild West form of medicine.

Those who were cured were believed to be exhibiting the common placebo effect. As one skeptical Web page[95] cites,

> The illusion of efficacy is also due to the power of suggestion. Belief in a particular remedy can help reduce pain and stress. This in turn enhances the body's own healing capabilities: the well-known "placebo effect." Unfortunately, such treatments may only mask the body's warning, and false hope can have dire consequences.

Serious[96] medical researchers and scientists became more and more alarmed at these bogus claims and the consequences.

In the early twentieth century, medicine became regulated and restricted by governments. No longer could anyone claim to be a healer. No longer were all modalities accepted. The medical schools adopted a well-defined curriculum, and in this curriculum there was no room for the practice of electromagnetic healing. Research followed only two paths: research on the nervous system and the electrical communication made possible by the nerves, and research on the chemical system and the drugs that affected the chemical functions in the body.

Economics is a fact of life. When an opportunity arises to earn money, people take advantage of that opportunity. The emphasis on the chemical model of the body created a big economic opportunity. One of the greatest successes of modern medicine is in this field of inquiry. The twentieth century saw huge advances in our understanding of how the body works chemically. Understanding the

---

95 The Committee for the Scientific Investigation of Claims of the Paranormal at www.csicop.org.

96 Who defined "serious" science and medical practices is open for debate.

chemical interactions at the cellular level allowed new drugs to be discovered or invented, drugs that prevented many diseases. Antibiotics, anti-depressants, vaccinations, and many more substances became the target of research because they were so good at fixing problems. Drug companies naturally funded even more research in these areas. It was not long before virtually all the research conducted in medicine was chemical in nature. Mainly governments or private sources funded research into the nervous system. Research into alternative modalities was virtually nonexistent.

Paradigms are established when the majority believe their current understanding and practice is the only correct way. Once established, paradigms are very hard to change. Through the decades of working successfully with the chemical models of the body, it became accepted that this was the only really viable approach to medicine. A good doctor had to understand the nature of an illness, look up the chemical cause of the problem, and apply a chemical solution to the problem. Most of the time, this worked. When it didn't work, it wasn't a fault of the paradigm; it was because we hadn't learned enough about the model yet. More research was needed.

Not all medical problems are solved by the current medical paradigm. People not successfully cured by Western medicine found themselves going in circles, visiting one doctor after another ... but since all doctors were working within the same paradigm, it is not surprising that no relief was obtained. If one doctor failed, it was highly likely that all doctors would fail. These patients began to seek solutions through different paradigms. The alternative modalities they tried are still looked at with ill-disguised contempt by many Western doctors, but not all. A few scientists, doctors, and researchers began to ask a bold question: what if the Eastern modalities actually did work ... and if they did work, *how* could they work? Their answers are exciting.

The economic returns from this line of inquiry are not large, especially compared to the returns from the chemical models of medicine. We should not expect large financial support from the corporate world for research into alternative models, because there are no large scale returns on these kinds of investments. Instead, we will have to rely upon private or government investment to broaden our understanding of these alternative models of medicine.

The good news in all this is … interest has resurfaced in models of communication within the body that are not just chemical or electrical in nature. Though this research is very small compared to the well-funded chemical models, which have done some remarkable things for humanity, alternative research is growing. The findings are fascinating. What is becoming clear is – the Eastern models of prana/nadis and Chi/meridians are not so subjective and fanciful as once thought. There are actual measurable, physical observations supporting these theories. This is where our journey takes us next.

New Paradigms

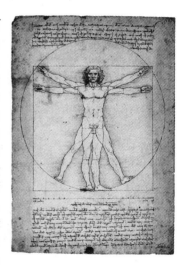

What is health? The word itself comes from wholeness. When we lack wholeness, we suffer; we are unhealthy. It follows then that healing is restoring the wholeness we are lacking. The body has an amazing ability to heal. What is surprising about all animals, all life, is not that we get sick from time to time or we aren't healthy. What is surprising is how healthy we are! There are so many ways we could become sick. There are so many interdependent functions and parts of the body that can fail. The fact that it works so well for so long is a miracle. For this miracle to occur the body must be extremely sophisticated.

Wholeness – health – requires communication internally and the ability to move energy. The cells of the body[97] need to communicate with each other. When this communication breaks down we cannot remain whole. The same point applies to transporting energy and materials within the body. Consider the example of a city during a blackout. When the power is down, transportation is shut down,

---

[97] And in one point of view that is all we are … a collective of billions of cells.

communication ceases, and the city stops functioning. The body is similar; we need information and energy to flow, whether this is chemical information in the form of substances moving from one area of the body to another or electrical information informing one area of what is happening in another area. Ill health can be considered, in this model, as a failure in the communication and transportation network of the body.

Disease and illness disrupt the flow of information and transportation within the body. For over five hundred million years complex life has been evolving and finding ways to improve the ability to communicate and transport energy and information within a body. Through trial and error[98] life has found ways to do this better and better. Better in this case means faster, more accurately, and with backup systems in case of problems. Nature and her laws of physics provide many possible methods and mediums to choose from. The most successful forms of life would naturally adopt as many of these mediums as possible.

The earliest multicellular life forms used chemical means to communicate. Materials were physically passed from one cell to the next. Then conduits were created within which these substances could travel farther, faster, and more surely. These conduits evolved into our blood system.

The nervous system evolved in a similar manner. On the surface of every piece of matter are atoms and their electrons. Some electrons are easily dislodged by a variety of naturally occurring events: sunlight, friction, chemical reactions, or nearby electrical activity. The atoms, when deprived of one or more electrons, are called "ions." Ionized atoms may attract and absorb an electron from a neighboring atom, thus becoming neutral again: but its neighbor is now ionized, so it borrows an electron from the next neighbor. Repeating this process creates a cascading wave of electrical energy. Our nervous system evolved by taking advantage of this physical process. But why would we expect nature to stop there? There are many other forms of information and energy transfer that we haven't considered yet. We use them in our machines every day: electro-

---

[98] And perhaps through some divine guidance, however, that topic is beyond the scope of the present investigation.

magnetic energy, photonic energy, infrared energy, microwave energy, gravity … this is not an exhaustive list.

A new paradigm is evolving in the West, one that broadens the scope of information and energy transportation mechanisms far beyond simple chemical and electrical models. This new paradigm includes many other forms of communication and energy movement, which could only be imagined in centuries past. With our modern, sensitive instruments, capable of detecting minute levels of energy, we are able to test these new models. We are going to explore just a couple of these new models, starting with electricity – not the electricity found in your home, but bioelectricity – the electricity of the body.

Bioelectricity

Have you noticed the shoes worn by children that light up as they run? Kids love the flashing light show put on by their shoes and parents love the fact that no batteries are needed. So, if there are no batteries, where does the electricity come from to spark the lights? The answer is "piezoelectricity."

Electricity is the movement of electrons. Electrons are the smallest and outermost part of the atom and thus are very mobile. A few moving electrons can communicate information precisely. A lot of flowing electrons can transfer energy in massive quantities. In our modern society we use electrons in both roles.

Piezoelectricity is electricity created by pressure. The word comes from the Greek *peizein*, which means to squeeze or compress. No batteries required. The piezoelectric phenomenon has been known for hundreds of years and was given its name in 1824 by David Brewster.

Certain kinds of crystals, when subjected to deforming stress, create electrical fields (measured in volts per meter) or cause electricity to flow (measured in amps). The reverse can also happen: when

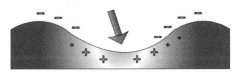

Piezoelectricity is created by deforming a crystal.

an electric field is applied to these crystals they will bend in response – the stronger the field the greater the deformation; the greater the stress – the stronger the field.

Piezoelectric crystals do not need to be recharged. When they resume their original shape the energy potential ends – when they are deformed again the field is regenerated. This wonderful ability of some crystals has been exploited in many technologies today – from the light show in shoes to lighting your barbeque, from electric microphones to sophisticated sonar systems – piezoelectricity has become commonplace

A crystal is a structured array of molecules repeated throughout the material. A crystal of salt is a simple cubic lattice of sodium and chloride atoms. Diamonds are arrayed in interlocking tetrahedral pyramids of carbon atoms. What is often overlooked is that tissues in our body are also aligned in structured, repeating patterns. The molecules of our muscles, bones, eyes, cell membranes, collagen, elastin, even our DNA … all have crystal-like structure.

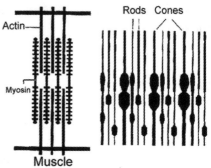

Our muscles and eyes under the microscope reveal their crystalline structures. Q

James Oschman, in his two excellent books summarizing scientific research into energy medicine, states that the living tissues of our bodies are best described as liquid crystals.

Liquid crystals, as he explains,[99] are "materials that are intermediate between solids and liquids and display properties of both." He goes on to explain that virtually the whole body is composed of materials arranged in a liquid crystal form and cites several studies confirming this model.

When our liquid crystalline tissues are subjected to deforming stress, they generate piezoelectric potential energy and tiny electric currents. Just like in the children's shoes, every move we make, ever

---

[99] Page 87 of *Energy Medicine in Therapeutics and Human Performance* by James Oschman.

breath we take (to paraphrase Sting) creates tiny currents of energy. Alternately, the presence of even small electrical potentials creates a small amount of movement or deformation in our tissues. This level of electricity is quite minute compared to the size of energy flowing in our nervous system. The voltage of the membranes of our nerve cells is in the range of millivolts.[100] The sizes of the piezoelectric voltages we are discussing are many orders of magnitude smaller than this – on the order of microvolts. It is no wonder that this very small amount of energy was never noticed before; our instruments were not sensitive enough and when they were, we just weren't looking.

If these piezoelectric energies we are discussing were expected to move materials in our body or affect us in large ways, we would be right to think they have no chance of affecting us. But consider this metaphor – you are cooking a big Thanksgiving turkey.[101] You know you need to preheat the oven, but you don't know how high to set the temperature. You call your mother on your cell phone and she tells you to try four hundred degrees.

The cell phone has at its heart a computer chip that consumes a very small amount of electricity, say fifty milliwatts. The oven produces a great deal of heat and requires a thousand watts to run properly.[102] And yet, until the small current in the cell phone gives you the information you need, all that power in the oven is dormant. Yes, certainly the cell phone could not hope to power the oven. An instrument set to measure the power output of the oven would miss the tiny energy flowing in the cell phone. But without the cell phone's intelligence, the power in the oven would never be activated. A small amount of information can create big changes. And this small amount of information requires very little power, especially compared to the large effect it stimulates.

If our bodies can be considered as liquid crystals, and if even small movements create electric fields and currents, this could provide a basis for scientific models of information and energy transfers beyond purely chemical or electrical mechanisms, which solely rely on our nervous or blood system. With such models we can

---

[100] Generally around fifty ~ seventy millivolts.

[101] Of course, since we are talking about yoga this would be a tofu turkey.

[102] That is twenty thousand times stronger than the cell phone.

begin to see how modalities that manipulate the body physically, such as yoga and massage, might have an effect on the functioning of our bodies, and therefore on our health.[103]

When an electron moves, as it does in an electric current, it gives rise to a magnetic field. How this electromagnetism can affect us is the next stop on our journey.

Electromagnetism

Every electron and every proton has an electric charge, thus an electrical field surrounding it. This is a field of force, just like the field of gravitational force we are so familiar with in everyday life. Compared to gravity, however, the electrical force is much stronger. In fact, gravity is a very weak force and is only noticeable because the earth is so huge.

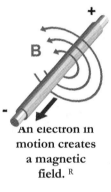

An electron in motion creates a magnetic field. [R]

Electrons are never still. When confined to the atom, electrons move constantly creating small magnetic fields. With many electrons, in many atoms, moving in random directions, these small magnetic fields cancel out and we do not notice them. But not always: sometimes the poles of the atom's magnetic fields become aligned, allowing the magnetic fields to become stronger and more noticeable. There are two basic kinds of magnets: permanent magnets and electromagnets. The permanent magnets are familiar to everyone; most fridges have at least one magnet attaching notes to the door.[104]

---

[103] An online paper discussing electrical flow across the skin, and piezoelectric effects, can be found at the Society of Electrodermology at www.electrodermology.com. There is a lot of research that indicates the body is indeed filled with crystalline piezoelectric materials. Oschman and the Society of Electrodermology have many references that can lead the interested reader to these studies.

[104] Only certain elements can be used as magnets. The elements include iron, nickel, cobalt, and also the rare earth elements of samarium and neodynium, which is the element most commonly used today in magnets.

Electromagnets have a magnetic field only when an electric current is present. When we pass a current through a wire, a magnetic field is created all around the wire. If we reverse the direction of the current, the orientation of the magnetic field also reverses.

A moving electron creates both electric and magnetic fields. It is therefore better to consider electric and magnetic fields as aspects of a more general type of field, known as the electromagnetic field. When we use this term we are referring to either or both of the electrical field and/or the magnetic field.

There are naturally occurring electromagnetic fields and artificially created ones in our environment. The earth has a very large magnetic field compared to the fields inside our body. The earth's field arises from many sources; lightening may create an even stronger electromagnetic field, albeit for a very short time. The electrical wires outside your home and inside your home all have their own electromagnetic fields. There are also magnetic fields arising from your fridge magnets and stereo speakers. These household fields are far stronger than the earth's magnetic field, but are not as pervasive.

The size of the earth's magnetic field ranges between 0.3 to 0.6 Gauss.[105] Our heart has an electric current regulating it, and it also has an electromagnetic field. The size of our heart's magnetic field is one million times smaller than the earth's magnetic field[106] and it too can vary from person to person, and indeed from time to time within the same person. Despite its weakness, the electromagnetic field of the heart is very measurable. Electrocardiograms (ECGs) are used to measure the electrical force at various locations throughout the body. While small, the heart has the largest, but not the only electromagnetic field in our body. Our brain is also a source of electrical activity, so it too has a measurable field. The brain's magnetic field is around a thousand times weaker[107] than the heart's and naturally was not detected until long after the heart's field was discovered.

---

[105] A Gauss is a unit of magnetism named after a famous mathematician.
[106] 10^{-6} Gauss.
[107] The brain's magnetic field is on the order of 10^{-9} Gauss.

As we have just seen, any electrons that are in motion will give rise to an electromagnetic field. What about those tiny piezoelectric fields we were discussing in the previous section? Do they too create tiny electromagnetic fields and, if so, can they be measured? The answer is … yes. These tiny fields, while too small to be detected until recently, do exist and their associated electromagnetic fields have been measured, thanks to the invention of a cool-sounding device known as a SQUID. Invented by John Zimmerman in the early 1970s, SQUIDs[108] are devices that allow magnetometers to detect very small electromagnetic fields. Zimmerman and others after him[109] were able to detect an increase in the electromagnetic field of a therapeutic touch practitioner's hands. The study of these generated electromagnetic fields is called "bio-electromagnetism."

Bio-electromagnetism

Our blood is mostly water with a lot of salts and minerals dissolved within it. Water saturated like this turns out to be an excellent conductor for electricity. It is not surprising that an ECG will pick up signals from the heart throughout the body. The heart's electrical field touches every part of us. Its magnetic field is also pervasive. The signals from the heart have been speculated to send information throughout the system. Unfortunately, the followers of the current medical paradigms have seen fit only to use the presence of the body's electric fields as a diagnostic tool, and have not worked out any therapeutic procedures that could tap into these fields. As we will see, alternative medicine practitioners have used this knowledge in a therapeutic way.

So far we have discussed only how an electron in motion gives rise to a magnetic field. The reverse is also true. A moving magnetic field can create an electric current. This is how an electric generator works: a magnet is placed within a coil of wires. When the magnet is rotated, electricity is created. Conversely, if electricity is run through the coil, the magnet rotates; that is the basis for an electric motor.

---

[108] SQUIDS stands for Superconducting Quantum Interference Devices.
[109] Such as Kusaka Seto of Japan.

Not only does our body create magnetic fields, our bodies can be affected by magnetic fields.

As mentioned earlier, John Zimmerman, the inventor of SQUIDs, began some interesting research in the early 1980s at the University of Colorado on the magnetic fields of touch therapists. A similar but more detailed study was done in 1992 in Japan.[110] The results of these studies showed that a therapeutic touch specialist emitted from her hands magnetic fields that varied at low frequencies, ranging from 0.3-30 Hz.[111] Most of the magnetic field frequencies centered around 7-8 Hz but the fields continuously spanned the range of frequencies. Of course, the therapists had no idea of what they were doing; they were just doing their thing.

The Japanese study included not just therapists but also Chi-gong masters, Zen masters, yogis, and meditators. Similar results were obtained. The strongest fields measured were a thousand times stronger than the field of the heart.[112]

Bio-electromagnetic Healing

All this could be considered fascinating but, so what? Why should this be important? Since the early 1800s, scientists and doctors have experimented with magnets for their possible therapeutic benefits. When medicine became standardized, this kind of research was stopped. Recently, however, it has begun again. The findings of these more modern researches have vindicated the earlier beliefs that

---

[110] See James Oschman's book *Energy Medicine,* page 78.

[111] A Hertz (or Hz) refers to the number of times each second that the magnetic field switches direction. Thirty Hz means the field switches thirty times each second. A 0.3 Hz measurement means the field switches every three seconds.

[112] Interestingly, at times the emitters of these fields would lose their abilities. One possible cause for this is the ever-changing frequency of the earth's magnetic field. Normally the earth's field switches at something known as the Schumann's frequency, which is in the range of 7-10 Hz. However certain events like solar flares can change this and may cause therapists and other Chi masters to have lesser or greater abilities at those times.

magnetism can help people heal in certain situations. One therapy is called "PEMF," pulsed electromagnetic field therapy.

One example of PEMF should suffice to explain its benefits. Occasionally, when someone suffers a broken bone, the bone doesn't heal. The break may remain for years or even decades. Somehow something has gone wrong with the repair mechanism in the body. The information needed to heal the fracture is not getting to the tissues responsible for fixing the break. In these cases today, a doctor is likely to recommend a small battery-powered magnetic field generator be placed around the broken bone. An oscillating magnetic field is applied for eight to ten hours every day. Clinical tests have shown that even for broken bones that have remained unhealed for forty years, the bones can be repaired with this technique.

The frequency of the magnetic field applied to a broken bone is seven Hz. This healing frequency is called the "frequency window of specificity" (FWS). Sisken and Walker in 1995 reported that various FWS's affect different tissues.

Frequency	Effects
2 Hz	Nerve regeneration
7 Hz	Bone growth
10 Hz	Ligament repair
15~20 Hz	Skin repair
25 & 50 Hz	Assistance with nerve growth

While Zimmerman's investigations of the magnetic fields emitted by touch therapists did not prove that healing was occurring, he did discover that the therapists were emitting magnetic fields, which spanned the same frequencies that other scientists discovered stimulated healing. Future studies are required to prove that healing touch can actually heal, but these results have pointed to a promising area of investigation.

Electrical activity in the body, beyond that which is found flowing through the nerves, has been found to be responsible for many of the body's functions. The mechanism by which cells lay down or reabsorb supporting materials (collagen) in bone and connective tissues is understood. Electric fields generated during movement signal cells[113] to lay down collagen, and thereby strengthen the tissues. With less loading or movement, the electric fields are weaker and less frequent and other cells reabsorb collagen. The other cells that are responsible for reabsorbing materials do not do this if an electric field is present.

The proof that electrical and magnetic fields affect and help the body is indisputable. Perhaps certain frequencies can even harm the body.[114] A question now arises … what does this mean for our models of the way the body works?

A Hypothesis for Further Study

A hypothetical model, which could be tested through rigorous scientific study, is that illness is caused by a blockage of information flow, while health is maintained by the proper flow of information. When the required information is not provided to an injured or sick area of the body, the body's own resources are not mobilized to respond or the body responds ineffectually or even inappropriately.[115] Alternative healing modalities such as yoga, Tai Chi, massage, energy manipulation therapies, and many others could be ways of injecting the missing information through very weak, low frequency electromagnetic field generation. Just as the cell phone was required to start the oven in our original metaphor, a small amount of electromagnetic information may be all that is required to stimulate healing. If this is possible, how could this energy flow within the body? Let's complete the construction of a possible model by looking more closely, at the cellular level, at how this information may be transmitted.

---

[113] Fibroblasts in connective tissues, osteoblasts in bone.
[114] We will address that question at the end of this chapter.
[115] Cancer could be considered an inappropriate response.

Integrins, Cytoskeletons, and Meridians

Blood vessels transport chemical energy stored in molecules throughout the body. Nerves conduct electrical energy. But what conducts the electromagnetic energies we have been discussing? Well, electrical and magnetic fields don't actually need pathways to propagate. They are transmitted through space itself. Unfortunately the fields diminish the farther away we get from their source and in some cases these fields can be shielded.[116] Over a very small region the fields will be strong enough to conduct energy or information, but over larger areas a different mechanism is required.

Electrical fields follow the flow of electricity. As we have seen, the nerves are not the only conductors of electricity in the body. An ECG measures the electrical activity of the heart in places far away from our chest. These signals are possible because the blood system itself conducts electrical information. So the circulatory system is one possible channel for electromagnetic energy, not just chemical energy. Interestingly, the Daoists long ago identified the blood system as a conduit of Chi. If Chi is not simply chemical energy perhaps they were sensing this conductance of electromagnetic energy through our blood vessels. Or, perhaps, the definition of Chi needs to be broadened to include all these forms of energy: chemical, electrical, and electromagnetic.

Does it stop there? Does our circulatory system feed every part of the body? What about inside the cells? How can information be transmitted to the insides of the cells themselves? To answer this question we need to look at the current and the evolving models of the cell.

---

[116] With metal plates, for example. See the section on Electropollution for a discussion on this topic.

The Bag of Soup Model

In most books that describe the anatomy of a cell, you will find a diagram similar to the one shown here. This is a very detailed view of the components we find inside the cell body. Detailed, but incomplete. What is that water-like substance inside the cell? Soup! In the popular model of the cell all the internal apparatus float in this soup.

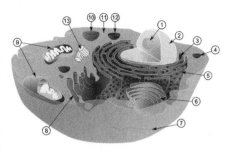

What is that stuff in the middle of the cell? s

Chemicals, from outside the cell, ease their way past the permeable cell membrane, and then drift around in the soup until they happen to bump into something important. The chemical energy model of communication requires a random movement of these chemicals until they find and latch onto their destination.

This is not a very satisfying model, relying as it does on random timing for information transfers to occur. James Oschman notes that many cellular activities happen much faster than a random walkabout would allow. Something is missing in this model.[117]

When we look in most anatomy books and see the way the body is depicted, we find a similar "something missing." The pictures will show in wonderful detail the circulatory system, or we may trace the skeletal system or the muscular or nervous systems. But all these models omit the material that these systems are embedded within. What is missing is the connective tissue. Connective tissues join the circulatory system to the nervous system to the muscular system and so on. Our connective tissues are ubiquitous and, as we have seen, are formed of collagen fibers, elastin fibers, and many other components arrayed in crystalline matrices. These matrices form the piezoelectric crystals that create and conduct the electrical energies we were discussing in the previous section.

---

[117] See Oschman's book *Energy Medicine*, chapter fourteen, for more details on this topic.

These matrices are exactly what are missing in the bag of soup cellular models. We need a new model that fills in the gaps and explains the cellular processes more completely.

The Integrins and Cytoskeleton

The newer models of the cell's anatomy recognize that the cell is not just a bag of goo. There is a structure inside the cell, just as there is outside the cell. The image shown here explains this nicely. As illustrated, the cell is filled with fibers and filaments, tubes and structure. Collectively this structure is called the "cytoskeleton" or the "cytoplasmic matrix" and, just like our body's bony skeleton, it provides rigidity and support to the whole cell. More than that though, the cytoskeleton also provides pathways for information to flow along. No longer do we have to imagine chemical information just floating around in the sea of soup waiting for a chance encounter. Now we find that chemical information can be guided to its destination by enzymes that line the cytoskeleton.

If you look again you will also see that these lines forming the cytoskeleton also extend out beyond the cell walls. These linking elements are called "integrins" and they connect the inner and outer worlds of our cells. We have already seen that the extra-

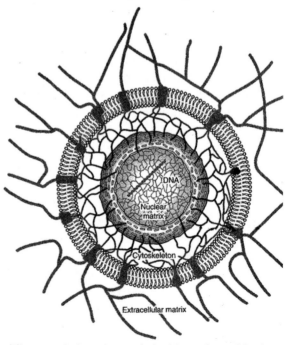

The cytoskeleton extends inside and outside the cell. T

cellular matrix is networked throughout our whole body. With each cell connected inside and outside, with the ground substance flowing everywhere throughout the body, we find that every cell has a connection to every other cell in our body. There is no place that is not connected to every other place within us.

In our human society we have a similar connection called the "Six Degrees of Separation" phenomenon: every human being is connected to every other by at most six connections through other people. With billions of people, there are almost an infinite number of ways we can connect to each other. With billions of cells in our body, there is also a virtually infinite number of ways[118] all of our cells are connected to each other.

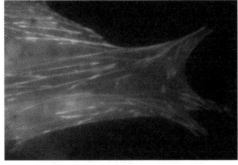

A micrograph of the cytoskeleton in fibroblasts. U

We have said this complete interconnection is potentially so. We have also postulated that illness is a blocking of information, an inability of the body to transmit healing signals to the affected area. If a problem isolates one region of the body from the others, information may not get through. Like a city suffering a power outage, communication lines may be out of service, transportation systems may fail. The city may survive for a short time but unless outside help arrives, the city is doomed. Our body is not very different. Health means wholeness. If one part of the body is cut off from the information flow throughout the body, illness arises.

---

[118] All right, to the purist, the number is nowhere near infinite and "virtually infinite" is a meaningless phrase. But the number is very, very large and would take far too many zeros to depict here.

Meridians Revisited

The Western scientists who originally investigated the Eastern claims of meridians and nadis went back to their dissection tables looking for physical manifestations of these channels. Their dissections discarded the supposedly inert connective tissues. They looked past these tissues searching for something that just wasn't there. They looked for channels and conducting tubes similar to nerves and blood vessels, and could not find them. Their conclusion: no channels, no meridians. Ironically, they discarded the very tissues that formed the channels they were seeking. The energies flow through the connective tissues, through the water-hugging fibers of the ground substance.

The ancient sages told us that there were seventy-two thousand nadis. Some said three hundred thousand. Some said three hundred and sixty thousand. They were wrong, of course. The number of connections between the billions of cells in our body is beyond counting. One estimate claims that there are over one billion trillion connections. That is likely to be a low estimate. These connections, of course, are the nadis and the meridians that the sages talked of. They are the conduits of the energies of prana and Chi. We can forgive these early sages for not getting the number right: but the point was taken. Calculators were rare two thousand years ago.

Chi Revisited

So far we have been looking only at the flow of information possibly encoded in the piezoelectrically generated energies of the body, and the associated electromagnetic energies that could travel along the crystalline structures of our connective tissues. The sages of ages past underestimated the number of channels; what about their claims that there are ten kinds of prana or thirty-two types of Chi? Were they exaggerating here?

The curious reader is directed again to James Oschman's books. We have only touched upon the research he has gathered relating to electromagnetism. In his studies, Dr. Oschman also investigates gravitational information, infrared, photonic, microwave, and many other forms of energy that the body seems to employ to communicate information. It does indeed seem likely that, over hundreds of millions of years of evolution, life on earth has adapted to, and adopted, everything Mother Nature has made available to us. When we add these forms of energies to the ones we have already talked about (chemical, electrical, and magnetic) the total exceeds the number the sages gave us. Once again, rather than finding that the Indian and Daoist yogis were exaggerating, we can speculate that they were being rather conservative in their descriptions of what is going on inside our bodies.

Models are Just Models

It is important to point out again that all these models are simply that: models. They are not attempts to describe the way the body really works, or to claim as fact anything posited. Models are simply tools to predict certain behavior and to assist us in developing interventions to correct malfunctions. Models are rarely one hundred percent accurate or complete. Models constantly evolve as new information is uncovered. It is part of the scientific method to test all models rigorously. Debate is not just welcomed, it is essential in order to push the boundaries of knowledge.

To be complete, the reader may wish to visit several Web sites that take issue with the Eastern models. Quackwatch[119] is one site that will offer a definite and strong counter viewpoint to many of the claims discussed above. The Committee for the Scientific Investigations of Claims of the Paranormal[120] also presents alternative views.

If the models we have reviewed do seem valid, they would also lead us to consider the impact of electromagnetic fields occurring around us, not just those inside of us. Every home that is wired for electricity has these fields. Whatever can heal also has the potential to harm, if misused. A complete list of the dangers that exist and how we could protect ourselves from these dangers is beyond the scope of our journey. But let's have a brief look into this area.

---

[119] At www.quackwatch.org.
[120] At www.csicop.org.

Electropollution

At very high levels, electricity can kill. Lightning kills sixty-seven people in an average year in the USA. At very low levels, electricity can heal. Electricity is the essential energy transmitted by our nervous system. Medical research has shown that very tiny amounts of electromagnetism, vibrating at low frequencies, can stimulate tissues to heal. Are there other levels of intensities or frequencies that could be harmful? Many people believe so, but there have been no studies definitely proving the case. There has been, however, a lot of anecdotal evidence supporting the fear.

Science can never prove something is *not* harmful. Studies can prove something *is* harmful. It takes only one case to show that something can hurt us. However, even if a thousand studies show that no harm has been caused, this does not mean that a procedure or device is safe. There may be another study, not yet conceived, that one day will prove a danger exists. Generally, after a sizable number of studies have been carried out with no evidence of harm, the scientific community will assess the danger as being low enough, the risks small enough, to endorse the procedure. But we will never receive an absolute benediction.

Can we be harmed by electric fields in our environment? Government and electric power company studies seem to show that we are not affected by being near high-voltage lines, but we can never be absolutely sure. Of more concern are the electromagnetic fields found inside our homes and offices. The concern is over frequencies higher than those we have looked at so far. While small amounts of energy flowing in the 2-30 Hz range can heal, the 50-60 Hz range appears to be dangerous.[121] Unfortunately, the electrical power used in our homes is in these frequency ranges.

A study by the United Kingdom Advisory Group on Non-ionizing Radiation states[122] the following:

---

[121] See Oschman's *Energy Medicine*, page 212.
[122] From the *ELF Electromagnetic Fields and Neurodegenerative Disease: Report of an Advisory Group on Non-ionizing Radiation.*

Laboratory experiments have provided no good evidence that extremely low frequency electromagnetic fields are capable of producing cancer, nor do human epidemiological studies suggest that they cause cancer in general. There is, however, some epidemiological evidence that prolonged exposure to higher levels of power frequency magnetic fields is associated with a small risk of leukemia in children. In practice, such levels of exposure are seldom encountered by the general public in the UK. In the absence of clear evidence of a carcinogenic effect in adults, or of a plausible explanation from experiments on animals or isolated cells, the epidemiological evidence is currently not strong enough to justify a firm conclusion that such fields cause leukemia in children. Unless, however, further research indicates that the finding is due to chance or some currently unrecognized artifact, the possibility remains that intense and prolonged exposures to magnetic fields can increase the risk of leukemia in children.

The interested reader can find many similar conclusions from even a cursory search on the Internet. The Manitoba Hydro Company's Web site[123] lists several of these studies, including the one cited above. A wider search will reveal, however, many very vocal groups who firmly believe that their own illnesses have indeed been caused by these local electromagnetic fields. Their evidence is anecdotal and thus cannot be considered valid for a scientific study. However, these individuals are convinced that electromagnetic pollution was the cause of their illnesses.

What to do? If you are concerned, there are many things you can do to reduce your risk. First, realize that the fields we are talking about decline in strength over distance rather quickly. The strength of the field between two magnets decreases by the fourth power of the distance. This means that if the strength of the field at one foot is one unit, at two feet the strength is only 1/16th of a unit. At three feet the strength has dropped to 1/256th. Generally if you are at least

[123] www.hydro.mb.ca/safety_and_education/emf/index.shtml.

three feet away from most household magnetic fields, you should be safe from their effects. Also, most appliances today like microwaves, TVs, and computers are shielded, which drops the strength of the fields even further. Most, but not all. Your toaster oven or an older model cell phone or cordless phone may have a very high level of electromagnetic radiation, much higher than any of the other appliances cited.

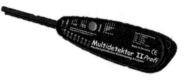

Another approach, which is more expensive than simply staying away from the devices that create these fields, is to buy filters for all your outlets. These devices will clean up stray fields and reduce the amount of electromagnetic radiation in your homes and offices.

Before making such a large investment, you may want to be sure this is a problem for you. A meter, like the one shown above,[124] can tell you for sure what the field levels are in your home, office, and even in your car (which may be the highest of all).

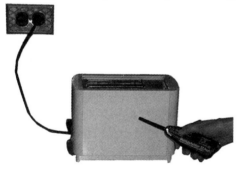

What may surprise many people is that an appliance need not be turned on in order to generate the fields of force. Simply having the device plugged in will create an electromagnetic field. The potential energy is still there even in a device such as a lamp or toaster that is plugged into a wall socket. To be completely safe, don't turn off the device; unplug it instead. Be careful of your laptop computer: if it is plugged in, its transformer may be generating a large electromagnetic field. Again, don't disconnect the power chord from the computer; disconnect it from the wall socket.

---

[124] This particular meter measures both electric and magnetic fields and can be obtained from Aaronia AG. Aaronia and other companies also sell filters and shielded cables that reduce or eliminate stray electromagnetic fields.

Manitoba Hydro offers a few more suggestions for the concerned consumer:

- Sit at arm's length from the screen of a personal computer and keep your distance from other monitors – particularly the back or sides where electric and magnetic fields are generally highest.
- Consider using hair dryers less since they create very high levels of electric and magnetic fields.
- If you have a portable fan or telephone answering machine in your bedroom, keep it away from your bed.
- The same applies to electric clocks, which produce much higher levels of electric and magnetic fields than battery or wind-up clocks.
- If you use an electric blanket or waterbed heater, consider using them to preheat the bed and unplug them before going to sleep.

Much more information on this topic is available at www.electropollution.com. For now, our journey takes us to look at a completely different place to measure energy. We are going to look at how to measure the energy that is flowing inside our bodies, without having to spend decades developing the sensitivities of a yoga master. We will see how modern instruments can be employed to peer inside our energy bodies.

Measuring Energy

SQUIDs are excellent at detecting magnetic fields. Not the squids you find in the ocean, the SQUIDs invented by John Zimmerman and employed inside magnetometers. Unfortunately, magnetometers of this sensitivity are still experimental and not widely available. They have been successfully used to discover the tiny electromagnetic fields emitted by touch therapists and other healers, but they are not available for use on a regular basis to evaluate everyone's energy health.

The classical approach by healers in the East to detect and monitor the flow of Chi in a patient has been to develop the healer's own ability to sense these flows of energy. Not everyone can do this. Nor can this be learned quickly. Ayurvedic or Daoist training to sense the multiple pulses of energy found in the wrists that indicate the health of the organs can take eight years or more. What would be ideal is a simple instrument, portable, and that can be operated with just a few weeks or months of training, not years. Such instruments have been created starting in the 1950s and the number of offerings has been expanding ever since.

The AMI

In 1971 Dr. Motoyama developed an instrument to detect and measure the function of meridians. He called the device the "AMI," which stands for "Apparatus for Meridian Identification." The AMI, as described in Dr. Motoyama's own words, is "a device developed to measure energy transfer through the meridians." The AMI electrodes are attached to both hands and feet and a small electric current is applied. Four electrical values are measured and recorded in a computer.

After analysis by the computer, normal or abnormal results are presented to the operator. The trained operator evaluates these readings in terms of meridian function, general physical health, and pathology (illness). The system also recommends specific points for optimal acupuncture treatment. Also detected is the functional status of the chakras. Based on all of the above, a diagnosis is possible with regard to the subject's physical constitutions and personality.

There is more information available on the AMI at the California Institute for Human Science (CIHS); however, for a full report on all the scientific studies of the AMI Dr. Motoyama's book *Measurements of Ki Energy, Diagnosis, & Treatments* is recommended. Unfortunately this book is hard to come by. Also, unfortunately, Dr. Motoyama has not built many AMIs; obtaining a reading is more difficult than getting an MRI scan.

Other Instruments

Dr. Motoyama was not the first person to measure energy flow in the body beyond the electrical energies of the heart and brain. In the 1950s, a German physician named Reinhold Voll merged his understanding of acupuncture and electricity to create an electroacupuncture system. His original instrument was later modified and simplified by his student Helmut Schimmel. The system was called the "EAV."[125] Later generations were called "VEGA." Since then dozens of variations from many companies have appeared. A more generic term has been adopted, electrodermal testing. Sometimes you will find another label applied: MSA or Meridian Stress Assessment.[126]

All these devices, like Dr. Motoyama's AMI, measure the galvanic response of the skin. Skeptics believe that, since these devices are just simple galvanometers that measure the resistivity of the skin surface, they have no diagnostic value. Proponents argue that the body's meridians are low resistance pathways along which Chi (i.e., electromagnetic fields) flow. When a pathway is no longer showing low resistance, the meridian has become blocked and the Chi is no longer flowing properly.

The more modern versions of these instruments combine well-laid-out and colorful reports and displays. The Prognos, claimed to be developed by the Russian Space Agency to aid their astronauts in self-diagnosing incipient medical conditions while enduring long periods in space, eliminates many of the skeptics' concerns.

These concerns include variations in results depending upon the operator and variations in interpretation by operators who have different levels of experience. In the EAV and VEGA devices, the degree of pressure being applied to the probe affects the strength of the signal received. If one operator pushes a little harder than another operator, the results will be very different. The Prognos avoids this problem by incorporating a feedback sound indicating when the right

---

[125] Electro-Acupuncture, according to Voll.
[126] More history on the EVA and Dr. Voll can be found at the VeraDyne Corporation at www.veradyne.com/electrodermal_analysis.html.

amount of pressure has been applied. The probe's spring-loaded tip ensures that a constant pressure is applied.[127]

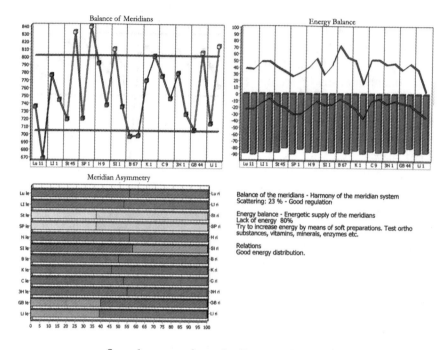

Sample output from the Prognos Software.

The Prognos software also interprets the readings directly, rather than leaving it up to the operator. Within its database the Prognos stores standard meridian readings that are used to calibrate the results and determine if the subject is being stressed due to a wide variety of causes: bacterial infection, parasite infection, toxicity due to metals, hormone or vitamin deficiencies, etc.[128]

---

[127] This question of variability and reliability of the Prognos was the subject of a study in 2004 by the University of Portland's Kaiser-Permanente Center for Health Research. The first objective of the study was "to characterize and calibrate an electrodermal screening device." The team concluded "Prognos performs accurately, against known resistors over the reported range of electrical skin resistance."

[128] Further details about the Prognos can be found at www.welnet.net. The most detail can be found at www.prognos.info. Unlike the AMI the

The whole area of measuring energy along meridians has engendered strong opinions by both proponents and skeptics. The interested reader may wish to investigate both sides of this debate further. For the skeptics' view, visit Quackwatch, which has compiled a good report on Quack Electrodiagnostic Devices.[129] From the other side, the CIHS has presented research it has been involved with and other's findings that support the case for these devices.[130]

Our exploration of the energy body, the second kosha, has revealed benefits of the Yin Yoga practice beyond those we discovered in the physical body. The Eastern understanding of energy was developed through centuries of experience: trials and errors. The maps written by the ancient yogis show within the body pathways of communication along which healing energies spread out and help maintain or heal the body. We discovered that recent investigations in the West have uncovered similar pathways for communication, and multiple energetic media that also nurture the body. The exercises and massages incorporated into our yoga practice stimulate these energies and open the pathways, allowing healing information to flow unimpeded throughout our systems. With this understanding in mind, our journey now takes us to the deeper koshas, where we will discover how Yin Yoga can assist in promoting our mental and emotional health.

Prognos is being offered to anyone so there is a good chance that the reader may be able to find a naturopath who uses the Prognos. The earlier VEGA devices are even more widely used but do suffer from the dual drawbacks of variability in results and interpretation.

[129] www.quackwatch.org/01QuackeryRelatedTopics/electro.html.

[130] At www.cihs.edu/whatsnew/research.asp.

Chapter Eight: The Mind Body

The Manomaya Kosha

On the physical level, we eventually come to realize that we are what we eat. What we put into our body becomes our body. On the mental level, we eventually discover that we are what we think. What we allow into our mind becomes our mind.

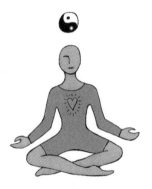

The Meditator V

In the computer world a term was coined that describes perfectly this process: GIGO – garbage in, garbage out. GIGO means that when you enter garbage into a computer, you get garbage out of it again. The same principle operates inside each of us. If we feed our physical body with garbage – we can't be surprised when our body turns to garbage. When we feed our minds with garbage, we should not be surprised at our thoughts also becoming junk.

What does it mean to think? We think we know, but do we? What is meant by mind? Again we think we know, but the closer we look, the less sure we become. The fact that we can even look for the mind makes us wonder…what is doing the looking? Can the mind find the mind? Can a fingertip touch itself? Can a subject be its own object?

These questions have been asked for thousands of years. The search for the mind, for our true nature, is ancient. It is useful to travel back to the beginning of some of these inquiries and understand the models that have been developed to help explain the mind and find our true nature. So let's embark upon another side trip – a journey to discover the models of mind and true nature, as seen in the ancient and modern yogic teachings, the Buddhist teachings, and some of the modern Western psychological models.

We have already been introduced to one ancient model of the self via the five sheaths of the koshas. We have examined the physical and energy bodies. The remaining three sheaths are the lower mind, the higher mind, and the bliss body. The lower mind, called "*manas*," is the home of our perceptions. The higher mind, called "*vijnana*," is the home of discrimination.[131] *Ananda*, or bliss, which forms the final sheath, is the ultimate or next to ultimate Self, a source of underlying joy.[132]

As useful as the kosha model is to begin to see how the body is layered, it was never accepted by the yoga community: the model is not detailed enough. The yogis adopted a more complete model that seemed much more accurate and useful. Philosophers of the *Samkhya* tradition developed this model, and it seemed to fit with the yogi's own experiences very closely. Let's begin by investing the Samkhya view of the universe.

Samkhya

Around 800 B.C.E. the age of philosophy arose almost simultaneously throughout the ancient world. In Greece, the Middle East, India, and China the sages, who were always the inward-looking psychonauts,[133] began to think about the way we think. Prior to this time, all religious practices were outwardly focused. The tools of religion, the rituals, and sacrifices were designed to barter and bargain with the elements of nature and the gods. The assumption was – if we conducted these sacrifices for the benefits of the gods, they would be pleased, and in turn would do us favors. The favors sought were of three kinds: rewards of health, wealth, and progeny. We all want to

---

[131] More precisely vijnana is knowledge and *jnana* is wisdom.
[132] There is debate over whether the anandamaya kosha is our ultimate Self or just the last wrapper around our true being.
[133] To borrow a term from Georg Feuerstein.

be healthy, to have lots of money, and lots of children. Enlightenment, three thousand years ago, was not a goal. At best one might hope to be taken to a heavenly reward after this life, but even this was a later religious invention.

Religion always distances the seeker from that which is sought. Religious rituals and sacrifices require intermediaries – priests, to act on the behalf of the petitioners. Direct connection to the divine is not possible, save for those very rare sages to whom the gods revealed the original truths in the first place.

In most of these ancient religions the gods, being metaphors for the elements of nature, were numerous, powerful, and capricious. They were not great examples of moral behavior. They were more like arrogant, narcissistic bigger brothers and sisters who could make life miserable for you if you didn't stay out of their way or keep them happy. Even in the earliest monotheistic religions, God was a stern taskmaster who had to be pleased and appeased in order for your life to be peaceful.

With the dawning of philosophy, the focus turned inward. The external powers of nature were seen as reflections of the inner world, and vice versa. External sacrifices and rituals became internalized. No longer were the gods out there; they were metaphors for what was happening in here. No longer did you need a priest to talk for you to the divine – the divine already resided inside you; you needed to do the work yourself. A map to self-realization, or more correctly Self-realization, was required to help guide you on the path, but you had to walk the path.

One such map became very influential in India around the time of the Buddha. It explained the inner and outer workings of the mind and the world. While the map didn't answer all the questions, and everyone did not accept some of the answers it did produce, it was the most comprehensive model yet devised. It became the foundation for yogic and Buddhist cosmology. It was the Samkhya psychocosmological model.[134]

---

[134] Samkhya literally means to enumerate or count. The name of this philosophy refers to its ontological enumeration of the principles of the universe.

We will leave it to the historians to argue whether Samkhya created this model, and thus can be considered the father of the yogic model that followed it, or whether there was an earlier version from which both Samkhya and yoga evolved, thus making the two brothers, rather than father and son. For our purposes it is enough to know that both Samkhya and Classical Yoga, from which all other yogas evolved (especially the Tantra and Hatha yogas most practiced today), share this same psychophysical view of the universe.

Our brief journey into the Samkhya philosophy begins with looking at the two great divides upon which the model is founded: *purusha* (soul) and *prakriti* (nature).

Purusha & Prakriti

Samkhya and the Classical Yoga of the Yoga Sutras are dualistic philosophies. Very few yoga teachers today realize this. In the West, dualism has been entrenched in our religions for over three thousand years. This dualism is easily seen in the metaphor of the clockmaker: God is the great clockmaker and this universe, and everything in it, is his wondrous invention, the clock. God is outside of the machine. In the Samkhya tradition there is purusha and there is prakriti, and these two are as separate as the clockmaker and the clock. Purusha is the soul, the Self, pure consciousness, and the only source of consciousness. The word literally means "man." Prakriti is that which is created. It is nature in all her aspects. Prakriti literally means "creatrix," the female creative energy.

Unlike in the Western religions, purusha did not create prakriti; in fact, if given a choice, purusha would prefer to have never met prakriti at all. But purusha is responsible for prakriti becoming animated, alive.

Samkhya philosophy holds that there are countless individual purushas, each one infinite, eternal, omniscient, unchanging, and unchangeable. There is no single purusha that sits hierarchically above any others. There is no creator god, no puppet master pulling any strings. Since purusha is pure consciousness, it follows that prakriti is unconscious. Prakriti is everything that is changing. Prakriti is not just the physical aspects of the universe that we can sense; it is our very senses themselves – our thoughts, memories, desires, and even our intelligence. Prakriti is everything that is that isn't conscious. Consciousness resides only in purusha, or more properly, as purusha.

Purusha, pure and distant, is beyond subject and object. One cannot understand purusha, for that would make it an object. Purusha cannot know or understand anything either, for that would make purusha a subject. Purusha simply just is. But, because of the presence of prakriti, purusha gets attracted to nature in the way a man is attracted when he watches a beautiful woman dancing. He cannot help but try to get closer. And then the disaster occurs: purusha becomes trapped inside prakriti. Like Brer Rabbit when he touches the Tar Baby, purusha gets more and more entangled in prakriti. Soon purusha forgets that it was ever separate and ceases to struggle to regain its freedom.

The union of purusha and prakriti was a horrible mistake. This unfortunate marriage should never have happened. The only remedy: a fast and thorough divorce! Like Brer Rabbit, the only way to be freed from the Tar Baby is to be thrown into the briar patch where we can scrape off prakriti and finally free ourselves. The briar patch is the practice of yoga.

Samkhya and Classical Yoga are *not* about union. The yoga of the Yoga Sutra is about getting a divorce, as quickly as possible. If you don't do it now, you will have to come back again and again, suffering countless new lives, until you finally get that divorce and are free at last.[135]

---

[135] It is curious how in the Eastern philosophies reincarnation is something to be avoided at all costs. To live again and again in this sorrowful world is unbearable. True joy, bliss, ananda is obtained only when we are free from the cycles of rebirth. In the West, reincarnation is considered a blessing. We are comforted with the thought that we won't really die when this body fails us. We are coming back again, and again, and again, to enjoy the cycles of life. The difference in these two views is the emphasis on what it is that is reincarnated. In the West we dearly hope it is our ego that survives to the next life. We are drawn to stories of how someone can remember her past life, hoping this means that something of the person that we are now will still be around in some future incarnation. In the Eastern view, nothing natural survives from one life to the next. By natural we mean nothing of nature, of prakriti. What returns is the soul, stained as it was by the karma

Purusha is easy to comprehend; we all seem to have an instinctive or intuitive understanding of the concept of soul or consciousness, even if we cannot describe it exactly. But prakriti is a bit more foreign. What is prakriti made of? Let's take a closer look at the underlying strands of prakriti.

The Three Gunas

Underpinning prakriti are three strings called "*gunas.*" These three strings combine in many ways to form the ropes of existence. The three gunas are *tamas*, *rajas*, and *sattva*. Tamas is passivity, inertia, heaviness, and dullness of existence. Tamas has been described as the cause of hunger, thirst, grief, fear, and confusion. Rajas is the opposite; it is activity, excitement, and passion. Rajas is the cause of lust, greed, and all desires – good and bad. In these two gunas, we find hints of the Daoist definitions of yin and yang. Sattva is neither. Sattva is wholesomeness, harmony, lucidity, and beauty. To the Daoist, sattva is the Dao.

These three gunas combine the way electrons, protons, and neutrons combine to form all matter in our universe. However, the gunas are more pervasive; not just our physical bodies, not just the earth and everything on it, but all of our thoughts, our personalities, our experiences, and our desires are manifestations of the gunas at play. Despite the numerous and complex ways in which the gunas can combine, they are still uncon-

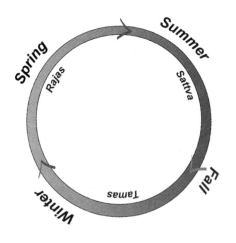

The three gunas are constantly in motion, never staying still.

of prior lives. Only once these stains are removed, through the discipline of yoga, can the soul truly be free to stay away from nature's clutches.

scious. Everything we see is "just the gunas acting on the gunas," and nothing more, according to Richard Freeman.[136]

Often students of yoga will confuse the role of the gunas and believe that sattva is the good gune, rajas is an okay gune, and tamas is the bad gune. Just as yin and yang are neither good nor bad, there are no attributes of good or bad inherent in the gunas. They are all part of prakriti, and the objective of Classical Yoga and Samkhya practice is to become free of prakriti completely – free even from sattvic states of being. Sattva can be harmful if you become attached to it and stop striving for freedom. Tamas can help release the attachment to sattva. Rajas can be good if you have become too tamasic.

The three gunas actually flow in a cycle: sattva replaces rajas, raja destroys tamas, and tamas develops out of sattva. We can see this flow every day. In the morning we are lying in bed not wanting to get up – tamas is predominant. We need desire, rajas, to motivate us and give us the energy to get going. We seek rajas in that morning cup of coffee or that lovely, sweaty Ashtanga practice. By evening, after a full day's work, we sit at night, a cup of herbal tea in hand, and relax with a good book. Rajas has ripened into a sattvic state of mind. But once the tea has been consumed and the favorite book has been read, our minds turn back to the tamas gune. We are ready for the oblivion of sleep once again.

The three gunas are constantly in flux; like the game of rock, paper, scissors ... as soon as one gets on top, the next one comes along and changes everything again. The cycle may turn quickly or it may take eons, but we know nothing lasts and everything changes. This is the nature of prakriti.

What still is unclear is how the three gunas manifest. How does everything that we see around us, that we experience within us, come to be? To answer this we need to look deeper into the model of Samkhya.

---

[136] Many of the analogies and metaphors in this discussion on Samkhya come from Richard Freeman's audio CD series *The Yoga Matrix*.

The Twenty-four Principles of Samkhya

Originally the three gunas were in complete balance. Prakriti was undisturbed. This original condition is known as *prakriti-pradhana* or *mula-prakriti*, which is the natural foundation. When purusha came near, prakriti began to change.

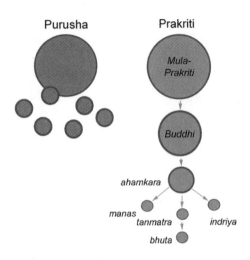

Purusha and Prakriti are completely distinct, making the Samkhya philosophy dualistic.

A good analogy of this is you and your car. While you are away, your car just sits there in its original state. Once you see the car, the desire arises to sit in it, to turn it on. When you and your car come together, things start to happen. You begin to drive and go places. Soon you forget your car is not you. It feels like you. You can sense exactly where it is on the road. The car reacts to the other cars on the road as if it had a mind of its own. It notices things like traffic lights and pedestrians, almost as if it was conscious. Soon you and your car are one and you have forgotten why you ever got in the car in the first place.

Once purusha activates prakriti, the first evolute arises; the first thing to appear out of the natural foundation of prakriti-pradhana is *mahat*, the great principle. This is also known as *buddhi* or the awakened intelligence. Mahat is intuition, or cognition, but it is not consciousness. Only purusha is conscious. But, because of mahat's great intelligence and luminosity, it is often mistaken for consciousness. Just as our car can sometimes seem to have a mind of its own, buddhi can seem to be conscious – it is an illusion.

From buddhi evolves *ahamkara*, the "I-maker." Ahamkara creates the sense of self (with a small "s"), also known as ego. In this respect, ahamkara pretends to be purusha (which is Self with a big "S"). So now your car starts to act as if it's the boss. Perhaps here our analogy begins to break down, but you probably know some people for whom their car is the boss. A small scratch on the fender can send some owners into great angst, and they act quickly to repair the superficial damage. It is at the level of ahamkara that subjects and objects arise. "I" becomes the subject, and the rest of the world provides its objects. At this level individualism arises because inherent in the subject/object duality there is separation.[137]

From ahamkara evolves manas, the mind, and the ten senses (the *indriyas*). Manas here is the lower mind, which we have seen in the kosha model. It is often described as the eleventh sense.[138] Also out of ahamkara arise the five elements (*bhuta*) and the five energy potentials (*tanmatra*). The elements we have seen before: space, air, fire, water, and earth. The five energy potentials are new to us. These are the tanmatras, the substances upon which the senses function. They are what is touched, what is tasted, what is smelled, what is heard, and what is seen.

What has not been explained yet are the other senses. Samkhya lists ten. Five we are very familiar with: these are called the "cognitive senses" – listening, feeling, seeing, tasting, and smelling. The remaining five are the conative senses: speaking, grasping, moving, excreting, and reproducing.

---

[137] While there are countless separate and individual purushas in the Samkhya philosophy, these cannot be said to be either subjects or objects. While individual and separate, they are connected because each purusha is eternal and infinite. This, however, is one area where Samkhya was found wanting. How can there be countless individual purushas, each one all-knowing and infinite, without each purusha running afoul of all the other purushas. Samkhya's strict adherence to its pluralistic purusha was one of its major downfalls. Another problem was its atheistic nature: there is no creator god in this cosmology. Every purusha is equal and equivalent to every other purusha. The final problem with Samkhya was its strict dualism. If purusha is distinct from prakriti, how can it ever become entangled in the first place?

[138] It is interesting to consider mind as a sense. What does the mind sense? Consciousness? But that is purusha! Perhaps the sages meant that the mind senses thoughts.

With these twenty-four principles, the Samkhya model is complete – a map of the inner and outer universe is offered to the psychonaut. While the map seems totally impossible to follow for us normal souls, this is a map blazed by those who have gone before us. Can we really critique what we have not experienced? But that raises the final question: how do we follow this map? What is the practice of Samkhya Yoga? How can we determine for ourselves if this map is accurate or not?

The Samkhya Practice

Liberation is freedom – freedom from prakriti. It is often called "*kaivalya,*" which means aloofness, aloneness, or isolation. To obtain liberation one must separate from the body because, despite all its wonderful qualities, the body is made from prakriti. Separation is needed from the mind as well. Remember, prakriti is not just the physical manifestations we see in life. Memories, thoughts, emotions, and even intelligence are all prakriti and need to be left behind. True liberation, in the Samkhya tradition, cannot be obtained while embodied. Only after leaving the body can one be truly and finally liberated. But, if the purusha is not cleansed of all its attractions to prakriti, then death is just the beginning of a new cycle, and the purusha once again becomes attached to prakriti.

To achieve liberation, the Samkhya yogis employ discrimination and renunciation. Discrimination (known as *viveka*) is a knowing that is gained through reasoning. Renunciation is a moving away from everything that binds us to this life. While similar to Classical Yoga, Samkhya practice does not focus on *samadhi* as the main tool for liberation. Both practices, however, require a fierce form of asceticism equaled only in the Jain religion.

In the fertile period, around 500~600 B.C.E., ideas were being developed and exchanged between many fields of inquiry. Samkhya philosophy informed pre-classical yoga, which borrowed from Jainism, which also influenced both Samkhya and Buddhism. Each philosophy borrowed, tested, adopted, and discarded ideas and practices from each other. Eventually a consistent psycho-cosmological model precipitated out for each philosophical approach.

In ancient Jainism we find a similar dualism to Samkhya; the purusha is called the *"ataman"* or the *"jiva."* Everyone has her jiva, unique and separate from all other jivas, just as the Samkhya philosophy believed purushas are separate. Your jiva is unfortunately stained or colored by its association with the world of nature. The Jains believed that the only way to clean the tarnish from the jiva is through fiercely adopting ahimsa: non-harming. Even breathing harms the molecules of the air; therefore, masks are worn to protect the air, and to avoid inadvertently swallowing an insect. The most extreme Jain saints would cease walking, because every step would harm some microscopic creature. Eventually the saints would just sit and wait for death to take them. This is a complete renunciation of the world and all its attachments.

This is similar to the fierce yogi practiced by the Samkhya and Classical yogis: this is total renunciation. But, in the Samkhya philosophy, renunciation alone will not free the purusha from prakriti's grasp. Viveka,[139] discernment, is also required. This is knowing the way of the universe, not intellectually, because the intellect is still prakriti, but at a deeper level. Viveka develops an inner knowing that discerns the ephemeral from the actual – separating the apparent nature of the world from its underlying reality. While it is gained through reasoning, viveka also develops the will to renounce all that is unreal.

Samkhya was a masterpiece of modeling the ways of the inner universe. The adoption of its cosmological structure by the Classical Yogis and Buddhists testifies to its power. However, the practice of Samkhya, and its underlying dualistic philosophy, was the basis for its eventual demise. Classical Yoga moved away from Samkhya, and replaced the emphasis on viveka with the practice of samadhi. Later yoga schools, starting with Tantra, followed the Buddha's path of renouncing the fierce renunciation practices of the Jains, Samkhya, and Classical Yoga paths. Eventually all that was left of Samkhya was the cosmology.

Let's move on now and examine how the two main yoga schools, Classical Yoga and Tantra Yoga, and understand mind and all that lies beyond mind.

---

139 Which also means to "separate out."

Chapter Nine:
The Yogic View of Mind

The model of the inner and outer cosmos created in Samkhya worked so well that the later schools of yoga adopted it with very little change. The Classical Yoga model changed the emphasis of the practice, but left the model virtually untouched. The Tantric school kept the twenty-four principles of Samkhya, but discovered that the Samkhya yogis stopped their inquiries too soon. On top of Samkhya's twenty-four principles, the Tantrikas added another twelve that served to bring together the dualistic universe into oneness. As time passes, it is natural that new ways evolve out of the old ways. Let's look first at the way Classical Yoga viewed the landscape of the mind, and how it taught the yogi to transcend the ordinary world. Then we will look at how Tantra moved on from there.

Classical Yoga

The Yoga Sutra, ascribed to Patanjali, is a concise summary of the Classical Yoga psychotechnology. We can call it psychology due to its deep delving into the shape and structure of mind, and the way we experience the world. We can call it technology because of the practical methods it offers to traverse the mind, and to make us ready for final liberation. In fact, the Yoga Sutra is so technical that it takes a lot of study to truly understand it. A guide is essential, for there are many important aspects of Classical Yoga technology that the Yoga

Sutra merely hints at. It is a map that, at times, gives only general directions; at other times it provides crystal clear explanations.

The second line of the Yoga Sutra sums up the purpose of Classical Yoga. It tells us exactly what yoga is: yogas-citta-vritti-nirodaha. These four words – yoga citta vritti nirodah – cannot be easily and succinctly translated into English; in general, the sloka tell us that yoga is the cessation of the fluctuations of the mind. Yoga is a way to stop the mind's movements ... but what is meant by mind and what is meant by fluctuation and just how do we stop them? These answers are provided.

The Yoga Sutra uses the term *citta* as the overarching term for what, in the West, we would simply call the mind. Iyengar[140] offers a detailed view of the various aspects of citta in his book *Light on Life*. Citta itself means consciousness, in its various manifestations. There are three major forms of citta. First, there is the lower mind's consciousness, called "manas." Manas is our perceptions, as we have seen in the Samkhya psychocosmology. Second, there is ahamkara. Ahamkara literally means "I-shaped," according to Iyengar. It is ahamkara that gives rise to our ego and our mistaken view of self. And third, there is buddhi or intelligence, which is the first manifestation out of the cosmic consciousness called "mahat." Manas and ahamkara are the outward-facing projections of consciousness. Buddhi turns us around and looks inward.

Vritti means whirlings, turnings, or fluctuations. Nirodah means restriction, death, or stillness. Although the Yoga Sutra provides a methodology for stilling the mind, before that is explored, an unspoken question is answered – "Why would we want to do this?" The answer is *tadadrastruhsvarupevasthanum*. When the mind is still, the seer can rest in her true nature. Now, before we learn how to still the mind and come to this rest, the Yoga Sutra provides a deeper view of the mind and the problems we face in trying to look behind it.

---

[140] B.K.S. Iyengar has written many books on yoga. His first book in 1966, *Light on Yoga*, was the first book many people had ever read on yoga, and was the only resource they had to learn the practice.

The Five Vrittis

Generally we can consider the vrittis as types of thoughts but they are broader than that. There are five main fluctuations that affect our outer consciousness:

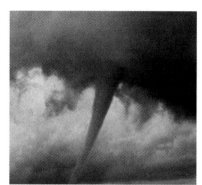

1. Correct knowledge (*pramana*)
2. Incorrect knowledge (*viparyaya*)
3. Imagination or fantasy (*vikalpa*)
4. Sleep (*nidra*)
5. Memory (*smrti*)

The vrittis are the whirlings of the mind. W

We all are subject to these five turnings in our minds, and they are not necessarily bad. Correct knowledge can help us do the right thing at the right time. But we can also do the right thing for the wrong reason; even incorrect knowledge can be helpful at times. The truth is, these fluctuations can be good or bad. Even right knowledge can be used in a harmful way. We have often seen things done with the best of intentions turn out drastically wrong. It not that these vrittis are good or bad that makes them worthy of study, it is their effect upon the state of our mind that is of interest. These turnings of the mind obscure the view of our real self and need to be calmed. Like the surface of a mountain lake on a clear moonlit night (our mind) when still, reflects perfectly the full moon (reality). But with even a small ripple, caused by a vritti, the moon's appearance is distorted.

Yin yogis, like all practitioners of modern yoga, can gain from understanding the Yoga Sutra's model of citta and the vrittis. Knowing that these five vrittis are operating during your practice, and during your life, can help you increase your ability to calm them. Being aware that the mind moves in notable, observational ways gives you a way to understand what is arising. Knowing that the vrittis exist gives you the opportunity to watch for them.

Kriya Yoga

The Yoga Sutra does not just offer one way to achieve the goal of yoga; it has several actions we can perform. At the beginning of the second chapter of the Yoga Sutra we are introduced to one particular form of yoga called "*Kriya* Yoga." Kriya means action, or in this case a ritualistic approach to yoga. It has only three steps: *tapas, svadhyaya,* and *ishvara-pranidhana.* Tapas is the dedicated effort or asceticism needed in order for our practice to bear fruit. Svadhyaya is the study of ourself, or self-study. This self-study includes knowing the scriptures and the practices recommended to help us achieve the goal of yoga. Ishvara-pranidhana is a giving up of all the fruits of our labor to a higher cause. It is surrendering to something bigger than our small self.[141]

These three steps of the Kriya Yoga are not physical. As described, anyone could undertake a complete yoga practice without doing a single asana. The Yoga Sutra offers the path of Kriya Yoga as one possible way to reach the goal of a still mind. This is a mental yoga; effort, or tapas, comes from a strong will. Tapas is an absolute requirement for success. Self-study is also essential and this comes from looking within, as well as looking without, for guidance. The last step, ishvara-pranidhana, is the one that may seem the most foreign to our Western minds: to act without regard for the results.

The Bhagavad-Gita, a small book buried in the midst of the epic poem of India, the Mahabharata, explains, with wonderful imagery, the reason for surrendering the fruits of all you do to a higher power. The Bhagavad-Gita contains the teachings of the Lord Krishna to his friend, the mighty warrior Arjuna. Krishna attempts to remove the delusions affecting Arjuna, and explains that Arjuna cannot do

---

[141] If you look back at the drawing of purusha and prakriti, on page 154, you may notice that there is one particularly large purusha shown. This larger purusha depicts ishvara: the first among equals. According to the Yoga Sutra, this is a special purusha – one that has never been tainted by prakriti. Ishvara is a lord, a particularly pure purusha, but not necessarily God. It is not clear in the Yoga Sutra whether this lord is the original creator of the universe or just the first among the many purushas. What is clear is that ishvara is not a personal god who will interfere in our personal life. However, ishvara does serve as an inspiration for us.

anything unless God wants it to be so. Do not feel pride when you accomplish something meritorious, for what have you really done? Do not feel depressed when things do not go according to your desire, for God's desire is always greater. Your only duty is to take the action; leave the results in God's hands. This is a hard lesson to grasp, and even harder to put into practice.

In our yoga practice, things may not always work out the way we hope. Some days we seem to be moving backward. But this is only a problem when we expect particular results. Give up the expectation and just do it. The will, the energy to do it, comes from tapas. Knowing *what* to do comes from self-study. The results are beyond your control. Offer them back to the source, or to anyone or anything else that may need assistance. Send the benefits of your effort to someone or something that needs special help right now. That is the power of prayer. That is the power of faith. Without faith, every spiritual practice flounders.

In Yin Yoga, the results may not be obvious for a long time. Yin tissues, such as our ligaments, have a lower blood supply to them than the yang tissues, such as our muscles. They don't strengthen or lengthen as quickly as our muscles. Our range of motion may take a long time to increase, or may not grow at all. But in the end, that is not the real point of the practice. Yin Yoga will help us to be healthy, strong, focused, and open. But all this too, is not the ultimate point. The ultimate result is outside of our control. If we succeed in our practice, it is because of grace from elsewhere. Our job is to simply do the practice.

The Obstacles to Yoga

The Yoga Sutra warns us about nine obstacles to our practice, called the "*antaraya.*" These will arise in our Yin Yoga practice just as they will in any yoga practice. These nine distractions of our consciousness[142] are:

---

[142] Also called the *citta vikshepa.*

1. Illness – *vyadi*
2. Languor – *styana* (or mental stagnation)
3. Doubt – *samshaya*
4. Heedlessness – *pramada* (or lack of foresight)
5. Sloth – *alasya* (fatigue)
6. Dissipation – *avirati* (or overindulging)
7. False views – *bhrantidarshana* (or illusions)
8. Lack of perseverance – *alabdhabhumikatva*
9. Instability or regression – *anavasthitatva*

If one is not healthy, strong, and dedicated, there will be no success in yoga. Although the Yoga Sutra spends very little time talking about asanas and physical practices, it is obviously essential that the body be strong enough to support the practice.

The Ways around the Obstacles

Chanting, or merely contemplating the sacred syllable Om, is one method to vanquish the nine obstacles. This is something that can be easily incorporated into the Yin Yoga practice. During the long durations of the postures, listen to the sound of the universe: Om. Hear the sound in your head, feel its vibration in your body.

Other ways around the obstacles include four additional practices:[143]

1. Friendliness – *maitri*
2. Compassion – *karuna*
3. Gladness – *mudita*
4. Equanimity – *upeksanam*

Equanimity is explained in the sutra as the state of being equally moved (or unmoved) by people who are in pain or happy, or by people who deserve merit or are unmeritorious. Jesus taught us that everyone loves her family and friends ... love your enemies too. That is true equanimity, true equality.

---

[143] We will see later that these four practices are also highly recommended in Buddhism.

Two other suggestions made in the Yoga Sutra for strengthening our practice are *sraddha* and *virya*: faith and energy. Faith is the best cure for doubt; energy is the best cure for sloth or languor. Also, *smrti* is recommended; memory – reminding ourselves of times when we were successful in the past – is excellent motivation to continue to work hard. Remembering solutions from our study, or other times in our life when we overcame obstacles, are also functions of memory.

The Five Kleshas

Right after the Yoga Sutra describes Kriya Yoga, it explains the five reasons we are bound. These troubles, or afflictions, are known as the *kleshas*:[144]

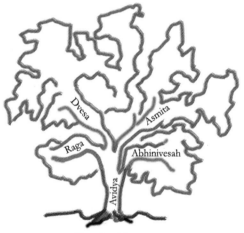

The Five Kleshas

1. Ignorance (*avidya*)
2. Ego (*asmita*)
3. Attachment to pleasure (*raga*)
4. Aversion to pain (*dvesa*)
5. Fear of Death (*abhinivesah*)

These five afflictions are often depicted as a tree. Avidya is the trunk of the tree, and the other four kleshas sprout from it. The Samkhya emphasis on viveka, knowing the real nature of the universe, is echoed in Classical Yoga's emphasis on avidya, or ignorance, as the chief affliction we suffer. Destroy avidya and all the other troubles go away.

Asmita is the ego. The problem with ego is not the fact that we have one; it is useful and even necessary to have an ego in order to function and live. The problem arises when the ego believes it is the

---

[144] We will see a similar list in the Buddhist philosophy called the five hindrances.

Self. If all we do is in service of the little self, our life will be sorrowful. When we serve our higher Self, liberation becomes possible.

Yin Yoga is especially good at giving us time to practice watching raga and dvesa. As we hold the poses, as we remain outside our comfort zone, aversion arises. We resolve not to move, and instead we simply watch the aversion come ... and eventually go. It goes away only to be replaced by some new aversion. As we finally release the pose we are flooded with pleasant sensations. The joy of coming out of a yin pose can create attachment. We want to stay and linger in this wonderful feeling. But, we again simply watch the pleasure, without reacting, and move on to the next pose.

The practice we do on our yoga mats prepares us to face challenges at other times. We begin to recognize our inner habits. We notice and remark to ourselves, "Ow ... this is aversion!" We notice, saying, "Ahhh ... this is attachment!" Knowing that these afflictions, or hindrances, are constantly arising, we can consciously choose to not react to them ... or perhaps *to* react to them, if that is appropriate. But now, because we are aware, the choice is consciously made. Our reactions are no longer automatic.

The final klesha is said to be the most difficult to overcome: abhinivesah. This is the clinging to life. Even the most advanced yogis may fail to let go of this last affliction. If at the time of death there is the slightest hint of the thought, "No! I don't want to go...," that person is doomed to return and try again.

Ashtanga – The Eight Limbs

Shortly after the Yoga Sutra explains the three stages of Kriya Yoga, a more extensive practice is given. This is the famous eight limbs of yoga, which has come to be called "the ashtanga."[145]

The eight limbs are:

1. *Yama*
2. *Niyama*
3. *Asana*
4. *Pranayama*
5. *Pratyahara*
6. *Dharana*
7. *Dhyana*
8. *Samadhi*

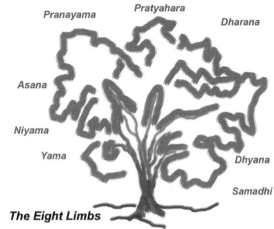

The Eight Limbs

There was a fondness in the philosophies of this era to create easy to remember lists: the five vrittis, the five kleshas, and the eight limbs. The Buddha also employed this technique, as we will discover.

The ashtanga begins with the yamas and niyamas, which are the ethical core of yoga. These are analogous to the Western Ten Commandments, with one important difference. Joseph Campbell points out that, in the West, the Ten Commandments are a bargain with God; if we conduct ourselves in accordance to these ten rules, we shall be rewarded in heaven. Religious people in the West strive and struggle to live according to these rules. Obviously we do not always succeed, and our failings can cause considerable grief and guilt.

---

[145] *Ashta* means eight and *anga* means limbs. Curiously, the Yoga Sutra does not mention this name, and some scholars feel that the ashtanga was added to the original sutra hundreds of years later, in much the same way that many religious texts in the West were edited and modified by copyists centuries later.

In the Eastern world, Campbell suggests, the ethical precepts of the yama and niyamas are ways that the spiritually advanced person acts. These precepts are not meant to be applied first, and then, once you master them, you are allowed to proceed with the other limbs of yoga. Rather, as you progress in your practice of yoga, you will find that your actions will become more and more ethical; more and more you will act in accordance to these precepts. With this understanding, we can strive to live ethically, but when we fail, we are not overcome with guilt or immobilized by grief.

The yamas are practices that govern our outward relationships.[146] There are five yamas:

1. *Ahimsa* (non-harming)
2. *Satya* (truthfulness)
3. *Asteya* (non-stealing)
4. *Brahmacharya* (living as God would live)
5. *Aprigraha* (non-greediness)

All of these yamas can also be found in our relationship to our yoga practice:

Ahimsa	– When we perform asanas, are we truly "non-harming" our body, or are we pushing too deep?
Satya	– Are we honestly watching what is arising, or are we telling tales to ourselves in order to con ourselves into going too far?
Asteya	– Are we stealing calmness from our breath?
Brahmacharya	– Are we performing the practice the way an enlightened master would perform?
Aprigraha	– Are we grasping after more than we really need right now?

---

[146] Many texts of yoga describe these yamas. *Light on Life* by Iyengar is recommended for students wanting to learn more. Also recommended is the *The Heart of Yoga* by T.K.V. Desikachar.

Following the yamas are the niyamas, which show up in our inward relationship with our self. Again there are five:

1. *Saucha* (purity or cleanliness)
2. *Samtosha* (contentment)
3. *Tapas* (austerity)
4. *Svadhyaya* (self-study)
5. *Ishvara-pranidhana* (surrendering to a higher power)

Once again all five niyamas can be developed in our Yin Yoga practice. The Hatha Yoga texts suggest that, before beginning your practice, the student should bathe, evacuate the bowels, and ensure the room is clean and free from bugs. This is saucha. Without a pure, clean body, our practice will not bear fruit. Samtosha, or contentment, is also to be practiced. With contentment, there is no grasping, no attachment or aversion. The final three niyamas we have seen before. These are the three stages of Kriya Yoga.[147]

The limbs of asana and pranayama will be discussed later in our journey. The final four limbs of the ashtanga are purely mental practices. Pratyahara develops the ability to focus; it is the closing of the sense doors, and a shutting out of all distractions. Yin Yoga provides many opportunities to practice pratyahara. We go deeply inside and are cut off from the distractions of the outer world. From here, dharana is possible. Dharana is concentration. This can be concentration upon an object, a sound, or even a sensation. The breath is a favorite object for concentration during asana or pranayama practice.

Dhyana[148] is meditation: in the state of meditation the object of meditation and the subject doing the meditation begin to merge.

---

[147] It is their repetition here that leads some scholars to believe that the ashtanga was added to the Yoga Sutra centuries after its original compilation.

[148] The evolution of the word dhyana is interesting. When the practices of yoga filtered into China, the words went with them. In the fifth century, the Bodhidharma arrived in China, practicing a special kind of Buddhist dhyana. The Chinese called this practice *ch'an*. In the tenth century, Japanese monks returning to Japan after studying this new practice, called

There are no thoughts arising to interfere with the perception of the object and the object itself. However, total oneness has not yet been reached. That occurs in samadhi.

Samadhi and Kaivalya

The Yoga Sutra states that samadhi is the ultimate *tool* of yoga. Note that this is not saying that samadhi is the ultimate *goal* of yoga. Where Samkhya practice involved discernment and renunciation, Classical Yoga involves samadhi and renunciation. But what is samadhi? That is not an easy question to answer.

Samadhi literally means "ecstasy." It is acquired through devoted practice and grace. Practice alone will not guarantee samadhi. The grace of the guru (or of God) is also required. In samadhi, consciousness itself shines forth as the object of concentration. This means that, in samadhi, the subject and the object become one: consciousness senses, and is absorbed in, itself.

In the state of samadhi, all perceptions are shut off. Nothing disturbs the immersion of the self in the Self. Iyengar warns that in the state of samadhi, no action is possible as there is no one to act. We cannot do anything while in Samadhi; to do requires someone to do, and something to be done. The presence of a subject (the doer) and an object (the thing we are doing it to) causes us to leave this wondrous state of samadhi, and come back to being a player in life.

The Yoga Sutra, being a very technical manual, offers a hierarchy of levels of samadhi. In fact, all yoga traditions expound upon the various levels of samadhi that the yogi will pass through. It is beyond the scope of this journey to examine these stages. However, it is interesting to note that the Yoga Sutra and other sages warn that the danger to the yogi is greatest at this stage. Samadhi is so pleasurable that many seekers get stuck here; instead of pushing onward to the ultimate goal, they become sidetracked in this ecstatic state.

The ultimate goal is kaivalya: aloneness or aloofness.

---

this practice *Zen*. Thus the Japanese word Zen is actually derived from Sanskrit dhyana: meditation.

Once a yogi has mastered samadhi and is back again in the ordinary world, what has changed? In samadhi there is no subject, no object, and consciousness is aware of only consciousness. When the yogi has left samadhi, she still knows the real nature of the universe. Once again she has entered the world of action, but now she acts out of the knowledge of the unity of everything. Iyengar says that kaivalya is samadhi in action. At this stage, the yogi is fully liberated. However, Iyengar is a modern yogin. The yogis of the classical era still believed in a dualist universe. Liberation is not possible while still trapped in the body. Kaivalya is not the final liberation. In modern times many scholars do interpret kaivalya to mean liberation, or *moksha*. Georg Feuerstein believes that, for the classical yogis, kaivalya meant only the ability to see without anything to be seen. This is the ultimate aloneness, but it is still one step removed from final liberation – the liberation that comes only with the release of the body.

Problems with Classical Yoga

Just as competing traditions dismissed Samkhya because it was dualistic, Classical Yoga too was considered flawed. It suffered the same problems as Samkhya. How could there be all these purushas floating about the universe, omnipotent and infinite, but separate? The rise of Buddhism, and its emphasis on the middle path, also created problems for Classical Yoga. Classical Yoga was fierce, its renunciation achievable by only a few. How could yoga ever be a spiritual practice for everyone, when it demanded such sacrifice? The Buddha tried earlier versions of Classical Yoga, mastered them, and dismissed these approaches.

Other yogis began to think in new ways. They began to ask, "If we can become liberated only through working while in our bodies, how can our bodies be part of the problem?" Surely the body must be part of the solution. The body should not be destroyed in order to achieve liberation; it must be honored, in the same way a temple is honored. In fact, the body is the temple in which we do our practice. This was the dawning of a new, radically different form of yoga. This was the beginning of Tantra Yoga.

Tantra Yoga

Chronologically, the early Samkhya philosophy arose just before the time of the Buddha, who died in 483 B.C.E. This was the time of pre-Classical Yoga. True Classical Yoga took form over the five hundred years or so after the Buddha. As now, very few people practiced this strict, severe form of yoga. While the ancient sages following this practice believed one could achieve true and final liberation only after leaving the body, there existed a belief within the Upanishads that living liberation was possible. This belief in living liberation[149] was quite attractive. After all, if there is only the Self, why should we have to get rid of anything else to recognize it?

At this time Buddhism was flourishing, but it was still steeped in the cultural biases of the day. Throughout the world at this time, the prehistoric matriarchal societies had died out. Civilization, technological advancements, and structured political hierarchies were all patriarchal. Women had few or no rights, and very little respect. Even the Buddha refused to allow his stepmother to join his sangha once her husband, his father, died. Ananda (the Buddha's cousin) pleaded with the Buddha, until the Buddha finally agreed, but only if his stepmother agreed to follow eight precepts that the men didn't have to follow. Everywhere the feminine was rejected and repressed.[150]

---

[149] Also known as *jivan-mukti*.

[150] See Karen Armstrong's book *Buddha* for a clearly written historical biography of the Buddha. On page 139 she lists the eight conditions the Buddha gave in order for his stepmother, or any female, to join the order: a nun must always stand in the presence of a monk; nuns must always spend retreats with monks (never by themselves); they must receive instructions every two weeks from a monk; nuns must not hold their own ceremonies; nuns must do penance in front of a monk for any offenses; a nun must be ordained by both a nun and a monk; she must never criticize a monk – however, she could be rebuked by a monk; and finally, a nun must not preach to monks. The Buddha only reluctantly allowed his stepmother, and other women, into the sangha, warning that, because he did this, his teachings would now last only five hundred years. Women, he considered, would "fall like mildew on a field of rice," destroying the order.

Tantra arose in reaction to the denial of the body and the denial of the feminine. Why do we have to consider the body or the mind as an enemy? Why do we deny the feminine energies? There must be a way to accommodate all these factors that are so obviously present in life! In Jungian terms, the Indian sages of the early first millennium were the first yogis to recognize and accept the *anima*: the female part of the soul. It would take European culture a thousand years to come to the same realization.[151]

Tantra arose out of the seeds of Samkhya, Classical Yoga, and Buddhism but it quickly surpassed all of these philosophies. Where the earlier schools were patriarchal and either dualistic or atheistic, Tantra embraced the feminine, the principle of unity, and offered a way for anyone to practice. Tantra ignored class structure, and as a result had many practitioners from the lower castes. This egalitarianism was unique and energizing.

---

[151] It wasn't until the eleventh century that the patriarchal imperative of the Catholic Church began to allow any hint of the feminine. Like the Buddha, the Church never fully embraced women in their hierarchy.

The Thirty-six Principles of Tantra

To the *tantrikas* (the practitioners of Tantra), the psychocosmological model of the universe created by Samkhya was good as far as it went, but it didn't go far enough. The model was good because, as in all spiritual realizations, the senses that show us the world present just a thin sliver of what is really there. However, the Samkhya yogis didn't realize that they were a victim of Maya; they failed to see deeply enough into the real situation. On top of Samkhya's twenty-four principles were another twelve.

Just above the great divide of purusha and prakriti sit the illusionary layers of Maya. Maya has several possible meanings, ranging from illusion to relative existence.[152] Tantrikas believe that there are five forms of Maya.

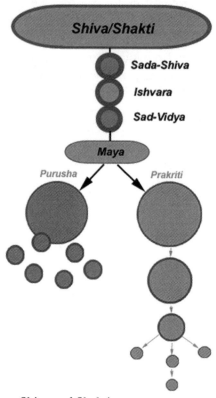

Shiva and Shakti are one, not two; thus the Tantra philosophy is non-dualistic.

Above these manifestations of Maya are the three pure principles of existence: *Sad-Vidya, Ishvara,* and *Sada-Shiva.* And finally, above these three pure principles is the ultimate reality of Shiva/Shakti.

Like two sides of one coin, Shiva/Shakti can never be separated. They co-exist as one, but they can be seen as two, depending upon which side you are looking at. As we descend the left side of the diagram, down from Shiva, we unfold the subjective aspect of existence. As we descend the right side, down from Shakti, we unfold

---

[152] As opposed to the actual reality, which is hidden behind her.

the objective aspect of existence. In Tantra we find a different view of God, the clock maker, and his creation, the clock. We discover that God *is* the clock; God is part of his own creation. And we are the clock too … we are part of his creation – and part of God at the same time.

It is far beyond our scope to delve deeper into the ontology of the Tantra model. Interested students may find Georg Feuerstein's book *Tantra: the Path of Ecstasy* to be helpful. The point of what we have explored so far is that, according to Tantra, the One unfolds into the Many. Liberation, then, is achieved when we traverse this path backward: from the seemingly many we find in our everyday life, we go all the way back to the One.

Liberation, this finding the One behind the Many, is possible while we are in the body. In fact, the body is a necessary tool to reaching this liberated state. Only incarnate beings can become enlightened and liberated. Even the gods are jealous of humans; only humans can become truly free. The path to liberation is the Tantric Practices.

Tantric Practices

The goal of the practice of Tantra Yoga is, fundamentally, to release Shakti, and move her up the central channel of the body, to meet with Shiva who is waiting for her just above the crown of the head. Of course, like all yogic teachings, there are some schools that claim the exact opposite is what must happen; Shakti must descend to the waiting Shiva. In either case, the tools mostly used to awaken and move the sleeping Shakti are the tools of pranayama.

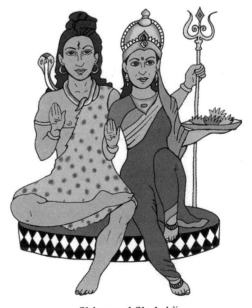

Shiva and Shakti [x]

Tantra also describes in detail the subtle body anatomy, which prana animates.[153] Pranayama, however, is not the only tool available. Tantra has a broad offering of techniques and practices. They include:

- *Mantra*
- *Mudra*
- *Yantra*
- *Pancha-Makara* (the Five-M's)

Our journey takes us now to look at these Tantric practices.

Mantras

The reciting of *mantras* (which are syllables, words, or texts) has been performed since the Vedas were revealed over five thousand years ago. In Tantra, mantra recitation (also called *"japa"* or repetition) reaches a grand height. The word mantra itself has several meanings. Manas means mind or thinking. *Trana* means liberation. Thus a mantra can channel thoughts into liberation. Another interpretation suggests that a mantra protects the mind. Mantras are sounds charged with the power to gain favors, to appease the gods, and to identify with the ultimate reality.

There are countless mantras. Hindu life is surrounded by mantras; from birth to death mantras are chanted. Mantras can be recited out loud, which gains one a certain amount of merit. When the mantras are whispered, greater merit is gained. The highest merit is gained when the mantra is heard silently inside. This silent hearing of mantras must never be rushed or done incorrectly; merit is lost in those cases.

Beyond seeking favors, mantras can be used as an object of concentration, helping to still the mind. Mantras can easily be incorporated into the Yin Yoga practice. A yoga teacher can generally

---

[153] We have already reviewed this energy anatomy in the section The Yogic View of Energy. The practices of pranayama are described in more detail in Chapter 15: Moving Energy.

recommend an appropriate mantra for a student to use.[154] Many mantras include the syllable Om. The Tibetan Buddhist mantra *Om mani padme Om* is a wonderful way to still the mind. Mantras praising the source of energy, the sun, are quite common and favored. The *Gayatri Mantra*[155] is often recited every morning and there are many CDs available with wonderful renditions of this homage to the sun.[156]

Mudras

Symbolic gestures are called *"mudras."* Mudra derives from the word *mud*, which means to delight. Basically mudras are seals that lock in energy and awareness. They can be formed by the hands or the body itself. The shapes represent inner states. This is easy to verify for yourself. Fold your arms in front of you and notice your inner state. Now release the arms and open them wide, joining the tips of your forefingers to your thumbs. Notice the changed inner state. Yogis who employ mudras can sense the energetic differences of even minor changes.

There are at least one hundred and eight hand gestures.[157] When we add all the body seals, we find there are a lot of mudras available. Some of the commonest hand seals are the *anjali* (prayer) mudra and the *jnana* (wisdom) mudra.[158] The jnana mudra is sometimes mistaken for the *chin* (consciousness) mudra. Swami Satyananda Saraswati, who has written many of the excellent books published by the Bihar School of Yoga in India, explains that the jnana mudra is done with the palm facing down, while the chin mudra has the palm facing up. Since jnana means wisdom, when we perform the jnana mudra we are sealing in wisdom. When we perform the chin mudra we are sealing

---

154 The mantra *so'ham* is discussed later, in the second half of our journey.

155 Gayatri is one of many names of the sun's energy.

156 Deva Premal, who has a hauntingly lovely voice, has two versions of the Gayatri Mantra available on two of her CDs, *Essence* and *Satsang*.

157 One hundred and eight is a magical number signifying wholeness. When you see a claim that there are one hundred and eight of something or other, you can be assured there are probably a lot more than that.

158 Pronounced ghee-yana, and sometimes spelled gyana or gian mudra.

in awareness or consciousness. These mudras are formed by touching the tip of the forefinger to the thumb. The jnana mudra is just one of many therapeutic mudras, and is said to be good for curing insomnia, nervous tension, and a weak memory.

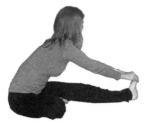

There are many books available on mudras. In Swami Satyananda Saraswati's book *Asana Pranayama Mudra Bandha* he has provided a full description of the five kinds of mudras: hand mudras, head mudras, postural mudras, lock mudras (bandhas), and perineal mudras. The book gives many examples of each kind of mudra, including a description for making the whole body into one big postural mudra: the maha mudra.[159]

Mudras are easily practiced in Yin Yoga. While in most of the postures, we can hold our hands in mudra or clasp our feet. Once the mudra is formed, the practice is then to sense the energetic effect of the mudra. That is a complete meditation all on its own.

Yantras

Tantra may also use geometrical devices as the object of meditation or concentration. These objects are *yantras*, and can be considered visual mantras. The yantra is a representation of the universe, and its contemplation leads to realizations about the universe's nature. The word yantra literally means a machine or device. While a yantra is similar to a *mandala*, the yantra is square and contains interlocking triangles. A mandala, however, can be of various shapes.

The *Shri Yantra*, shown on the facing page, contains five downward-pointing triangles representing Shakti, and four upward-facing triangles representing Shiva.[160] Together these nine triangles form forty-three individual triangles. Toward the outside are found

---

[159] As shown in the picture above, sit down with one leg forward, the other knee bent so that the foot is brought to the inner thigh, press the heel into the perineum, and clasp the extended foot with both hands.

[160] Shiva's lingam is always shown pointing upward, indicating virility, and Shiva's triangles also point upward, in the direction of his phallus, which is a good way to remember whose triangles are whose in these yantras.

two circles of lotus petals. The inner eight petals represent Vishnu, and the outer sixteen petals represent the attainment of the desired object. Vishnu's consort is Lakshmi, who is also known as Shri. She is the goddess of good fortune, and it is after her that this yantra is named.

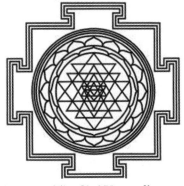

The Shri Yantra Y

At the center of the yantra is a dot, called a "bindu" or seed point. This is the focal point. In this one infinitely small point is found the infinitely large universe. Whatever exists outside is found inside, and vice versa. This single realization is at the core of many religious esoteric teachings. The macrocosm is a reflection of the inner microcosm, and what happens in one realm affects the other.

The practice of yantra visualization is not easy, and its mastery depends upon the student's power of concentration and her ability to feel and control the subtle energies. Tantra also employs visualization of a chosen deity. Similar to a yantra, the objective of this practice is to completely identify with the form being visualized. Every nuance should be experienced completely, especially when the eyes are closed.

The use of mantra, yantra, and mudras are far from the only, or even the most well known, forms of Tantra practice. Of more notoriety are the Pancha-Makara: the Five-M's.

The Pancha-Makara of Tantra

Remember, Tantra evolved in the midst of a repressive culture, one that kept people of lower castes subjugated through cultural bias, devalued women, and saw the body and the mind as an evil enemies to be overcome. Life was very hard for people who were not males of the Brahman caste, or kings and princes. Anything that could suspend the everyday worries and concerns of the masses would be welcomed. Tantra offered a path to people who had no other means to experience joy. The path included rituals; the rituals included the Five-M's.

The *Pancha-Makara* were ways to cleanse and transcend the mind. Each "M" stands for a particular practice:

- *Madya* or wine
- *Matsya* or fish
- *Mamsa* or meat
- *Mudra* or parched grain
- *Maithuna* or sexual intercourse

In our Western culture today, these five practices seem rather mundane and unremarkable. But a thousand years ago, this was quite shocking to conservative society. The use of alcohol was frowned upon by virtually all religions. The adoption of the non-harming ethic in Jainism and Buddhism was carried into *Vedanta*,[161] which had become the most common belief system in India at the time Tantra was flowering. Non-harming, or ahimsa, meant being vegetarian; no meat or fish was to be consumed. Mudra, in this context, is not the practice of seals, or gestures; it is speculated this meant the use of drugs.[162]

The final practice is one that has given rise to most of the misunderstandings about Tantra – sexual intercourse. The first misunderstanding arises due to the existence of two very different schools of Tantra: the right-handed school, and the left-handed school. The right-handed school believed that the Pancha-Makara were to be interpreted symbolically. One did not actually drink alcohol, eat meat, or get high. Instead, one used the imagination to simulate the effect of such a practice, in order to transcend the ordinary world. The left-handed school disagreed, believing that each practice was indeed meant to be actually performed.

To appreciate the effect of the Pancha-Makara today, we would need to adapt them to suit today's culture. Today eating meat,

---

[161] Vedanta is the major branch of Hinduism, and arose out of the Upanishads.

[162] Obviously if mudra comes from a root word meaning delight, drugs would be a good way to be delighted. Even today ganja and bhang (marijuana) are quite popular in India.

drinking alcohol, engaging in freely available sexual relations, or indulging in drugs does not shock us. These don't jar us out of our normal state of mind. To understand the intent of the Five-M's, we would have to change these to practices that are not only cultural taboos in today's society but are things that we would find personally revolting to do. If a spiritual school existed today that required you to ingest live maggots, and then publicly perform ritual incest with your grandmother or grandfather, that school would quickly gain a reputation similar to the one Tantra was tarnished with for centuries.[163]

Due to the misunderstandings about the less commonly practiced left-handed school of Tantra, and due to the fact that anyone, regardless of gender or class could practice Tantra, both the right-handed and left-handed schools were driven underground. Remember, Tantra is really trying to free and raise shakti energy so that living liberation can be achieved. The tantrikas were not indulging in the Pancha-Makara for simple pleasure. In fact, during maithuna, orgasm was not allowed. And besides, there were many other Tantric practices that didn't involve any of the Pancha-Makara. Pranayama and physical exercises had no stigma in and of themselves. But they were guilty by association.

---

[163] Please note: This is not to suggest Tantra promoted incest! In fact, it was always very clearly stated that sexual relations with one's mother was never allowed. (However, the women participants in such sexual rituals were generally older and more experienced in the ceremonies than the men.)

Hatha Yoga

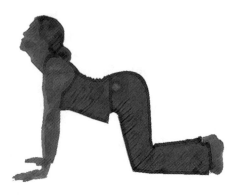

Society's disgust for Tantra's teachings resulted in the evolution of a new school of yoga: Hatha Yoga, which arose from Tantra Yoga. Hatha kept many of the practices that Tantra developed, but just as Tantra discarded what it didn't like of Classical Yoga, Hatha also dropped the unsavory parts of Tantra. Hatha Yoga focused its practices on building a healthy body, one that would be perfect for the higher practices of mediation and samadhi. In this respect Yin Yoga is just one of many branches of Hatha Yoga. The objective in the Yin Yoga practice is also to prepare us for the deeper spiritual inquiries into reality, and eventually enlightenment. Along the way many physical, emotional, and mental benefits are obtained.

Hatha Yoga is often called the ladder to *Raja Yoga*. Raja means kingly or royal. Raja Yoga contains the higher limbs of the Yoga Sutra: dharana, dhyana, and samadhi. Yin Yoga also prepares us to work with the mind at progressively deeper levels. To do so requires insight and dedication. These are qualities that yoga shares with the ancient practice of the Buddha, who was also an accomplished yogin.

Chapter Ten:
The Buddhist View of Mind

A young man came to visit the Buddha one day. He was filled with questions. He asked the Buddha about the nature of the universe, about the meaning of life, about death, and about many other things. The Buddha paused, and then in reply asked the man a question of his own. "Did someone tell you that I would answer these questions for you?" "No," replied the young man, "I am just eager to learn." The Buddha regarded him closely, and then taught an unexpected lesson.

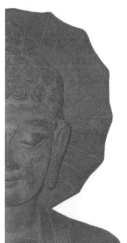

"Once there was a man who was wounded by a poisoned arrow. A doctor was quickly summoned. The poison was deadly, and the man had little time left. As the doctor began to extract the arrow, the wounded man stopped him and asked, 'Wait. I must know who shot me! Why did he do this? What kind of man was he? Was he angry or jealous? Did he shoot me out of rage, or by mistake?' The doctor explained that the man had a choice: allow the arrow to be removed right away without any answers, and live, or wait for all his questions to be answered, and die."

What he taught, the Buddha explained to the young man, was a way to end suffering. That was far more important than knowing the structure of the heavens. Why would you want to waste one minute on unimportant details when the most important work in your life has not even started? Learn to free your mind, end your delusion, and end your suffering before worrying about all these other questions.

The Buddha lived in a time when the Samkhya philosophy was becoming widely accepted. However, the Buddha was a very pragmatic man. He did not bother with models of the cosmos. He wanted everyone to explore his or her own situation in minute detail. The Buddha's teachings gave specific advice on how to avoid suffering and obtain release.

There are few hierarchical models of mind and consciousness in the Buddha's teachings. If there is a psychology at all, it is an applied psychology. It resonates today closely to the schools of behavioral psychologies, which we will address in the next part of our journey. For now we will explore a brief vignette of the life of the Buddha, his realizations, and his main teachings as they can be applied to our practice of yoga.

The Historical Buddha

There are many wonderful stories about how the Buddha's birth was accompanied by celebrations by the gods, about how he came into the world in an unusual way,[164] and his first steps and his first words. Like all the founders of major religions, stories and myths grew and multiplied. But, like all mythic heroes, the historical facts are far less available. Karen Armstrong's book *Buddha* is a concise presentation of what we really know of the historical Buddha. The proven historical facts are few and can be summarized quickly.

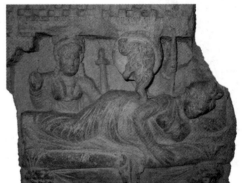

Siddhatta Gotama of the Shakya tribe was born in

The Buddha arriving from his mother's side. z

---

[164] He exited from his mother's side at the level of the heart.

Kapilavatthu in the small country of Shakka.[165] Shakka was in a very remote area of what is now the western edge of Nepal. Shakka was squeezed between the larger kingdoms of Magadha to the southeast, located in modern Bihar, India, and Kosala directly west. It was a time of political strife and physical danger.

The generally accepted year of birth for the Buddha is 563 B.C.E., although some Chinese scholars put this one hundred years later. The Buddha lived for eighty years. Siddhatta was a prince, his father one of the many aristocrats who participated in governing Shakka. When he was twenty-nine, Gotama left his family, including his newborn son, to search for the answer to why life was so filled with suffering, and to find a way to end suffering.

The future Buddha first studied yoga under two masters; he became an adept at all the yogas his teachers taught. This included mastery of the deepest meditations and the highest levels of samadhi. Gotama became a very accomplished yogin, but he found that the real answers he was seeking still eluded him. The highest knowings offered by his teachers were not the ultimate realization. He left each teacher and, living with five other devoted yogins, practiced on his own. His yoga was fierce; he almost died from his austerities.

Six years after his renunciation of the privileged life in Shakka, Siddhatta renounced this new life as well. Extremism, he declared, was not the answer. From now on he would practice only the middle way, a path of moderation. He decided, as Armstrong writes, "to work with human nature and not fight against it." This meant he would steer a path between giving into the pleasures of the world self-indulgently, and the extreme, body-denying asceticism of the yogis and Jains.

Sitting down under a tree, Siddhatta vowed not to move until he achieved enlightenment. He succeeded and then, after a time of internal debate over what he should do next, he decided to share what he had learned with the world. For the next forty-five years, the now awakened one, the Buddha, taught. Although he taught, he knew that ultimate realization cannot be taught; the way can only be

---

[165] We are using the Pali version of these words. Often we may see the Buddha's name written in the Sanskrit language as Siddhartha Gautama.

pointed to. The individual must walk the path personally. All a Buddha could do was point the way to the path.

The Buddha left the world in 483 B.C.E., after suffering a fatal and painful case of dysentery, an unfortunately common disease of the time.

This much is known about the Buddha. Also known is where he taught, whom he taught, and the way the teachings were passed down through the generations. But, beyond these dry facts, there arose many wonderful stories and metaphors, each with its own value to the student of the mind. Joseph Campbell warns us that whenever we read mythic stories, we must not read them as if they were facts. To believe these myths are historical truths would be to reduce them to the equivalent of dry headlines in a newspaper. The proper way to digest these stories is to ask what they mean to you! Personally! What does the fact that the awakened one is said to have sprung from his mother's side at the level of the heart, and not in the normal way, mean for you?[166]

What motivated the Buddha to seek enlightenment was his observation of the conditions of life. He saw sickness, he saw aging, he saw death. In the midst of all this suffering, he saw a holy man attempting to free himself from the afflictions of life. Siddhatta decided to personally seek the solution to suffering. Upon his enlightenment he realized he had indeed found the way. He called the way the Four Noble Truths.

---

[166] A wonderful and enjoyable side trip is to visit these mythical stories about the Buddha. Many of Joseph Campbell's books have several illuminating tales. You may want to read the *Transformation of Myth through Time* for several illustrative stories. A more extended side trip would lead you to the works of Campbell's good friend Heinrich Zimmer and his weighty book *Philosophies of India*. Right now our journey takes us deeper into the main teachings of the Buddha.

The Four Noble Truths

The Buddha decided to use a process commonly used by doctors in his day to describe the problem of our life and its solution. A doctor, visiting a patient in distress, will first determine what the problem is. Once known, the doctor goes on to discover the cause of the problem. Next, she tries to see if there is a cure for the problem. Finally, she prescribes for her patient the way to effect the cure. This is a very simple, effective, and pragmatic approach. The Buddha, being very pragmatic, followed these four steps as well. He called this first teaching the Four Noble truths. These truths are:

1. Suffering exists
2. There is a cause of our suffering
3. There is a cure for our suffering
4. The cure is the Eightfold Path[167]

In these simple truths, the Buddha added nothing superfluous. There is no metaphysical tradition; there is no psychocosmological model; there are simply these four facts.

1 – Suffering Exists

If you are alive, there will be times in your life when you will experience pain. Pain can come in many guises. There is physical pain, emotional pain, psychological pain, and spiritual pain. These are the inevitable consequences of simply being alive; it is part of the deal. This does not mean that life is painful all the time. Certainly there are times when we are not in pain, and we feel neutral or happy. But pain is a part of life, despite our attempts to deny it or run away from it. No life is free from pain.

Suffering is different from pain. The Buddha explained the difference with a story.

---

[167] We will look at the Eightfold Path in detail in a few moments.

"Once," the Buddha told his followers, "there was a man who was shot by an arrow.[168] How do you think the man felt?" asked the Buddha.

"Hurt! In pain!" replied his followers.

"Right," agreed the Buddha. "Now this unfortunate man was soon struck by a second arrow. Now how do you think he felt?"

"Much worse!" replied the followers.

"Just so!" agreed the Buddha again. "The name of that second arrow is suffering."

Pain, as we have seen, is inevitable. It is a part of the bargain of being alive. But suffering is optional! Suffering, according to the Buddha, is that second arrow. Suffering is the reaction we inflict upon ourselves when we are subjected to the first arrow of inevitable pain.

In his book *Who Dies?* Stephen Levine suggests many ways to examine this truth for ourselves. Levine is a Buddhist counselor who has studied for many years with Elisabeth Kubler-Ross and Ram Dass. He has worked with people who are dying and in constant pain. His practical, meditation-based teachings help the terminally ill come to recognize that they are not their disease, they are not their pain, and there is someone beneath the pain who is creating the suffering they are experiencing. It is not the sensations that create the problem, but rather the stories we add on top of the sensation that create the suffering. Once we recognize how we create our own suffering, the original sensations, which we call pain, are made more bearable. Levine's meditations help us see the difference between pain and suffering.

Our Yin Yoga practice is also an excellent time to notice the truth of this first of the Buddha four noble truths. As we hold the posture for a longer and longer period of time, sensations begin to increase. We leave our normal comfort zone, and we become distinctly

---

[168] Arrows, as you will notice, are a common metaphor of these times.

uncomfortable. We may even be on the verge of experiencing pain.[169] This discomfort is the first arrow – it is simply a sensation. How we react to a sensation is the interesting part of the practice. Do we add mental stories and judgments to a sensation? Do we tell ourselves how much we dislike the sensation, and wish it would end?

If this is your normal reaction to discomfort, whether while in a Yin Yoga pose or at any time in your life, study the discomfort. Get to know it. What is really going on there? This is the place where the practice can yield the greatest insight. Learning to watch and study the sensations arising in our yoga practice prepares us to also watch these arising at other times in life.

This common reaction to stress or challenging situations leads us directly to the Buddha's second noble truth.

2 – There is a Cause of Suffering

Suffering exists because we cause it to exist. Remember that sensations are inevitable. Pain is a part of life, but suffering is optional. How do we cause suffering? The Buddha recognized that we do this in two ways: we cling to things that we find pleasant, and we run away from things that are unpleasant. These two reactions are called attachment and aversion. We have seen these before; they are the third and fourth klesha of Classical Yoga, raga and dvesa.

The *Issue at Hand* by Gil Fronsdal explains that there are four kinds of clinging we subject ourselves to. The first is a clinging to a particular spiritual practice or routine – thinking that if we just follow the rules, that will suffice, and we will be happy. Unfortunately, we do not have to look very far to see the damage caused by intolerant and strongly held religious or spiritual practices. The second form of clinging is grasping certain views. These are all the opinions we hold, and the stories we apply to ourselves. We can be so strongly attached to a particular self-view that, if it is damaged or lost, we are also lost. There are many examples of men strongly attached to their self-view of being successful businessmen and family providers. When a personal financial crisis arises, such as a crash in the stock market,

---

[169] Hopefully you are not going so deep that you *are* in pain.

this self-image is destroyed, and these men become so lost that their only solution is suicide. The third form of clinging is the grasping to the sense of self; this is a form of asmita (ego), which was described in Classical Yoga. Everything that occurs in the world is interpreted in terms of how it affects or doesn't affect me (the ego or small self).

The final clinging is the first one the Buddha actually mentioned. Fronsdal lists it last because it is the one people least understand, and are the most afraid of giving up. It is the clinging to pleasurable sensations. The Buddha did not say that pleasure was bad; he made no moral judgment about pleasure or pain. What he warns against is the clinging to pleasure. Just as there will be times in life when pain is present, there will be times in life when pleasure is present. Enjoy those moments, but when they go, let them go. Learn to enjoy the moments as they arise, and leave them in the past once they are gone.

Aversion is the flip side of the clinging to pleasure. It is natural for animals to seek that which feels good, and avoid that which feels bad. Natural, but not necessarily the best strategy if your goal is true happiness. The pleasure of this moment may not lead to sustained pleasure in the future. We must rely upon a deeper intelligence to guide us. Is the pleasure of that extra dessert really going to make you truly happy – especially when you succumb to that temptation every night, and eventually develop diabetes and heart problems? These are small short-term pleasures that cause us a great deal of delayed pain.

There are small short-term pains as well, which, when we avoid them, create long-term suffering. Is the putting off of the meeting with your boss over an uncomfortable issue really going to make you happier in the long run? If we only follow our animal nature when presented with pleasure or pain, then we are giving up real happiness.

When pain is present, as Stephen Levine eloquently explains, it is only present in the moment. These moments change. Once the moment is gone, let this moment be gone. Don't worry about when the pain will return. Don't allow your mind to relive the past episodes of uncomfortable sensation. Learn to live in this moment.

3 – There Is a Cure for Suffering

Here is the good news: the Buddha diagnosed our condition. Understanding what was causing our suffering, he looked for and found that a cure does indeed exist. This cure is often referred to as *nibbana*,[170] but this is not always a preferred designation. Nibbana can be easily mistaken for just another state of being, which in itself becomes desirable. Once attachment arises again, the cure does not work. In this respect, nibbana can become as much of a trap to a Buddhist seeking liberation as samadhi can be a trap for the yogi.

States of calmness, joy, and happiness do arise, but if we become attached to them we are still subject to suffering. It is possible to end our suffering, even if it is not possible to end the sensations that precede it. The cure the Buddha discovered is described in his last truth.

4 – The Cure Is the Eightfold Way

Often to help understand the eight steps the Buddha taught, they are grouped into three categories. The first category is *panna*,[171] or wisdom.

1. Right View (or understanding)
2. Right Intention (or thinking)

Next comes the second category of *sila,* or ethics. This is similar to the yamas of the Yoga Sutra's ashtanga. These three steps are:

3. Right Speech
4. Right Action
5. Right Livelihood

---

[170] Or *nirvana* in Sanskrit.
[171] Or *prajna* in Sanskrit.

Finally the last three steps are called meditation, concentration, or samadhi.

6. Right Effort
7. Right Mindfulness
8. Right Concentration

You will find slight differences in the names assigned to these eight steps. This is due to the difficulty in precisely translating the Pali words into English. The *Buddhist Bible* by Dwight Goddard, for example, translates the second step of Right Intention as Right Mindedness and the seventh step of Right Mindfulness as Right Attentiveness.

These steps, like the eight limbs of the Yoga Sutra, are not meant to be done sequentially. One works toward all eight, almost in a spiraling manner. One way to understand the importance the Buddha assigned to these steps is with another story.

A man is holding a knife in his hand. He pushes the knife into a woman. She dies from the wound.

A simple and tragic tale; however, let us look deeper. The action is horrific, but what was the intention behind the action? If the man in the story is a thief, and the intent is to harm the woman, the action is indeed heinous. If the man is a surgeon, and he inserted the knife into the woman with the intent of saving her life, the action was tragically heroic. The intention is more important than the action. This is the flavor of Right Intention or Right Thinking.

Worse than wrong action is wrong speech. Worse than wrong speech is wrong thinking. Even if you refrain from acting out the thoughts in your mind, the harm is done just by the thought's presence. It is the thought that counts! Put another way, if the thought never arises, there will be no need to watch for wrong speech or wrong action. It always comes back to how and what we think.

The cure for our suffering lies in the way we think. We need to train our minds to no longer cling to pleasure, and run away from pain. This doesn't mean we avoid pleasure, or seek out pain, but rather that we treat both of these conditions equally. This is not easy, as we know. Just as the yogis have noticed that we must overcome the five kleshas, or afflictions, the Buddha also pointed out we needed to overcome five hindrances that get in our way of non-clinging and non-avoiding.

The Five Hindrances

In the Yoga Sutra we were told of the five kleshas, or hindrance to our practice. These were ignorance (avidya), the ego or I-making (asmita), attachment (raga), aversion (dvesa), and the fear of death or the clinging to life (abhinivesah). The Buddha taught that there are five mental hindrances, called the "*kilesa*,"[172] that serve to distract our minds and prevent us from living in this moment. The five are:

1. Desire, which leads to clinging and craving
2. Aversion, which leads to anger or hatred
3. Sleepiness or sloth
4. Restlessness
5. Doubt

We will visit each hindrance more closely starting with desire.

Desire

Desire, in the context of meditation or yoga practice, is the clinging to pleasant thoughts or sensations. Similar to raga in yoga, desire can create attachment, which causes suffering. It is not the pleasure that is the problem, but rather our craving for pleasure that enslaves us. When we try to hang on to pleasant moments, ignoring the fact that everything changes, we create a fear internally, the fear of the moment ending. Of course, the moment passes and the pleasure ends. This is one of the realities the Buddha talked about constantly. He called it "*anicca*," or impermanence. Everything ends; good times and bad times all have their time, and they pass away. So

---

[172] The Sanskrit version of this Pali word is "*klesha*."

even if we attain our heart's desire, even when we are basking in pleasant feelings or situations, this kind of pleasure is an illusion because it is transient. Desire creates suffering, and hinders us from realizing the true joy of being.

Desire can be watched. In our yoga practice we will experience pleasant sensations frequently. Coming out of a long-held Yin Yoga pose can often create sensations that are extremely pleasurable. Enjoy these sensations when they arise, but don't cling to them. At the end of the practice there is also a very pleasurable buzz throughout the body. This good feeling may last for hours afterward. For many people this is the reason they return to the practice; they want to feel that sense of well-being over and over again. There is nothing wrong with enjoying the feeling, and if that is the motivation you need to keep doing your practice, that too is perfectly fine and all right. However, just recognize that this is a craving, this is an addiction. Watch these desires come into existence – don't react to them; just notice them. Eventually the desires will recede, and you will be able to enjoy the sensations of pleasure when they arise without the clinging or the hidden fear of their passing.

Aversion

When we are faced with situations outside our normal comfort zone, we tend to react in one of three ways:

1. We run away from the situation as fast and as far as we can, or
2. We try to change the situation as quickly as possible, or
3. We just give up and, usually in a sullen, self-pitying way, surrender

The first two ways are very yang ways of dealing with life. Many people will hide or run away from uncomfortable situations. Of course, this never changes the situations or ourselves, so when we are faced with another challenging situation, we do the same thing again. The second strategy is to change the situation. We are taught early and often in our culture to change the world, to make something of ourselves, to make a difference – to become yangsters. And certainly there are times that these are totally appropriate things to do. If we see a child being beaten, we take action; we try to stop the beating. At times, a yang response to the world *is* the proper reaction. But not always, and not all the time. Harmony is the balance between yin and yang. If we are always trying to change the world (including changing our friends, our spouse, our boss, our coworkers …), we are going to burn out.

There is a difference between acting to right a wrong, and acting to end sensations that we don't like. The difference is found in our motivation. If we are trying to avert harm to another being, that can be considered Right Mindfulness or Right Intention or Right Action. This action is skillful and helpful. If we are simply trying to end any uncomfortable sensations we are experiencing that are not harming us,[173] that is aversion.

The third way we avoid challenging situations is very yin-like – we give up. This type of surrender is also not skillful, if it involves thoughts that include the word "should." For example, we give up trying to change the situation but think that life really *should* be something other than it is right now. We surrender to what is happening, but we dearly want something else to be happening.

There is a fourth way to react to situations that take us outside our comfort zone. Accept what is happening, and simply watch, with great curiosity, what is going on. This is not giving up and wallowing in self-pity. This is not crying to the world, "Oh, why did this happen to me!" This is calmly observing what is really going on. This is looking for *what* is creating the sensation of discomfort.

The Yin Yoga practice is excellent for providing opportunities to watch the arising of aversion. As we hold the postures, and as the sensations increase in intensity, aversion arises; we want to move. As long as we are not in pain, and not harming ourselves by remaining still, we don't move. We remain in the pose and simply watch the arising of sensations. We watch how these sensations morph and change. We ask ourselves, "What is there about this feeling that makes me want to move?"

---

[173] Such sensations could include boredom, anxiety, or the dull achy feelings that arise in our Yin Yoga practice.

Learning to be non-reactive in the midst of challenging situations while on our yoga mat helps to build strength, resilience, and flexibility. Later, when challenges arise at other times in our lives, we can draw on these skills. Instead of reacting as we would normally, instead of running away, or trying to change the world, or instead of even just giving up, we find we have another powerful option: we can simply watch and observe what is really going on. Once we can really see what is happening, then a better way to respond may be revealed to us.

Sloth

We all feel tired from time to time. During meditation or yoga practice, our mind and body may become very sluggish. We don't want to move, we don't want to concentrate; our will is sapped; we may be physically or psychically exhausted; we may be in pain or in extreme discomfort. If we mechanically proceed with the practice, we may sleepwalk through it, or space out entirely. This robotic activity is not skilful and little benefit will accrue to you if you persist in the practice while in this state.

In yoga this state is often termed tamasic – this is inertia, a dullness that steals the will to perform. The cure is rajas or activity. If we are meditating with eyes closed, we may need to open them and sit a little taller. If we are practicing yoga, we may need to add more vigour to the poses; do several vinyasas.[174]

However, what the body may need is rest.

We can tell only by really paying attention to what is happening. Are we sluggish because we have exhausted ourselves? If this is really the case, further effort will make the situation worse. If you are depleted from too much yang activity, rest. However, if you are just feeling a cycle of inertia, notice this and react accordingly to wake yourself up. Too much yin is not good. The cure is a bout of brisk yang activity; this can be mental or physical activity.

---

[174] See Chapter 15: Moving Energy for several suggestions.

Restlessness

The flip side of sloth is an inability to calm down. Restlessness is too much yang. Restlessness is the buzz of too much caffeine, or the mind churning constantly while we try to sleep at night. Restlessness can manifest physically as constant movement, or agitation, or mentally as constantly dwelling on the same thoughts over and over. Guilt is a great cause of restlessness. We relive our sins, and never allow ourselves to forgive and move on. Guilt itself is a terrible sin, one that many Jews and Catholics subject themselves to.

The restless urge to move is often found in the Yin Yoga practice. We ask ourselves to remain still, but we can't. We fidget – we feel an itch, and immediately react and scratch it. We just can't settle down and be still. Usually when the body is moving, it is a sign that the mind is moving. And when the mind is moving, usually the breath is also fractured. Smoothing the breath, and watching it calm and slow is one excellent way to calm the mind. Once the mind is calmer, the body will move less. Once the body is quiet, there will be less need to breathe fast, and the cycle will positively reinforce itself.

Restlessness in meditation often arises due to the mind constantly being draw back to plans or inventories of our life, or our failings. We obsess – we can't let go of the cycle of planning and evaluating our plans. We make judgments over and over again; we judge who we believe we are and how we are doing. The cure here is to allow our mind to come back to simply watching the breath. The harder this is to do, the more we need some support, or tools. An excellent tool is to count the breaths. Start at one with the next inhalation, two for the exhalation, three for the next inhalation ... keep counting until you reach ten, and then start over.

If several minutes of counting breaths doesn't work, perhaps feeling the breaths will be more fruitful. Notice the way the air feels as it passes your upper lip and enters the nose. Feel the air in the throat or chest. Or notice the way your belly or chest moves up and down with each breath.[175]

---

[175] We will be introduced to several other meditation techniques in the second half of our journey.

Doubt

In yoga, doubt is called "samshaya." The cure prescribed is *shraddha* or faith. The Buddha defined doubt as indecision or skepticism. This can be a healthy, skillful thing to do. The Buddha often asked his students to question everything. Never accept something as true simply because an authority asserted it is so. You must walk the path for yourself, investigate everything personally, and ask questions.

But, when questions overwhelm us, indecision arises. We may become stuck, unable to make a choice. Like the hungry donkey, halfway between two piles of hay, that can't decide which one to go to, we remain rooted and eventually suffer for our indecision. Too many people use doubt as an excuse for living. There is a time to evaluate, to question, to gather information, but then there comes the time to act. Life is not a spectator sport – no one can make this journey for us. Do not let doubt become a hindrance – we need to take action in life.

How did the Buddha recommend we take action? Fortunately he had many suggestions on how to behave. Five suggestions, called the five precepts, form the ethical foundations for living.

The Five Precepts

Every religion and spiritual practice has a code of conduct. We have seen how the Yoga Sutra laid down five yamas and five niyamas to govern our inward and outward attitudes. Buddhists follow a similar, but shorter list that we have seen are called the Five Precepts.[176] These suggestions are to:

---

[176] Thich Nhat Hanh has updated these precepts for our times and culture. He calls these "the Five Mindfulness Trainings." Details can be found at his Plum Village Web page, http://www.plumvillage.org/practice/html/5_mindfulness_trainings.htm, or at http://www.deerparkmonastery.org/our_practice/fivetraining.html.

1. Refrain from killing
2. Refrain from stealing
3. Refrain from sexual misconduct
4. Refrain from idle speech, lies, and rumors
5. Refrain from intoxicants

The first four have a direct correlation to the yamas and niyamas of ahimsa, asteya, brahmacharya, and satya. As we noted earlier, these practices are not the Ten Commandments; there is no deal with God that if you follow these rules, your place in heaven is assured. In fact, the Buddha never liked to talk about heaven or life after death. His interest was to end suffering in this life, right now. The five precepts are tools that can help one stay out of trouble, until enlightenment is finally obtained.

While we become more mindful, we will naturally act in accordance with these precepts. Until then, we make the effort to follow these steps, even if it is not in our current nature to do so. Refraining from killing has the benefit of building a sense of identity with others. We are not referring to simply killing other people – any killing or harming creates a sense of separation from others. While we become aware of the interconnection between all beings, and all things, we are less likely to cause harm. So too with stealing, sexual misconduct, or lying; when we know that everything is connected, we have no wish to spread harm or negative energies.

If you decide to follow these precepts, and fail, do not fall into the familiar pit of despair and guilt. Only enlightened beings act with total enlightenment. We just do our best, and when we do come up short, as we will, we resolve to do better next time.

Isn't this the way we would like to practice our yoga too? We can't possibly do all the poses. We can't always be present all the time. Even the most advanced yogis have postures that elude them, or have postures that they can do now, but won't be able to do in twenty years. We simply work toward whatever goals we set for ourselves, and do our best. If, or rather when, we fail – we don't beat ourselves up; we don't allow ourselves to become discouraged. We just move on and try again. After all … it is the journey that counts, not the arriving.

The Buddha spent little time philosophizing or developing cosmological models of the universe. His concern was the mind. To be complete we could investigate the Buddhist dissertations on the psychological levels of the mind, the five *skandas,*[177] or the eighteen factors of cognition. But this would move us away from the most valuable teachings the Buddha left us.[178]

The real jewels of the Buddha's teachings are the methods for calming and controlling the mind. Remember that the Buddha was a yogic adept; he mastered all the most advanced practices, and found them wanting. His practical advice focused on following the Eightfold Path and meditation. It is through the various forms of Buddhist meditations that our journey becomes shorter.

Buddhist Meditation Practices

Buddhist meditation is the focusing of the mind onto a single object, or range of objects, with the intent of building awareness. Another name for meditation is mindfulness: we are simply present, aware of what is happening. When we can really notice what is going on, all the things we imagined were happening drop away until finally, what is left is the truth.

There are many different types of meditative techniques offered by the various schools and styles of Buddhism. Despite these differences, the most common anchor for the mind is the breath. The breath is completely portable; is always with us and always available to bring us back to this moment. One of the Buddha's teachings on using the breath is in the *Anapanasati* sutra. Here the Buddha tells us:

---

[177] The five aggregates of personality: form, the body of sensations, perceptions, mental activity, and consciousness.

[178] For an excursion into these psychological features of Buddhism the reader may wish to visit an overview by Dr. C. George Boeree (http://webspace.ship.edu/cgboer/buddhapers.html) or a detailed dissertation by Silva Padmal (http://ccbs.ntu.edu.tw/FULLTEXT/JR-ADM/silva.htm).

The meditator, having gone to the forest, to the shade of a tree, or to an empty building, sits down with legs folded crosswise, body held erect, and sets mindfulness to the fore. Always mindful, the meditator breathes in: mindful, the meditator breathes out.[179]

Formal meditation practice does involve sitting in a comfortable posture. The Yoga Sutra offers the same advice: your seat (your asana) needs to be comfortable and stable. However, this does not mean you must be in the Lotus position. If Lotus is an easy posture to maintain, without undue discomfort, for thirty minutes or longer, it may well be your ideal posture. For most Westerners, however, the pain is neither conducive to the practice nor is it good for your knees; it is better to adopt an easier posture that can be maintained for long periods. Sitting cross-legged, or even sitting in a chair, is okay if your back is straight and tall and your knees are below your hips. Sitting on a cushion, rather than right on the floor, is recommended even if your hips are very open. Regardless of which way you are sitting, or even if you are meditating while in a Yin Yoga posture, ultimately, in the words of Larry Rosenberg, "it is the mind that must sit."

Often the student will find one teacher requests that the eyes be closed but the next teacher will tell the student that her eyes must be open. These edicts come from different traditions. In the Theravada tradition, which employs the practice of vipassana (or insight) meditation, the eyes are closed.[180] In the Zen and Tibetan traditions, the eyes are open or half open but cast downward.[181]

Each tradition has reasons for its choice. Closed eyes create less visual distraction but can induce sleepiness. Open eyes may be subjected to many distractions but it is harder to dream when the eyes are open. Since both ways are offered by various traditions, there is obviously no right or wrong way to have the eyes. Choose the

---

[179] From *Breath by Breath* by Larry Rosenberg.

[180] An excellent online resource through which one can learn the *vipassana* practice is www.vipassana.com.

[181] Details of the Zen methods can be found in Philip Kapleau's rigorous book *The Three Pillars of Zen* or in the gentler approach offered in Suzuki's *Zen Mind, Beginner's Mind*. Or you can go online and visit www.zenspace.org.

option that works for you; if studying with one teacher, follow her guidance while you work with her.

What should be avoided is a constant switching between the two modes while meditating. If you believe you are allowed to open or close your eyes at any time, the danger is that thoughts will arise. You begin to debate if now would be a good time to switch modes. In our meditation such thoughts are acceptable and perhaps inevitable, but we do not wish to *react* to such thoughts. We simply note them and go back to our anchor, watching the breath. Meditate with your eyes open or closed, but once you have chosen an approach, stick to it.

This, of course, is just a guideline. It doesn't mean you won't be allowed into heaven if you close your eyes while meditating once in a while. There may in fact be times when switching is the best choice – if you find you are getting really sleepy, and suffering the full body jerks with your eyes closed, it may be better to open them. If you find your mind is just too wild with your eyes open, close them. But during a short yin pose of three or five minutes, you should endeavor to stick to one mode.

Watching the Breath

There are many different ways to watch the breath. In the Zen tradition we may be asked to simply count the breaths. Begin with the inhalation ... that is one. The exhalation is two. The next inhalation is three. Keep counting until you reach ten, and then begin over at one with the next inhalation. If this becomes easy, and you can count to ten without getting lost, without reaching twenty, or without counting mechanically in the background, then try to count only the exhalations.

This approach is sometimes called "*shamatha*" with support. Shamatha is one permissible way to meditate in all schools of Buddhism and other spiritual paths, as well as in the yogic schools.[182] Shamatha means calm abiding, tranquility, or meditation – as we sit

---

[182] However, *vipassana*, or insight meditation, is unique to the Theravada school of Buddhism.

and breathe, we just sit and breathe. Nothing special is happening, nothing special will ever happen … that is what makes this practice so special.

In the vipassana tradition you may be asked to follow the sensation of the breath – notice how it feels to breathe in and out. Where do you feel it? You may be asked to follow the feeling of the air on your upper lips as you breathe, or to follow the feeling in the throat, belly, or chest.

Please note: we are not trying to change the breath in any way. Our approach is very yin-like: we accept the breath the way it is. In very active yang styles of yoga, we do try to change the breath – for example, when we perform ujjayi breathing. In pranayama, we very obviously try to change the breath. But, in shamatha or vipassana, we want the breath to be whatever it wants to be: we accept it as it is. This is not easy! As soon as the mind tunes into the breath, it tries to control it, perfect it. Drop the effort and just watch. Watch the beginning of the inhalation, notice the exact moment the inhalation ends, the moment the exhalation begins, and the exact moment the exhalation ends. Notice the slight pauses, if any, between the in and out breath, and the out and in breath. Don't try to create, force, or do anything.

Of course, you need not only follow the breath while meditating in a sitting posture; you can do this while walking as well. In Zen this is called "*kinhin*." Walk slowly or quickly. Walk indoors or out in nature. However you choose to walk, watch the breath. Every time you notice your awareness has wandered away, simply bring it back to this breath.

The Anapanasati Sutra

The Anapanasati Sutra provides sixteen contemplations, or places to direct awareness. These are set into groups of four with the first group focused on the body, the second on feelings, the third on the mind, and the last group focused on wisdom. Larry Rosenberg suggests that, although the Anapanasati Sutra is used mainly in the Theravada tradition that he teaches, the Buddha's teachings in this sutra can be of value to meditators following the Zen or Tibetan traditions. Those drawn to watching the breath, as the basis of their meditation, can benefit from knowing what may arise while they practice.

The sixteen contemplations can be very briefly summarized:

1) Breathing in long
   Breathing in short
   Sensitive to the whole body
   Calming the whole body

2) Sensitive to rapture
   Sensitive to pleasure
   Sensitive to mental processes
   Calming mental processes

3) Sensitive to the mind
   Gladdening the mind
   Steadying the mind
   Liberating the mind

4) Focusing on impermanence
   Focusing on fading away
   Focusing on cessation
   Focusing on relinquishment

The process is breathe in and out, and focus awareness on each contemplation. For example, you may think "breathing in long" while you are breathing in long, and think "breathing out long" when you are breathing out long. When you master one contemplation, move to the next.

Along with a full description of the Buddha's teaching, Rosenberg offers the following five, very mundane ways to practice meditation:

1. When possible, do just one thing at a time
2. Pay full attention to what you are doing
3. When the mind wanders from what you are doing, bring it back
4. Repeat step number three several billion times
5. Investigate your distractions

You will quickly notice that this advice is something that need not be left on the mat or on the zafu.[183] This is instruction for everyday life. We practice doing all this while we meditate, or while we practice our yoga, but we practice so that it will be easier to do this at *all* times.

In Yin Yoga we have lots of opportunity to watch the breath, and investigate distractions. The asanas generate a lot of distractions. So what to do when the distractions are so strong that they take us away from the breath, and we just can't come back? In these cases we switch the object of meditation to the sensations.

Awareness of the Body

"If the body is not cultivated, the mind cannot be cultivated," said the Buddha. "There is one thing that when cultivated and regularly practiced leads to deep spiritual intention, to peace, to mindfulness and clear comprehension, to vision and knowledge, to a happy life here and now, and to the culmination of wisdom and suffering. And what is that one thing? Mindfulness centered on the body."

In the book *The Issue at Hand*, from which the above quotation comes, Gil Fronsdal tells us that his teacher once said, "Do not do anything that takes you out of your body." This simply means, don't go away. Don't do anything that will take you away. Stay present, and pay attention to the body.

Not only are physical sensations present in the body, emotions are also felt in the body. Thoughts may be heard in the head, but feelings, physically or emotionally, must be noticed in the body. This

---

[183] A zafu is a cushion used for meditation.

is one of the big reasons that all forms of yoga are so great at taking us down the path to meditation. In yoga we feel the body, we feel the breath, and we notice anything that distracts us or takes us away from this moment of sensation. Consider a time when you felt a strong emotion – wasn't there an accompanying tension or sensation somewhere physically? That knot in your belly, that quiver in your voice, the flush in your cheeks, the pain at the base of your neck … Buddhist psychology teaches that emotions are embodied: we just need to notice them.

The Buddha was quite clear that there is a big difference between a sensation and our reaction, between pain and suffering. When we really pay attention to what we are feeling, we start to notice that what we thought was suffering is something else. In his book *Who Dies*, Stephen Levine uses this difference in a very helpful and skillful way for those who are dying or in constant pain. He teaches his clients to really investigate the sensations, to ask themselves to note exactly what they are experiencing. You can ask if the sensation is sharp or dull. Is it burning or cool? Where exactly is it? Does it move around, or does it stay in one place? Does it come and go, or is it constant? Does the size and shape of the affected area change? The more we can notice, the further away we take the sensation from any associated suffering.

As we meditate, we ask the same questions. If our original anchor is the breath, we seek to return to awareness of the breath. However, if a sensation in the body constantly arises that is so powerful that it pulls our awareness away from the breath, we change the object of our concentration and go with that sensation. We watch the sensation with the same curiosity and commitment that we were watching the breath. Curiosity is a wonderful gift to use in meditation. Strive to be as curious and as focused as a cat. What are you actually feeling at this moment?

Drop any ideas of what you *think* you are feeling. Often we allow a memory or some past pain (or pleasure) to replace what is really being felt. Or, without our noticing, a fear that we may begin to feel a new pain replaces, in anticipation, the actual current sensation. We imagine a feeling that hasn't arrived yet. Don't fall for these old tricks of the mind. Notice what is present right now.

Yin Yoga is an excellent time to develop our skill in watching sensations; there will be lots of sensations all over the body. If one becomes predominant, and prevents you from focusing on the breath, go with that predominant sensation. Notice everything, as Levine suggests. Also notice if, along with the physical sensation, emotions have arisen. This is not uncommon when we do any work with the hips. Often emotions such as anger or irritation will arise when we open this area. Be open to this arising.

Not all emotions need to be strong or overwhelming, of course. Most of the time, the emotions are so mild we don't even notice they exist. But, they are there if we look for them. It is rare that we are not experiencing any emotion. The emotion may be contentment or mild joy, unease or mild anxiety. Irritation can arise for a moment. A common emotion, for students just beginning Yin Yoga, is boredom. The mind is used to being stimulated, and rebels at doing nothing.

Fronsdal tells us that there are four aspects to being mindful of emotions:

1. Recognition – we first recognize that an emotion has arisen
2. Naming – once we know an emotion is present, what is it?
3. Acceptance – this is yin-like! Allow the emotion to be present
4. Investigation – drop any judgments about the emotion, and look at it with fresh eyes

Fronsdal then goes on to suggest ways to become mindful of our thoughts. This is a much deeper and more challenging practice.

Mindfulness of the Mind

Our breath is always with us. Sensations are also always present, even if not noticed. So too, emotions are there for the finding, if one chooses to search. Any of these objects can be used as the foundation for mindfulness training. As we progress from watching the breath to sensations to emotions, the challenge grows to stay focused. The sensations come and go, sometimes here, sometimes there. The emotions are ephemeral at times, and are often very difficult to detect and watch. The biggest challenge, however, is to watch our minds.

Many beginning students believe that the purpose of meditation is to stop all thoughts. They have heard the definition of yoga from the Yoga Sutra[184] and believe that meditation too has the goal of ending the whirlings in the mind. And sometimes this may actually happen: the mind may become so calm that fewer and fewer thoughts arise, until there is complete stillness. But this is never a permanent state, so the Buddha said this couldn't be the real goal.

We do not try to stop our thoughts from arising: we do not wrestle with them. As Fronsdal offers, "Mindfulness of thinking is simply recognizing that we are thinking." Certainly when we watch the mind we can become calmer. But this is not the calmness of torpor, a drugging or dulling of the mind. This is an active calmness, the yang within the yin.

When we do more than simply watch each arising thought, we get caught up in it. We struggle with it. The thought creates some emotional response and this is manifested somewhere in the body. This cycle is endless – the mind affecting emotions, emotions affecting the body, the body affecting the breath, and then the breath affecting the mind again. Sometimes the cycle begins with a sensation in the body or an arising emotion. Any arising can in turn create new thoughts. We can interrupt this cycle by not reacting to, or struggling with, the thoughts.

Rosenberg discusses the third tetrad of the Anapanasati sutra[185] in detail in *Breath by Breath*. This is the grouping where we breathe with the mind. He warns us:

> The point is to change our mind from a battlefield, where we're always fighting these (mind) states, or getting lost in them, to a place of peaceful coexistence. Then these visitors, these guests in consciousness, don't have such power.

His prediction on when we succeed: "When that happens, these states start thinning out, falling away."

---

[184] Yoga citta vritti nirodah.
[185] The mind group.

The Buddha told us long ago that it is our attachments that cause our suffering. The way to end attachments is by simply watching them arise. We observe and get to know our cravings. Instead of just instinctually reacting to them, trying to obtain whatever it is we want at that moment, we just let the thoughts or feelings come. Rosenberg says that there is something false about *trying* to let go. Often it is an attempt to push away, which means a struggle is occurring. The practice is not to struggle or push away desire or attachment, but simply to observe it.

Wishing our states of mind don't happen is pointless; it doesn't work to force them away. All our states of mind need to be accepted as part of our consciousness. Let them come, let them blossom, look at them closely and when they go, let them go. Thich Nhat Hanh suggests an even more radical approach. Echoing Jesus, he suggests we learn to love our kilesas.

Whether we meditate while formally sitting for thirty minutes, or use the briefer periods of a Yin Yoga pose, we can always come to the deeper level of mindfulness – watch the mind itself! We have found four acceptable anchors to our mindfulness practice. We can begin by watching the breath, we may choose to watch sensations in the physical body, we may watch emotions arise and flow, or we may choose to watch our minds. There is another effective anchor we can also use. We can simply listen.

Listening

"Yoga begins with listening. When we listen we create space." So states Richard Freeman in his CD set, *The Yoga Matrix*. As an example, when we listen to a good friend, we give her space to be whoever she needs to be in this moment. We don't begin to think of our response or interrupt. We fully listen. We are fully present and aware of her.

Recall that space, akasha, is the most subtle of the five elements in the Samkhya cosmology. And the sense associated with space is listening, which implies that it is the most subtle sense. There exist complete meditative practices that focus solely on listening as the technique; the anchor is sound. With practice, we can learn to discriminate minute details in all the sounds around us. We drop any judgments that this is a nice sound, or an annoying sound. Meditation centers are often very noisy places; there are lots of sounds to work with. Or we can go on retreat to a very quiet part of nature, but even here, there will be lots to hear.

Listening can be done anywhere, and at any time. Like our breath, our ability to listen is always with us. During our Yin Yoga practice we have lots of time, and many chances to practice this form of mindfulness. Settle into your pose, and then listen. Hear the sounds close to you. Notice the sounds far away; notice the brightness, the tone, the pace, and timbre of each sound. Notice your reaction to the sound; do not attempt to stop these reactions. At first you may find you don't like certain types of sounds: the music in the background may seem distracting; the teacher's voice or the breathing of another student close by may get on your nerves. Just notice these emotions, and let them be. Return to simply listening.

When your practice has ended, notice if your ability to really listen stays with you as you prepare for your next activity. Remind yourself to come back to simply listening throughout the day. When we listen, thoughts tend to recede or stop. We naturally pause when we are in input mode. We are open to noticing whatever there is to be noticed. Erich Schiffmann suggests buying a digital watch with a count down timer. Set it to chime every twenty minutes, and each time it chimes, pause – listen – just for a moment, drop whatever activity your mind is engaged in, and come back to this moment with full awareness. Listening is a very quick and effective way to regain this moment.[186]

---

[186] A very nice program you can download onto your computer is a bell that sounds throughout your day, reminding you to come back to the present moment. You can find this program at the Washington Mindfulness Community Web site: http://www.mindfulnessdc.org/mindfulclock.html.

Red Lights and Telephones

Whether we are on a zafu or on a mat, how do we begin our meditation? How do we end the session and take the mindfulness with us? These are practical considerations that are important for transferring the practice of mindfulness into everyday life.

Often teachers will suggest beginning your practice with an intention. One of the highest intentions is that of the *bodhisattva*. The bodhisattva is an enlightened master, a buddha who has forsaken final liberation, choosing instead to remain with us for the benefits of all the other beings who have not yet reached enlightenment. They have four qualities referred to as the *Brahma Vihara*.[187] These are:

1. Loving kindness to all creatures
2. Compassion for all who suffer
3. Sympathetic joy for all who are happy
4. Equanimity, a pervading calm

This grand intention may be a bit over the top for most students. Stephen Batchelor in *Buddhism without Beliefs* offers a more tractable resolve. He suggests our intention include "aspiration, appreciation and conviction." For example, he offers these words to begin our practice:

"I aspire to awaken, I appreciate its value, and I am convinced it is possible."

The resolve to awaken may at first seem a selfish one but all Buddhists assure us that if we awaken, everyone benefits. Sarah Powers has adapted Batchelor's phrasing and uses a similar intention at the beginning of her classes. She will often say,

"I vow to awaken to awareness for the benefit of all beings. I appreciate its immeasurable value and believe it is possible, as I am now, without condition."

---

[187] Similar to the Yoga Sutra's teaching of *maitri*, *karuna*, *mudita* and *upeksanam*.

You may wish to copy this phrase completely or develop words that resonate with your own intentions. A common phrase, short and succinct, is *lokah samasta sukhino bhavantu.* This simple and beautiful chant is a wish for all beings everywhere to be happy.

Once your practice on the mat has ended, the real practice begins, bringing mindfulness to every minute of your day. Of course, we cannot be truly mindful every second, but we can intend to be. Bringing mindfulness to our lives is the subject of many books and teachings. Buddhist teachings in all their forms are very practical and pragmatic. Wonderful authors abound. Taste the teachings of Charlotte Joko Beck with either of her excellent books *Everyday Zen* and *Nothing Special.* Or dip into any of the ninety or more books by Thich Nhat Hanh (also affectionately called Thay) such as *Peace is Every Step.*

Thay has several excellent suggestions for bringing our awareness back to the moment. One practice is the *Telephone Meditation.* When the phone rings, most people's first instinct is to answer it right away; we have some hidden fear that the person on the other end will hang up if we don't answer in the first two rings. Thay points out that the other person really wants to talk to us, so we don't need to rush. First, when the phone rings, we should pause, stop whatever we are doing, and just notice the phone. On the second ring we should think about who the other person is and smile. On the third ring we should think about ourselves talking with this person and again smile. On the fourth ring we move toward the phone. Finally we pick up the phone and say "hello" with a smile.

Another wonderful everyday meditation Thay offers us is the *Red Light Meditation.* He has noticed that many drivers – when they get stopped at a red light – get angry or upset with being delayed. So many people have allowed their lives to become so busy that they resent their time being wasted in traffic. Being slowed down easily irritates them. But that reaction is a choice: we can choose to react another way. Thay suggests we see each red light as an opportunity to do a mini-meditation: we can thank the light for turning red, for giving us a chance to check back in with our life, to notice our breath or sounds, our body or feelings. We can win back another precious taste of this moment, the only time we can actually be alive.

All these techniques of building mindfulness help us in our daily life. The more we practice, the easier it becomes to practice. As noted earlier, the Buddha was not concerned about models and science – he didn't care why the world is the way it is. His concern was to help end suffering now. The yogic models of Samkhya or Tantra didn't concern the Buddha. His advice was always practical and pragmatic.

In the West many brilliant minds have pondered the mind, and have developed a wide array of models and theories about how the mind works and how we can end our suffering. Many of these thinkers have independently rediscovered methods that the Buddha described two and a half millennia ago. Their models also echo the divisions of mind noted by the psychonauts of early yoga. Our journey down the Yin River now takes us toward some of these Western viewpoints of mind. We will learn how these too can assist our practice of yoga.

Chapter Eleven:
The Western View of Mind

To many people in the West, investigating the mind conjures images of lying on a couch, while behind them sits a man looking suspiciously like a Viennese doctor holding a notebook: Herr Doctor Freud's reputation persists as the archetypal psychiatrist. Many are familiar with his early psychological model of the mind – the id, the ego, the superego surrounded by the libido, which thrashes around causing all sorts of suffering. Freud blazed a pioneer's path, but one that we will not journey down. Rather we will follow the path laid by Freud's friend and disciple (at least until their famous falling out), Carl Jung.[188]

There are many possible psychological models of the mind we could investigate that have become popular in the West, just as there are many esoteric models of the mind in the East. Philosophers have looked deeply into the way the mind works for centuries. Rene Descartes developed his famous axiom from these investigations. He hoped to solve the basic existential quandary with the phrase "I think, therefore I am." As we have seen from the Eastern point of view, this axiom is backward. In the East, it is more a case of "I am, therefore I think … now how can I calm down all those thoughts and find out who I am?" Carl Jung's approach to the mind is chosen for illumination due to his efforts to find a bridge between the Eastern and Western views of the psyche.

---

[188] Jung was born in 1875 and died in 1961.

We will begin by looking at the models found in Jungian psychology.[189] After seeing how Jung developed many similar realizations about the mind to those we have seen developed in the East, we will look at a more practical, pragmatic approach for dealing with the mind. This school of mental practice is "Cognitive[190] Behavioral Therapy" or CBT. CBT deals with *how* we think, and how *what* we think affects what we feel and how we act. CBT psychologists would also modify Descartes' axiom: "We are what we think."

The Jungian Model of the Mind

Jung, like all yogis, based his concepts of mind on personal experience: his was not a theoretical model void of any practical reality. Through his own crises and mental breakdown and his long climb back to wholeness, he observed the landscape of the psyche up close and personally.

Simply stated, Jung's model of the psyche has three main parts:

1. the ego, which is the home of our consciousness
2. the personal unconscious into which we stuff everything we have seen and forgotten or would like to deny exists within us
3. the collective unconscious, which we share in common with all human beings and which holds the many archetypes that are symbols of life situations

The ego must exist, according to Jung, for without an "I" to witness, there can be no consciousness. Unlike the Eastern models where the ego presents a false "I" that needs to be shown as a sham or an illusion, to Jung, the ego needs to continue. It is an unavoidable

---

[189] A term Jung himself did not fancy. He believed each patient needed a specialized approach tailored to his or her own unique situation. In this manner he mirrored the yoga teaching philosophy of Krishnamacharya and his son Desikachar.

[190] The word "cognitive" may seem foreboding but basically it means thinking.

part of the psychic landscape, and has as much right to be recognized as the unconsciousness aspects of our psyche.

The personal unconscious is the "matrix of all potentialities." Jung believed the unconscious is able, just like the conscious mind, to think and feel, to have purpose and intention. He described its contents as

> … everything of which I know, but of which I am not at the moment thinking; everything of which I was once conscious but have now forgotten; everything perceived by my senses, but not noted by my conscious mind; everything which, involuntarily and without paying attention to it, I feel, think, remember, want and do…[191]

Jung's recognition of the collective unconscious was a crowning achievement, and one often misunderstood and rejected by other psychologists of the time. The collective unconscious is hereditary, not personal. It is not created by the individual's experiences in this life, but is shared as a repertoire of instincts across every human being. These instincts take the shape of archetypes or images that arise in cultural myths or personal dreams; they are the demons and angels within but reflected or projected outside onto events and people around us. These are the images that the Tibetan Book of the Dead[192] warns will appear in the first few moments after death. Unless we recognize them as simply parts of our own mind and do not fear them, we will panic and rush foolishly into our next cycle of birth and death.

According to Jung, archetypes are only alive when they are meaningful to us. Since the symbols of another culture have little meaning to us, those images do not awaken the archetypes in our Western psyche.[193] Just take note of your dreams, the ones that are

---

[191] Jung: *The Structure and Dynamics of the Psyche* – page 185.
[192] The Bardol Todol.
[193] Hindus and Buddhists in India and the Daoists in China used metaphors based on their culture. Jung was adamant that people in the West should stick to the images of the West in order to understand their own situation. Of what value to a Swiss bricklayer is an image of Shiva dancing on top of a dwarf named Avidya?

most vivid, disturbing, or memorable, to find how your archetypes are clothed.

There is a fourth part of the psyche not mentioned above: the Self. This can be considered just one of the many archetypes Jung introduced us to, but this is the ultimate archetype. It is the organizing principle within each of us that guides us and gives us a direction to follow. In Jung's own words:

> It might equally well be called the "God within us." The beginning of our whole psychic life seems to be inextricably rooted in this point, and all our highest and ultimate purposes seem to be striving toward it.[194]

Jung's description of the Self sounds distinctly Eastern. He claims it is both unitemporal and unique, just as the yogis described purusha. The Self is universal and eternal, just as the Tantrikas believe. It expresses both our human image and god's image.

With this model in mind, let's turn to look at what Jung wanted us to achieve through his work.

The Goal of Jungian Psychotherapy

The goal of the spiritual practice of yoga is liberation from the cycles of birth and death. The goal of the Buddha's meditation is to end suffering. The goal of Jung's psychotherapy is "individuation," which means the integration of our unconsciousness with our consciousness, allowing the Self to arise.

Jung was unique in the West. He not only sought to end the suffering of his patients from their illness, he also wanted to help healthy people realize their full potential. His therapy was not limited to those afflicted, as were all the other psychotherapies of the day. Like his ancient Eastern counterparts, he wanted to cure his patient's present problems and make them strong enough to face the real existential problem – he wanted them to become whole.

---

[194] Jung: *Two Essays on Analytical Psychology*, page 67.

The Self, according to Jung, is the source in the beginning – and this same Self is the goal in the end. Between these, there is unfolding a continual development, an integration of the personality. That is the process of individuation. This transformation occurs through the interaction of the ego and the unconscious.

Around the middle of his life Jung was introduced to the teachings of Daoist alchemy through his friend Richard Wilhelm and Wilhelm's translation of the book The Secret of the Golden Flower. Jung realized that alchemy was a metaphoric approach to the transformation he was seeking. The alchemists, in trying to transmute base elements into gold or silver, were really attempting to liberate God from the dark matter of the universe. To Jung, this was the whole psychic process of liberating our Self from the dark matter of our unconsciousness.[195] Many spiritual teachers, throughout the ages, have sought this same goal.

The Tibetan Buddhists believe that we can become liberated only if we shine a light on our inner darkness, so that, at the moment of death, the darkness' metaphoric apparition does not overcome us. Jesus, in the Gospel of Saint Thomas, preached, "If you bring forth what is within you, what you bring forth will save you. If you do not bring forth what is within you, what you do not bring forth will destroy you." These teachings are the same as Jung's exhortations to achieve individuation: the fractures within us must be healed and a new being will emerge…the original being, the Self.

How to achieve individuation is the next understanding we need to gain.

Individuation

Just as a sick person, weakened by illness, cannot perform advanced yoga or meditation, neither can the person with a fractured personality achieve enlightenment. Integration of the whole person is required. Georg Feuerstein says this in another way, "enlightenment

---

[195] Yoga itself is an alchemical process … see Tim Miller's article using this metaphor in his *The Alchemy of Yoga* at
www.ashtangayogacenter.com/alchemy.html.

is no substitution for integration of the personality." The history of yoga is full of highly advanced gurus who mastered many esoteric practices but did not heal their own psychic schisms. Their deep imperfections caused great pain and suffering to their disciples and followers.

Individuation is possible only when consciousness heeds the unconscious. The opposites within us must meet in order to complement each other. Isn't this exactly what we mean when we name our yoga "Ha" and "Tha" yoga? The opposites of sun and moon, the opposites of yin and yang, the opposites of light and darkness need to come together, to be unified or yoked.

Radmila Moacanin tells us, in her book *The Essence of Jung's Psychology and Tibetan Buddhism*:

> Jung postulates that on a psychological level the union of
> opposites cannot be achieved by the conscious ego alone – by
> reason, analysis – which separates and divides; nor even by the
> unconscious alone – which unites; it needs a third element, the
> transcendent function.

With this observation, Jung denies the claims of the Samhkya yogis: viveka is not sufficient for achieving liberation. We must go beyond reason or understanding. We must go way beyond dualism and follow the teaching of the Tantras. We seek wholeness.

In 1916 Jung wrote a book on this topic, which he called *The Transcendent Function*. The function, the task, is transcendent because we need to go beyond both the rational and the irrational. We need to bring them both together and this can be done only from outside both.

Jung used two main methods to help his patients:

1. dream interpretation
2. active imaging

Interpreting dreams is an ancient practice. The Bible praised Joseph's skills when he interpreted his Pharaoh's many dreams. It is also a modern practice, employed by Freud as well as many others before and after Jung. Dream Yoga has also been popular in the last century. Swami Sivananda Radha wrote a book on this topic called *Realities of the Dreaming Mind: The Practice of Dream Yoga.* In Jung's hands, dreams were deconstructed into the archetypes of the personal and collective unconscious. He brought their stories to light.[196] But this is only viveka; this is understanding the message. More than understanding is needed. To truly change, action is needed.

Active imagination is one of Jung's original and unique contributions to Western psychotherapy. He uses the alchemist's approach to transform the psyche, to reconcile the opposites deep within us. He begins the process with calming the mind. Moacanin describes the task as being very similar to basic meditation.

> ... to induce a calm state of mind, free from thoughts, and merely to observe in a neutral way, without judgment, just to behold the spontaneous emergence and unfoldment of unconscious content, fragments of fantasy...[197]

This is no different than what we have been asked to do in our Yin Yoga practice during the periods of meditative holding of the poses. This is the teaching of the Buddha, to simply watch what is arising without judgment. Jung suggests we record in some way the symbols that arise during this meditation: record them in writing or by drawing them or by dancing them. Give them a life of their own.

Now that suggestion is new.

This next stage of active imagination brings the conscious mind to the activity: let it join the dance. Both the unconscious and conscious become active together. If the therapy, if the practice is successful, the patient, the student, is now able to live her life consciously. No longer is she subjected to the confusing, hidden urges of the unconscious mind that drives her actions without her conscious awareness or cooperation.

Active imagination has many similarities to the practices of cognitive behavioral therapy (CBT), which we will look at more

---

[196] See his collection of writings in the book *Dreams*, translated by R.F.C. Hull.

[197] *The Essence of Jung's Psychology and Tibetan Buddhism* by Radmila Moacanin

closely later. In all these practices, the objective is the same: to use the mind to program the mind. We use our conscious mind to affect the unconscious mind and change the patterns of our behavior, our deep samskaras.

Jung Meets the Buddha

The Western approach to studying the mind is empirical; our science is based upon observations that are verifiable. The Eastern approaches are metaphysical but the Buddha insisted his followers observe for themselves everything he taught. Buddhism is also completely empirical. Yoga too requires the student to see for herself – follow your guides but take nothing for granted; check it out personally.

Everything that works is real.

Do you doubt your own experiences? Don't. Reality is there within what you are seeing, experiencing. But we can get fooled; that is why we need the guides. They help us look behind the disguises; they help us interpret the symbols. But again and again, they will warn us that we are the ones who must do the looking.

There are numerous similarities between Jung's psychological methods to achieve individuation and those of the Buddhist traditions. Active imagination has its counterpart in the Tantra practice of yantra. Yantras are symbols that are concentrated upon until the energies of the unconscious are released into conscious awareness. Jung's desire to understand the meaning of the unconscious symbols is the same desire to discern the real (*sat*) from the unreal (*asat*). This is the goal of an ancient mantra:

> *Om asatoma sat gamaya*
> *Tamasoma jyotir gamaya*
> *Mrithyor ma amritam gamaya*

Lead us from the unreal to the real
Lead us from the darkness to the light
Lead us from the fear of death to immortality

The Buddha and other Eastern teachers taught a radical transformation of consciousness. Jung taught us how to sacrifice our ego in order to allow the emergence of our Self (the God within). Both approaches require a guide; there are dragons at every turn along this path. Even though these dragons are symbols of our own inner darkness, they are dangerous creatures nonetheless. They can devour the unprepared and cause grave psychic and even physical harm. The practice of deep meditation, advanced yoga, or individuation is not to be done alone.

There are differences as well between Jung's approach and the Eastern ways. Jung absolutely requires the ego to maintain its existence. We do not transcend the ego – we incorporate the ego; the ego simply becomes subordinate to the Self. The ultimate goal for Jung is not total consciousness with an absence of problems or strife. With each new level of consciousness achieved comes a new burden. The process of individuation is never complete. Remember Jung is an empiricist; he deals only with what can be known, and this prevents him from entering the realm of metaphysics. We cannot bring to consciousness everything that is unconscious; we can only work toward that goal.

For the Buddha, everything that needs to be known can be known and liberation can be achieved. With liberation comes bliss and an end to suffering. Tantric Buddhists believe this liberation is achievable in one lifetime. Ananda (bliss) can be found right here, right now. Jung, by contrast, did not believe complete individuation, attaining complete wholeness, is possible.

But one thing Jung and the teachers in the East would agree upon. Jung complained, "...still too few look inward ..."[198] Today there are many people suffering psychic pains who are advised to seek solace in drugs. Taking an antidepressant, or even stronger drugs, is a lot easier than svadhyaya, looking inward. And for some this may be helpful, but there are many who have turned inward – many of these people are using the modern tools of *cognitive behavioral therapy* to help them cope with the challenges in their lives.

---

[198] Jung: *Two Essays on Analytical Psychology*, page 5.

Cognitive Behavioral Therapy

Understanding our dreams or understanding our habitual behavior can certainly help us understand why we face challenges in our lives but this knowledge alone will not help us deal with the challenges. If our hope is to change the way we are feeling, to end our suffering, we need other tools to assist us in changing our habitual patterns.

The eightfold path that the Buddha described twenty-five hundred years ago proclaimed we needed to do things right: right thinking, right speaking, right actions … Conversely, what can make life more difficult is wrong thinking, wrong speaking, wrong actions … Correcting these wrong habits is where the tools of CBT are very useful.

CBT is a merger of two distinct therapies. At his Web site,[199] Dr. John Bush explains the two precursors to CBT.

> Behavior therapy helps you weaken the *connections* between troublesome situations and your habitual reactions to them. Reactions such as fear, depression or rage, and self-defeating or self-damaging behavior. It also teaches you how to calm your mind and body, so you can feel better, think more clearly, and make better decisions.

> Cognitive therapy teaches you how certain *thinking patterns* are causing your symptoms – by giving you a distorted picture of what's going on in your life, and making you feel anxious, depressed or angry for no good reason, or provoking you into ill-chosen actions.

Together these two therapies form a powerful, clinically proven approach to achieving a more satisfying life. CBT is very different from psychoanalysis, which can take years of work, and has, in Dr. Bush's words "not much science behind it." Even the early client-centered therapies of pioneers, such as Rogers, were based on the

---

[199] www.cognitivetherapy.com. If that is not working, try http://suicideand mentalhealthassociationinternational.org/cognitivether.html

personal intuition of the therapist. The clinically proven benefits of CBT have caused it to become the preferred approach to dealing with emotional and behavioral problems.

Behavior Therapy

Bush lists the three main approaches of Behavior Therapy, which appeared in the 1950s. These are:

1. Desensitization
2. Behavior modification
3. Behavior activation

Desensitization seeks to reduce the troublesome emotions by allowing these emotions to arise while in a relaxed state. Behavior modification aims to replace undesirable behaviors with desirable ones. It requires knowing the cues that we use to initiate behavior, interrupting these cues, and replacing them with more appropriate behaviors. The final approach aims to pull the client out of her depressed state by restoring everyday habits or pleasurable activities that may have been lost or forgotten.[200]

---

[200] Another school of behavioral modification is called Neuro-Linguistic Programming or NLP. NLP became prominent in the 1970s and '80s through the work of Richard Bandler and John Grinder. They modeled brilliant therapists, such as Milton Erickson and Virginia Satir, and distilled from these experts the essential tools they used to help their clients. While NLP has grown in popularity through the years, its teachings spread most widely through the work of Anthony Robbins and his first book, *Unlimited Power*. Robbins, however, did not use the name NLP for the procedures he adopted from Bandler and Grinder, much to their annoyance. For insight into their approach, the reader may want to read their initial book *Frogs into Princes* or visit Robert Dilts' NLP University at www.nlpu.com.

Cognitive Therapy

Cognitive, or thinking therapy, arose in the 1960s. Dr. Bush describes two main approaches:

1. Rational Emotive Therapy (RET)
2. Dr. Aaron Beck's Cognitive Therapy

RET simply wants us to act or think more rationally. The work is to identify our irrational thoughts as they arise and lead to problems, and correct them. Dr. Beck's cognitive therapy has the same goal as RET. He began to identify many different types of cognitive errors, and developed many ways to correct these thought patterns.[201]

An example of a cognitive problem could be – someone cuts you off in traffic; the thought arises in your mind that that person hates you. From this faulty thought, you begin to have thoughts about how many people in your life don't like you. You become depressed. This depression has no reality behind it. You don't know why the person cut you off ... most likely it was because she was not paying attention. If you change your thoughts to how the other driver may have been having a bad hair day and was easily distracted, your chain of reasoning would lead you to a completely different conclusion. Rather than being depressed, you may instead send a wish to the other driver; you may wish for her to calm down, put on a hat, and enjoy her day in peace and safety.

CBT begins with the premise that outside events and other people are not what cause us problems; what causes all our problems is the way we react or think about these outside situations. It is the way we respond that makes all the difference in our life. This is akin to the Buddha's statement that life contains pain, but our suffering is optional. Once we recognize our response, we work to change it.

---

[201] Dr. Beck is considered the father of CBT and has written many books on the topic. *Cognitive Therapy and the Emotional Disorders* is an excellent introduction to the subject. Dr. Beck works today with his daughter Judith, expanding our understanding of cognitive centered therapies. More information can be found at www.beckinstitute.org.

And it is work! This is not easy, but if the student or client is determined to change suffering into joy, the work will bear fruit.

Newer Approaches

Dr. Bush describes more recent advancements in this whole field that come very close to what we have been investigating in Eastern metaphysics. These approaches, which arose in the 1990s, include

1. Mindfulness Meditation
2. Acceptance and Commitment therapy

The typical goal of these approaches is to become less affected by our thoughts, by any sensations or events, or by our mental fantasies and imaginings. Included in the second approach is a holding true to our personal values in all we do and think. The methods are very similar to meditation techniques, which we will investigate in the section Meditation on Energy.

The typical approach to cognitive behavior therapy includes observing and changing the way we react to situations, our thoughts about these situations, and the emotions that arise. One powerful tool to use to do this is "recording thoughts."

Recording Thoughts

We have seen earlier that thoughts affect our emotions, which in turn can affect us physically, which in turn can affect our thoughts. Our physical, emotional, and mental bodies are completely interconnected; doing something to one kosha affects all the others. We can call the process "connecting the dots." If we can interrupt these connections, we can stop the avalanche of thoughts, emotions, and physical feelings from continuing their destructive cycle.

A very valuable tool offered in CBT is the "Thought Record." The book by Edmund Bourne, *The Anxiety and Phobia Workbook*, and the book *Mind Over Mood* by Dennis Greenberger and Christine Padesky both have a series of tables that can be used to record thoughts, and help change the way thoughts affect our emotional state. The thought record assumes that the cause of our emotional unbalance, or any suffering we are experiencing, is preceded by thoughts that unconsciously and automatically arise when certain situations occur. If we can detect this flow, and interrupt it or substitute different conclusions, we can change the emotions or the suffering we are experiencing.

To make a thought record, create a table with the following seven headings across the top of the page, beginning with:

Situational Analysis

The first step in compiling a thought record is to note a situation you were in when an upsetting emotion or suffering occurred. Note whom you were with, what you were doing, where you were, when this happened ... be as detailed at possible. Write it all down in point form.

Mood Analysis

The second step is to describe the moods you were feeling in that situation. Use one-word labels such as sad, mad, glad, anxious, impatient ... then quantify the intensity of the mood in percentages. Really intense moods might be rated eighty or ninety percent. Weak moods might deserve ratings of only ten or twenty percent.

Automatic Thought Analysis

The third step is a bit more challenging, but can be fun. Ask yourself what was going through your mind when the situation arose, before you started to feel the moods. What thoughts came unbidden? Then ask yourself, "What do these thoughts mean about who I am?" What do these thoughts imply about your future? What is the worst thing that could happen because of this situation? How would this make other people think about you? What specific images arose in your mind at this time? Write these down. Circle or highlight the thoughts that seem to be the most powerful ones. These are called "hot thoughts."

Evidence that Supports the Hot Thoughts

List any evidence you can think of that would prove the hot thoughts to be true. Be factual here ... don't mind read, or assume you know what other people are thinking.

Evidence that Does Not Support the Hot Thoughts

Now, search for reasons why these thoughts are perhaps mistaken. This is a critical part of the process. Take each thought one at a time. Mull them over slowly: don't rush this. Ask yourself, "Are there other reasons why this situation could have occurred?" Consider what you would say to a friend who sought your advice, what evidence you would offer her for why these hot thoughts are wrong. Think of past times when you knew the hot thought was wrong. Think of as many reasons as possible why these thoughts are not true. Write these down.

Alternative Thoughts

Since you have many reasons why the hot thoughts may be wrong, come up with some more appropriate thoughts or conclusions that you *could have* reached in this situation. Look for balance. At the end of each alternative thought, rate how strongly you believe this thought to be true by assigning a percentage to it. A very believable thought may rate a ninety or one hundred percent.

Moods Revisited

After doing all this work, pause for a moment, and look again at the moods you listed earlier; rerate their intensities. How strong are they now? [202]

---

[202] Further information on creating thought records can be found at Advances in Psychiatric Treatment: Identifying and Changing Unhelpful Thinking at http://apt.rcpsych.org/cgi/content/full/8/5/377?eaf.

The thought record not only shines a light on the cause of our suffering, just as psychoanalysis or viveka does, but it also unhooks the causes from our reactions. By looking at how irrational our reactions are, and by accepting new thoughts, we can completely change the way the dots are connected. We can change the suffering we experience even though the pain, or the situation, is unchanged.

Yoga and CBT

What is happening to us is often outside our control; changing our *reaction* to what is happening to us – is controllable. The key to this is awareness. This is same intention that advanced yoga students have for their yoga practice. They want to become keenly aware of their experience. They don't want to just notice the physical feelings they are having – they want to also notice the thoughts these feelings are creating, and the resulting moods. Once they can see how the physical is connected to the mental and the mental to the emotional, they are ready to alter these connections.

Holding a Yin Yoga pose for three or five minutes gives us time to really look deep and see what is happening. We start to see these connections forming. We become keenly aware of emotions like irritation, anger, fear, or even boredom, surfacing. We can start to trace these emotions back to certain thoughts and sensations. We can then choose, if we like, to change the way we are reacting. We can choose to awaken ... or to A.W.A.K.E.N.

A.W.A.K.E.N.

We call yoga a practice for a reason. Practice prepares us for the real work ... the work of living our life. Practice consists of rehearsing, over and over, the actions and reactions we want to master, so that, when the time comes, we are ready to perform skillfully. Yoga practice builds awareness, which leads to choice. When we practice coming face to face with challenging moments, we learn how to slow down, and notice what is really going on. We learn how to decide the right way to act or react. We awaken to all the possibilities that exist in that moment, rather then default to one habitual, and perhaps inappropriate, action.

This awakening can be achieved through a six-step program combining both yin and yang elements. In cognitive behavioral therapy a similar program is offered to help people cope with anxieties, phobias, and debilitating fears. There are fears that help us to live, and there are fears that stop us from living. These fears may be consciously recognized, or they may live deep inside us, directing our behavior and reactions without our conscious awareness. All these anxieties are stimulated by situations or thoughts, real or imagined. When faced with a challenge, our unconscious mind often sends us subliminal directives (activated by the samskaras). When we deliberately create challenges, such as during our yoga or meditation practices, we get a chance to rewire the unconscious mind, to reprogram new and more appropriate responses. We can undo the karmic defaults we live under.[203]

The six-step program that helps us conquer our fears and anxieties,[204] and awaken to the moment, is called A.W.A.K.E.N. Each letter represents one stage of the program:

1. **Allow**
2. **Watch**
3. **Act**
4. **Keep at it**
5. **Expect the best**
6. **Now**

When these steps are followed, over and over again, they become a healthy, healing habit. Once the habit is established, the fears we experience are reduced to only those that are appropriate for the situation we are in. To make these six steps into a habit, do them during your yoga practice or at any time you recognize unease creeping into your body, mind, or heart.

---

[203] Thich Nhat Hanh would call these samskaras "weeds," which we tend to water mindlessly. We water weeds when we could be watering beautiful flowers.

[204] These would be called "*dukha*" in the Yoga Sutra.

Allow

Allow: this is the yin practice of acceptance – allowing things to be as they are in this moment. In our Western culture, the drive is to change the world. At a very early age we are exhorted to be active, to do something, to make something of ourselves. We are told to go out and change the world. This is the essence of yang – all our heroes and role models are yangsters.

And there is nothing wrong with being a yangster! There are certainly times in life when the most appropriate thing to do is to take action. As we already discussed, if we see a child being beaten, we take action to change that. But if we are constantly in yang mode, we will soon burn out. Stress without rest is not balanced living. We need, at times, to just let the world be the way it is.

In reality there are actually very few times we can change the world or change the situation we are in. Our ego would like to believe we can always do something, but this is simply not true. There are many times when the appropriate action is inaction, because there is nothing we can do, except perhaps make things worse.

Allowing things to be as they are is an important skill to learn. This is not one that is prized or taught in our culture. Maybe for one or two weeks of the year, we are told to take a vacation, to take a break and rest. But then we fill those two weeks with all sorts of yang activities, and we get no closer to really balancing our inner and outer worlds. Two weeks, of course, is hardly enough to balance fifty weeks of feverish living. We need to learn to allow every day. Practicing Yin Yoga is an excellent time to learn to allow, to accept, what is happening without reacting or trying to change the world.

King Canute was famous for trying to change the world. He tried to stop the tide from coming in. He failed, of course, and as a consequence got all wet.[205]

---

[205] By the way, the mythical king knew what he was doing. He was proving a point to his flatterers and attendants. They were the ones saying that he was so great and powerful that he could command the very oceans of the world. To teach them a lesson he ordered his chair to be placed in the path of the oncoming waters. The rest is mythic history.

Practice allowing; begin with your breath ... allow it to be whatever it wants to be. This is not easy! Once our ego becomes aware of the breath it thinks it can do a better job and tries to control it. But practice ... allow the breath to just be.

When a fear sneaks upon you ... allow it in! Welcome it, as King Canute welcomed the water. The ego is the attendant flattering you with false praise. Ego is whispering in your ear, "Push the fear down! Keep it hidden ... just command it and it will go away!" Show the ego that you don't have to fight the fear. Resisting fear is fruitless – let it come, just as we allow the waves to come ashore. [206]

When we learn to allow what is happening we take power away from whatever is happening. This is a principle of martial arts practice: do not resist. When we resist what is happening, we weaken ourselves and give power to that which we resist, making it stronger. According to Jung, "What we resist, persists." Instead ... practice allowing.

Watch

Once we have allowed the world to be the way it already is,[207] our next practice is to observe it – simply watch. Watching does not have to be done with the eyes: listen: feel. Observe what is happening in any way you can – but really notice what is happening.

So often we assume we know what is going on; we don't really, but we think we do. We note quickly what is happening, think we have it all figured out, and then move our attention somewhere else.

---

[206] Jung noticed that there exists a frightening part of our psyche that he called "the shadow." The shadow is formed by resistance: everything that we deny about ourselves we throw into a dark bag we carry behind us. But what we resist doesn't go away or become weaker: it hides and grows stronger. The shadow is very scary. We will do anything to avoid facing it; including projecting its attributes onto others and blaming them for the very weaknesses we deny exist in ourselves. It is unfortunate when a person projects his shadow onto another person. It is catastrophic when a country projects its shadow onto another country: war is often the result. This is the price of not allowing.

[207] And that includes allowing ourselves to be the way we already are.

Really watching is hard work. It requires a commitment to remain present and really look at what is going on.

Cultivate a sense of curiosity. Imagine you are a cat waiting by a mouse hole. Don't let your attention waiver for even one second. Watch for the mouse. When a mouse appears, because we are yogi cats and vegetarians, we let the mouse go and wait for the next one.

When we really watch what is happening, we start to notice things we never saw before. In your Yin Yoga practice, begin to pay more attention to the sensations you are experiencing. Where exactly is the sensation? Ask yourself questions. Is it moving or constant? Does it come and go? Provide one- or two-word labels for the sensations. Is it hot or cool? Is it dull, or achy, or sharp, or piercing? The more you watch closely, the more you will see – the better you will be able to describe exactly what you are experiencing. The more you watch, the more you will notice that you really didn't know what was happening at all! You have been living your life blind.

Watching by listening can be a complete meditation all on its own. Many monks prefer this mode of meditating; they become quite accomplished at detecting very subtle nuances of noises. You may choose to do this as part of your practice as well. As you hold a yoga pose, or sit in meditation, allow the sounds around you to come to you. This too is the essence of yin. There is no need to chase after the sounds – they come to you. There is no need to do anything about them. You don't have to judge them as nice or irritating: all you do is allow them to come and listen to them. You become a yinster.

When fears, or anxieties, or other challenges in life present themselves to you, allow them to come and watch them as you have practiced. Notice what exactly the challenge or fear or anxiety consists of. Don't judge it as good or bad. Just notice what is happening. The more information we have about a situation, the more skillfully we can make choices. Then the time may come to take an action, if that is appropriate.

Act

Look again at the yin and yang symbol. See that white yang dot in the middle of the dark yin portion? There is no way to completely separate yin and yang. They are both present in every situation. Even in this six-step process of dealing with life, by allowing and watching events to unfold, there is a 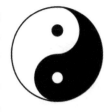 need for yang energy. Taking action is also present. This is not, however, the normal action of doing for the sake of doing; this is the action that arises naturally from the previous stages of allowing/accepting and watching.

In Daoism the term "*wu-wei*" literally means "without action." It contains this paradox of action without action. This is often seen in the masters of the martial arts; with a minimum of action they achieve everything. This is a fundamental tenet of Daoist teachings: water is the most yielding of all elements and yet the most powerful. Gentle rains can wear a mountain to the ground.

In our practice we also act without acting. When fears or anxieties root us, make us unable to do anything, we act, we do what we must do. Despite the fear, despite the challenges facing us, despite our ego's cries, we act. Because we have allowed the world to be the way it is, because we have accepted what is, and because we have watched and observed what is really going on, our action becomes skillful.

This sounds very reasonable but it is not very common. As we have seen earlier, normally we do one of three things when we are faced with challenges in our lives. Many people, when they are outside their comfort zone, will try to change the world. They will struggle to make the world become the way they want the world to be. Other people will recognize that they cannot change the world and instead will run away from it. They will figuratively hide under their beds and hope the challenges looking for them will pass them by. The world changers and the ostriches soon find out that these strategies don't work very well. They may then join the third group of people, the people who simply give up. In a sullen, self-pitying funk, they submit to the pains of life and take every opportunity to let everyone around them know just how unfair life is.

Changing the world or running away from it are yang reactions that don't work. Giving up is a yin reaction that also doesn't work. Allowing, watching, and acting is a yin/yang way to meet life that does work.

For example, in the winter the weather becomes cold. If we were driven by our yang impulses we would try to change the weather or we would run away from the weather by moving to a warmer climate. Other people may stay put but they will complain bitterly about the fact that no one seems to be doing anything about this awful weather. The skillful way to deal with this unchangeable challenge is to allow the weather to be what it is, to watch how we feel because of this weather, and then to take appropriate action – to dress more warmly.

For people afflicted by phobias the same approach works: when facing a challenge that has taken you outside your comfort zone, allow the waves of fear to flow over you. Accept these feelings without judgment. Then watch; pay attention to what is really going on. Don't imagine what is happening or try to color it in any way, just notice what is. Then take the action that your fear doesn't want you to take – live your life – act skillfully, but do act.

When we practice yin yoga or yang yoga, we do the same things. We move outside our normal comfort zone; we allow the postures to flow around us, through us. We watch and notice the sensations arising, ebbing, and flowing. And, when appropriate, we take action, perhaps coming out of the pose if we have gone too deep or going deeper if the body mind has opened to that possibility.

Allow, watch, and act ... that is basically the process – except we can't just do it once.

Keep At It

Tapas is dedication, the sticking to your practice, as described in the Yoga Sutra. It is the first step of Kriya Yoga. It is the third of the niyamas. One of the earliest definitions of the word yoga was discipline. It is tapas, or

June 2006	June ▼	2006 ▼				
Sun	Mon	Tue	Wed	Thu	Fri	Sat
28	29	30	31	1	2	3
4	5	6	7	8	9	10
11	12	13	14	15	16	17
18	19	20	21	22	23	24
25	26	27	28	29	30	1
2	3	4	5	6	7	8

discipline, that we need now. Once we have learned how to allow the world to be the way it is, once we have learned how to watch all the sensations flowing through our minds, hearts, and bodies, once we have learned to take appropriate action, we need to keep doing this. Over and over again, we build a habit. A habit of allowing, watching, and acting.

Habits are built through repetition; if you can repeat an action every day for twenty-one days, it will become a habit. If you can practice your yoga every day for three weeks, it will be difficult for you to stop doing yoga. If you can practice allowing, watching, and acting for three weeks, it will be difficult to stop allowing, watching, and acting.

Twenty-one days is not a long time!

Each cycle of allowing, watching, and acting takes very little time. Each succeeding cycle will take less effort as well. The more we practice, the easier the practice becomes. But, it does take effort, especially in the beginning. Establishing any new behavioral habit takes effort.

Expect the Best

The Yoga Sutra warns that there are nine obstacles (the antaraya) on our path. The third of these obstacles is called "samshaya." The Buddha also warned of five hindrances, called the "kilesas." The fifth of these hindrances is the same as samshaya; it is doubt. Doubt can cause all your efforts to be in vain.

The cure for doubt is shraddha or faith. Faith is the basis for every religion and every spiritual practice. If one has no faith, all sacrifice is in vain, all effort is wasted. Faith is found in every aspect of your daily life. We have faith when we go to bed at night that we will awaken in the morning. We have faith that when we go to work in the morning, our business will still be there. We have faith that when we are hungry, food will be available. These seem obvious, but … what if this faith was lacking? If you were worried about not waking up tomorrow morning, your effort to sleep would be drastically affected. If you doubted that food would be available for your next meal, all your attention during the day would be focused on that concern.

Faith is not always rewarded. There are times when things don't work out the way we expected, but, considering how often faith is rewarded, those few times are the exceptions that prove the rule. Faith allows us to function skillfully; faith leads toward the world we desire.

When we work to A.W.A.K.E.N., we do so with the faith that it will succeed. We can increase this faith through visualizations and affirmations. During your next meditation create a picture, sitting across from you, of your older self. Picture the "you" that you will be in five years from now. Notice how good you look, notice how strong and healthy you appear … notice that glow of wellness all around you. Notice too how happy you will be in the future, how calm and wise you will be. Notice all the other attributes you wish you had today, but think you are lacking.

Your future self has all those attributes – notice them. Don't just see them in your mind's eye but feel them; hear them too. When you have a complete picture of your future self, including sounds and feelings, allow your future self to approach you, bless you, and teach you. Hear your future self tell you that all will be as you expect it to be. Feel yourself give you a big, tight hug … and merge into you. You are already that future self; within you, right now, are the seeds of all these future attributes. Sense these seeds deep inside, already beginning to germinate. Know that, within a few years, these seed will have grown.

Now!

There is no time like the present. We have all heard this saying before, but we miss what it is really saying. Another catchy phrase helps explain this more clearly:

The past is just a memory,
The future is just a fantasy,
This moment is a gift … that is why it is called the present!

Live in this moment. If you need help read *The Power of Now* by Eckhard Tolle or visit his Web site.[208] This moment is the only time you can actually live your life. The future doesn't exist, the past also doesn't exist; the only moment that has ever existed is this moment, the eternal now.

In the gospel of Saint Thomas, Jesus was asked when the kingdom of heaven would arrive. Jesus responded that "the kingdom of heaven is spread out over the earth but men do not see it." People often confuse infinity and eternity. Eternal life means to live in this moment because this moment, now, is eternal.

A similar sentiment was echoed by a Zen master who said, "This world with all its squalor, poverty and pain, this *is* the golden Buddha realm." Do not wait for some time in the future to be happy, to be present, to be awake. It is all here right now, waiting to be recognized.

Allow, watch, act, and keep repeating these steps while expecting the best to happen. But do all this right now. Make A.W.A.K.E.N. into a habit, and you will awaken to this moment.

Do it now!

Our exploration of our deeper koshas has reached an end. We have seen that the earliest explorations of this mysterious realm of the mind envisioned our consciousness (purusha) as very distinct and separate from the rest of the universe (prakriti). The Samkhya and Classical Yoga schools believed that the process of liberation required us to rescue our consciousness from its prison inside of nature. However, the later school of Tantra Yoga felt that consciousness and nature were simply two sides of the same coin and could not, and

---

[208] At www.eckharttolle.com.

should not, be separated. Through practice, liberation could be achieved right now, in this very lifetime.

The Buddha shared the same realization and described a path to achieve this liberation in the here and the now. The practices that the Buddha gave us have been rediscovered and applied in some of the Western practices of psychotherapy; again we have seen the Eastern realizations mirrored in Western thought.

The first part of our journey down the Yin River has come to an end. We leave behind the waters that have illuminated for us the various models of our body mind: ancient and modern, Eastern and Western. We take with us the knowledge of why Yin Yoga is so valuable for us, and the realization that we can come back and revisit these streams of learning at any time. For now, we float on to the second half of our journey. It is time to learn the actual practice of Yin Yoga.

Part Two – Practice
Chapter Twelve:
The Practice of Yin Yoga

The Hatha Yoga Pradipika tells us

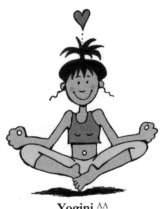

Yogini [AA]

Success comes to him who is engaged in the practice. How can one get success without practice; for by merely reading books on yoga, one can never get success.[209]

Swami Swatmarama, the fourteenth-century sage who wrote the Hatha Yoga Pradipika[210] might well add today "or by reading a Web page." Still, for many people, a book or a Web page may be their only means to learn a yoga practice, and so our journey down the Yin River reveals to us some guidance for the practice of Yin Yoga.

---

[209] Hatha Yoga Pradipika, I-67.
[210] Which means "Light on Yoga."

Please Note! Before embarking on this practice please make sure you are able to do so. Check with your doctor or health care professional before starting any yoga practice. The guidance given in this book is not meant to replace medical advice, and should be used only as a supplement if you are under the care of a health care professional. While care has been taken in compiling the guidance, we cannot take any responsibility for any adverse effects from your practice of yoga. When you are not sure of any aspect of the practice or feel unwell, seek medical advice. For more information on precautions before practicing yoga please check the Before You Practice section.

We will begin by looking at *how* to practice Yin Yoga, and then proceed to describe the postures (also called "asanas" or poses) most commonly used in the practice. There are not nearly as many asanas required in the yin style of yoga as are found in the more active practices. There are perhaps three dozen postures at most (excluding variations). The yin areas of the body generally targeted in the practice are between the knees and navel, the lower body. Since the poses are held longer, there are fewer poses that one can even attempt in one session, compared to the yang styles of yoga where one pose may be held for as little as five breaths. We will discover the most common poses and see them in detail, including their variations, options, and some contraindications.[211]

After viewing the most common asanas we will discover several flows; a flow is simply a linking together of asanas in a logical sequence. These flows have been created with a central theme or purpose in mind. Just as the asanas presented will not exhaust the

---

[211] Contraindications are indications of when not to attempt a specific pose.

possible poses one can do in Yin Yoga, the flows will be even less exhaustive.[212]

The last section on practice will concern the moving of energy. Suggestions will be offered on various movements, breathing patterns, and meditations designed to affect and stimulate the flow of energy (Chi or prana) in the body.

Finally, as Swami Swatmarama warns us,

Success cannot be attained by adopting a particular dress. It cannot be gained by telling tales. Practice alone is the means to success. This is true, there is no doubt. [213]

The Swami must have been looking ahead 600 years and saw the modern desire for matching yoga outfits and coordinated colored mats. How one looks is certainly not the key to success. Said another way, this time by Pattabhi Jois,

Practice! All is coming…

---

[212] In the www.YinYoga.com Kula Web page other teachers and students will be offering their own favorite poses and flows – you may wish to check there for more on these topics. Or you can add your favorite ones.
[213] Ibid, I-68.

How to Practice Yin Yoga

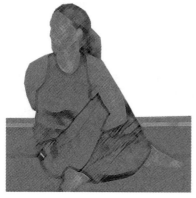

Having seated (himself) in ... a room and free from all anxieties, (the student) should practice yoga, as instructed by his guru.[214]

Straightforward advice. What type of room, you may wonder? Well the room is easy to come by. Simply find for yourself

... a small room of four cubits square, free from stones, fire, water and disturbances of all kinds, and in a country where justice is properly administrated, where good people live and food can be obtained easily and plentifully... The room should have a small door, be free from holes, hollows, neither too high nor too low, well plastered with cow-dung and free from dirt, filth and insects.[215]

Well, finding a place like this can't be too difficult, can it? Cow dung is plentiful and probably available at your local Safeway. Justice is universal today. That is all easy ... but what the heck is a cubit?[216]

The above teaching shows us that advice given in ages past may not be the best advice for us in our current age. Having a good teacher who can interpret the teachings and intentions of the gurus of the ages and bring the teachings to us in a modern manner is invaluable.[217]

---

[214] Hatha Yoga Pradipika, I-14.

[215] Ibid, I-12 and 13.

[216] Actually, a cubit was considered to be the length of a man's arm, from the elbow to the tip of the fingers, or about eighteen inches. So this would mean you need only about six feet of space (assuming you are not more than six feet tall).

[217] For my own part, I am indebted to Sarah Powers and Paul Grilley, who have guided me and so many others in our learning of Yin Yoga. When I

The Three Tattvas of Yin Yoga Practice

A tattva is the reality of a thing, or its category or principal nature. Sarah Powers offers us three very simple and very effective principles for the yin practice.

1. Come into the pose to an appropriate depth
2. Resolve to remain still
3. Hold the pose for time

Remembering these three principles as you practice will simplify everything. We will look at each step of *how* to practice in more detail in a moment. Knowing *when* to practice is a different matter.

When to Practice Yin Yoga

There are no absolutes. The question of when to practice Yin Yoga has no absolute answer. There are many possible answers, and each one is simply different from the others, not better or more correct. We find we have many options for when to practice Yin Yoga, depending upon what we would like to achieve through our practice.

We could do our yin practice:

- When our muscles are cool (so they don't steal the stretch away from the deeper tissues)
- Early in the morning (when the muscles are more likely to be cool)
- Last thing at night (to calm the mind before sleep)
- Before an active yang practice (again, before the muscles become too warmed up)

---

open my mouth to teach or sit down to type this book, it is their voices that come out.

- In the spring or summer (to balance a natural yang time of year)
- When life has become very hectic (to balance the yang energies in our lives)
- After a long trip (traveling is very yang, even if we are sitting down a lot during the trip)
- During your moon cycle (to conserve energies)

Yin Yoga deliberately targets the deeper connective tissues. To be most effective we want the muscles to be relaxed. If the muscles are warm and active they will tend to absorb most of the tension of the stretch. When we do our Yin Yoga practice early in the morning, the muscles have not yet woken up; this is why we feel so stiff when we first wake up. In the same way, doing our yin practice before an active yang practice allows the stretching to settle deeper into our tissues.

By the end of the day our muscles have been warmed up and are at their longest. The physical benefits of a yin practice will be fewer at this time; however, the psychological benefits may be greater. The daytime is yang. A yin practice, before going to sleep, may balance this energy. Similarly the spring and summer are yang times of year. When life is busy, when we spend many hours traveling, these are all yang times of our life. Balance is achieved when we cultivate yin energies. During a woman's menstrual period she may naturally find a yin practice beneficial.

On the other side of the coin, a yin practice is not recommended when we have already been very placid. After sitting at a desk for eight hours in the dead of a dull winter's day, a more active practice may create balance much better than a yin practice. Listening to your inner guide may give you the best answer to the question: is this a time for yin or yang?

Before You Practice

Virtually every yoga studio has a list somewhere of the general precautions their students should take before practicing yoga. Sometimes these precautions, or guidelines, are posted on the studio's Web sites. Many books on yoga 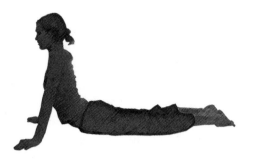 have similar cautions. Even though Yin Yoga is considered a gentler practice than its yang brother, these guidelines still apply. Below is a summary of many of the most common precautions. Once again, this is not an exhaustive list. Please take note and adapt your practice accordingly. If you have any questions, please talk to a teacher or your health care professional.

- If you are pregnant or have serious health concerns such as joint injury, recent surgery, epilepsy, diabetes, or any cardiovascular diseases (especially high blood pressure), be sure to discuss your intention to practice yoga with your health care professional.
- Don't wear perfume or cologne when you practice. Deep breathing is part of the practice and you do not want to be deeply inhaling these fumes.
- For Yin Yoga, do not eat anything for at least one to two hours before class. And no big meals at least three hours before class. Give yourself time to digest before your practice. (For a yang practice you would extend the waiting times before practicing.)
- Before you begin it is nice to have a shower. Be fresh. Evacuate bowels and bladder.
- If you are already physically exhausted, keep the practice very brief and gentle.
- Avoid practice if you have had a lot of sun that day. Prolonged sunbathing depletes the body – let it recover before stressing it further.

- Remove wristwatches and anything metallic that makes a complete circle around the body.[218] If practical, remove glasses too.
- Wear loose, comfortable clothing, so that the body is not restricted.
- In Yin Yoga, you will not generate heat internally. Feel free to wear extra layers of clothes and socks: keep the room a little warmer than normal.
- Have cushions, blocks and blankets handy for padding, and to sit up on for most forward bends and meditation.
- Remove obvious distractions: unplug the phone, put out the cat, tell family members that you need some quiet time now.
- Avoid drafts and cold flowing air.

Above all, practice in a relaxed manner. If you have something to do right after your practice, decide up front to finish earlier than necessary, so you don't feel rushed at the end. Don't expect to have a "great practice" … that kind of expectation can be counter-productive. Expect to do the best you can do and … just be present to what arises.

Now … on to how to practice Yin Yoga.

---

[218] Metal circles will distort and interfere with electromagnetic energy flow, which is one of the forms of Chi. Electric motors and electric generators are possible because of the magnetic effect of electricity flowing inside a metallic circle.

Playing Your Edges

The first principle of Yin Yoga is – every time you come into a pose, go only to the point where you feel a significant resistance in the body. This advice applies to all styles of yoga – yin or yang. Don't try to go as deep as you possibly can right away. Give your body a chance to open up and invite you to go deeper. After thirty seconds or a minute or 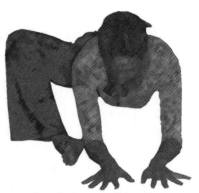 so, usually the body releases and greater depth is possible. But not always. Listen to the body and respect its requests.

Consider your will and your body as two dancers. When you watch two dancers in a wonderful performance, they move in total unison. You cannot tell who is leading and who is following. The dance flows with an ease and grace that seems impossible given the effort that must be there somewhere; and yet it is effortless. Too many beginning (and, unfortunately, even experienced) yoga students make their yoga into a wrestling match – the mind contending with the body, trying to force it into postures that the body is resisting. Yoga is a dance, not a wrestling match.

The essence of yin is yielding. Yang is about changing the world; yin accepts the world for the way it is. Neither is better than the other. There are indeed times when it is appropriate and even necessary to change the world. As we have already observed, yang is a quality much admired and modeled in our culture. We are taught at an early age to make something of ourselves, to change the world and leave our mark on it. And that is perfectly normal … some of the time. However, we are rarely taught how to balance this quality with the quality of acceptance. We are not given the chance to learn how to not struggle and just allow things to unfold. Part of the yin practice is learning this yielding.

This philosophy is reflected well in a prayer, which has uncertain roots. It has been circulating the world for perhaps one hundred years.[219] It speaks to this very challenge of balancing yin and yang. The prayer is:

God grant me the serenity to accept the things I cannot change
Grant me the courage to change the things I can change
And grant me the wisdom to know the difference.

Accepting the things we cannot change is the serenity of yin. The courage to change what needs to be changed is yang. Harmony or balance in life comes from having the wisdom to know the difference. This wisdom cannot be given to you or taught to you. It must be earned and learned through your own experience. Our first tattva is the opportunity to gain this wisdom. Listen to your body, go to your first edge and when, and if, the body opens and invites you in deeper, then accept the invitation and go to the next edge. Once at this new edge, again pause and wait for the next opening.

In this manner we play our edges, each time awaiting a new invitation. We ride the edges with a gentle flowing breath, like a surfer riding the waves of the ocean. The surfer doesn't fight against the ocean, she goes with it. Fighting the ocean is a silly thing to do.

When you come into the pose, drop your expectations of how you should look or be in the pose. There is a destructive myth buried deep inside the Western yoga practice. This myth is that we should achieve a model shape in each pose. That is – we should look like some model on the cover of a yoga magazine. To this end we use our body to force ourselves into a required shape. To dislodge this myth we should adopt the following mantra:

We don't use our body to get into a pose – we use the pose to get into our body.

Once we have reached an edge, pause; go inside and notice how this feels. You know the pose is doing its work if you can feel the body being stretched, squeezed, or twisted. Those are the three things

---

[219] It has been adopted by the Alcoholics Anonymous and is called the Serenity Prayer. Wikipedia claims that the theologian Reinhold Niebuhr originally wrote it in the 1930s or early 1940s.

we can do to ourselves in a pose: we are compressing tissues, stretching tissues, or twisting (shearing) tissues.[220]

Another mantra to adopt in our practice is:

If you are feeling it, you are doing it.

You do not need to go any further if you are already feeling a significant stretch, compression, or twist in the body. Going further is a sign of ego; it is not doing yoga. Staying where you are is embracing yin.

This is not an excuse to stay back and not go deep into the posture. When we play our edges we come to the point of significant resistance. This will entail some discomfort. Yin Yoga is not meant to be comfortable; Yin Yoga will take you well outside your comfort zone. Much of the benefit of the practice will come from staying in this zone of discomfort, despite the mind's urgent pleas to leave, to move, to do anything but stay. This too is part of the practice.

As long as we are not experiencing pain, we remain. Pain is always a one-way ticket out of the pose. Pain is a signal that we are tearing the body, or close to tearing the body.[221] Burning sensations, deep twisting or sharp electrical-like pains are definite no-nos – come out immediately. Dull, achy sorts of sensations are to be expected, however. But, no teacher can know what you are feeling; be your own guru at these times and develop your wisdom. Come out when you are struggling to stay at this edge. If you feel your muscles tensing, you are struggling!

Be aware that our edges are not only physical ones; we have emotional and mental edges too. You may find that you are unconsciously holding back from going deeper because if you went one millimeter further you would be flooded with painful memories, thoughts, or feelings. You may not be ready for these yet. Honor your edges wherever they appear. Honor them, but above all … notice them!

---

[220] See section The Physical Body for more on this topic.

[221] We have an unfortunate saying in the West, "No pain, no gain." If you translate this saying into the yoga language of Sanskrit, it is rendered, "*bullshitihi!*"

Playing the edges is not always a "go further ... go further ... go further" process. Often we go forward ... pause ... go ... pause ... maybe back up a little ... wait ... then go again or maybe just stop there. Our edges are always changing: yesterday they may have been quite different than today. Our bodies change. Some days we retain more water in our tissues than other days.[222] Water retention affects our flexibility. We cannot expect that every day our edges will be in the same place. Accept these changes and just take what is offered.

Acceptance: that is the essence of yin.

Resolving to Be Still

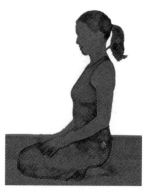

The second tattva of the Yin Yoga practice is stillness. Once we have found the edge, we settle into the pose. We wait without moving. This is our resolution, our commitment. No matter what urges arise in the mind, no matter what sensations arise in the body, we remain still.

There are two exceptions to this advice. First, we move if we experience pain or if we are struggling to stay in the pose. And the second exception is – we move if the body has opened and is inviting us to go deeper. Unless these two reasons arise, we remain still. This is not a time to fix our pedicure, to look around and check out what the other students are wearing. This is the time for stillness.

Sarah Powers teaches that we seek three kinds of stillness:

1. Stillness of the body ... like a majestic mountain
2. Stillness of the breath ... like a calm mountain lake
3. Stillness of the mind ... like the deep blue of the sky

---

[222] Especially for women whose bodies change so much over their monthly cycles.

Stillness of the Body

The body becomes as still as a great mountain. A mountain is unaffected by the winds and dramas swirling around it. Clouds come and go, rains pelt and snows melt, but the mountain remains.

Stillness in the body means the muscles are inactive. Every time we move, we engage our muscles. The muscles naturally want to take any stretch in the body. One of the muscles' jobs is to protect the joints. Only if we keep the muscles very quiet can we allow the effect of a deep stretch to sink into the joints. Fidgeting uses the muscles; fidgeting is a sign of a distracted mind.

When we move, we require energy. Energy is obtained by breathing. When we move, we affect the breath. Stillness of the body leads to stillness of the breath.

Stillness of the Breath

Stillness here does not mean cessation. The breath becomes quiet, unlabored and gentle. Like the surface of a mountain lake, unruffled by wayward breezes, the breath is calm. A calm breath is regular and even, slow and deep, and natural, unforced.

Some students prefer a soft ujjayi breath[223] during their yin practice. This is perfectly okay, as long as it is soft. The harsher ujjayi found in the yang practices may create waves on the surface of the lake. A soft rhythmic sound of the breath will assist with calming the mind.

The breath need not be shallow or short, but it must be regular and unforced. You may try to extend the breath to four seconds, or longer, on each inhalation and exhalation. There may arise natural pauses between the inhalations and exhalations. This is fine, as long as it is unforced and natural. In the pauses between the breaths is the

---

[223] The ujjayi breath is obtained by slightly constricting the back of the throat – the same way is it slightly closed when you try to fog a mirror with your breath. With lips closed, ujjayi has an "ahhhh" sound on both the inhalation and exhalation. The sound may remind you of the wind in the trees, or the waves on the shore. A yang ujjayi may sound more like Darth Vader.

deepest stillness. Allowing the breath to be long, even, and deep is part of allowing this stillness of the breath to arise.

Once the breath has become quiet, the deepest stillness arises.

Stillness of the Mind

The sky is always with us. Clouds may block our view, but we know with a certainty beyond faith that, behind the clouds, the deep blue sky is there. The sky is a metaphor for our true nature. We rarely see who or what we are, because there is so much drama in our lives, so many thoughts and distractions prevent us from seeing clearly what is really there. But on brief, wonderful occasions, the clouds momentarily part, and we get a glimpse of the blue sky behind the drama. As our practice deepens, these holes in the clouds come more frequently, and the gaps become larger. Eventually we see more and more of the sky for longer and longer periods.

This vision of our true nature is possible only when the clouds of thoughts have drifted away; stillness of the mind is required for this clarity. Stillness cannot be forced; the very act of trying to become still defeats itself. Stillness here must arise spontaneously of its own accord. We can, however, create the conditions for this arising.

To still the mind, the breath must be calm. To calm the breath, the body must be still. When these conditions have been met, deep awareness is possible. This state can be achieved only by commitment and dedication. Commit to stillness and allow whatever arises to be just what it is.

Holding for Time

When we have arrived at our edge, once we have become still, all that is left to do is to stay. The yin tissues we are exercising are not elastic tissues. They do not respond well to constant 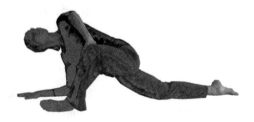 movement: they are plastic. Plastic tissues require long-held, reasonable amounts of traction to be stimulated properly.

Reasonable is a relative word. If you have ever worn braces you know that the pressure is not comfortable, but neither is it the maximum you could bear. Your orthodontist knows that applying twice as much tension in the braces does not mean you can get away with wearing them for only half as long. Yin tissues don't respond to maximum stresses for a short time.

Paul Grilley noticed that basketball players, who jump up and down, placing tremendous loads upon the ligaments of their feet, do not develop fallen arches. Their arches don't fall because the extreme strain is very brief. They are more likely to break bones, or tear ligaments or tendons in their feet, than to develop fallen arches. However, a one-hundred-pound waitress, who is standing on her feet for eight hours a day, is a prime candidate for fallen arches. She is experiencing a gentle pressure for a long period of time. That is the condition for changing our yin tissues.

Yang postures may be held for as little as five breaths, or as long as a couple of minutes, depending upon the style of yoga being practiced. All yang poses require muscular engagement to maintain the pose. Yang tissues require yang exercise. Yin postures are generally held for at least one minute, and for some people as long as twenty minutes. Yin tissues require yin exercise. It is the long, gentle pressure that coaxes yin tissues into being strengthened.

It can be dangerous to mix up these forms of exercise. Yang tissues can be damaged by being stressed in a yin manner – statically held in one position for a long period of time. No physical trainer would suggest you try to build stronger biceps by holding a heavy barbell in a half-curled position for five minutes. Muscles need repetitive movement to grow stronger. Similarly, being stressed in a yang manner can damage yin tissues. Repetitively dropping back from standing into the wheel pose can overwork the ligaments in the lower back, eventually wearing them out. We must make sure we exercise yang tissues in a yang way and yin tissues in a yin way. The yin way is to hold a pose under a reasonable, non-maximum stress for long periods of time.

If you are practicing on your own, use a timer or a stopwatch to set a constant length of time for the postures – three to five minutes may work well for you. If you are just beginning Yin Yoga, you may want to start with one- or two-minute holds and work your way toward longer periods. You may find that some postures allow you to remain in the pose longer than others – this is all right. Our bodies are not uniformly open. It may be better to stay in a challenging pose, like saddle, for less time than in an easier pose, like butterfly. If you are struggling to remain in a pose, come out – regardless of whether the timer has sounded or not.

The yin practice is very portable – you can take it with you anywhere – you don't need a yoga studio, you don't even need a yoga mat. All you need is four cubits of space on the floor. That is to say – all you need is enough room to stretch out. You can do these poses while doing other activities. While this may not provide you with the deepest benefits – the meditation practice you get with a dedicated practice – you can still affect your tissues physically. Sitting in yin poses while reading or talking on the phone, while eating at your coffee table or watching television, will help open the tightest hips.[224]

One last bit of advice: people love to do things that they love to do. Sounds obvious. Said another way, when you are in balance you will tend to keep doing things that keep you in balance. However, when you are out of balance, you will tend to continue to do things that keep you out of balance! Active people love to do active yoga. Calmer people (a nice way of saying less active people) love to do calming yoga. Don't always practice what you love; practice what you need! Active people probably need Yin Yoga more than anyone else. Calm people probably need to do more yang practices more than anyone else.

Now that you have some idea of how to practice Yin Yoga, the next step is to learn the postures, also known as the asanas.

---

[224] In fact, one strong recommendation for opening your hips and strengthening your lower back is to give away all the chairs in your home! Live on the floor whenever you can.

Chapter Thirteen: Yin Yoga Asanas

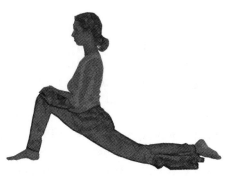

The Hatha Yoga Pradipika lists only sixteen postures. Of these, half are seated positions. Those postures are meant to be held for a long period of time. They are yin postures. In Paul Grilley's book *Yin Yoga*, he lists eighteen yin poses, along with five yang poses to be used in between the yin poses. If you are planning to hold each pose for five minutes, and if you allow a one-minute rest between postures, a five-minute meditation at the beginning of the practice, and a five-minute Shavasana at the end, in a ninety-minute class you will have time for only thirteen poses. There will be even fewer if you are doing two sides or other variations in each posture.

There is not a great need for a lot of postures in the Yin Yoga practice. Paul states in his book, "The more yin your practice the less variety is needed and the emphasis is placed on a few basic postures." The next section will list over two dozen Yin Yoga asanas. Each description follows a standard outline, which includes:

- A picture of the pose
- Benefits of the pose
- Contraindications (reasons for avoiding the pose)
- Alternatives and options (sometimes with pictures)
- Meridians and organs affected by the posture
- Joints affected by the posture
- Recommended hold time
- Counterposes to be done after the pose
- Names of similar yang asanas
- Other notes of interest

The picture of the asana will provide an example of the posture: sometimes a picture is worth a thousand words, but please remember that every body is different. Your body probably won't look the same as the student in the picture. The shape is not what's important. As David Williams[225] helpfully advises, "The real yoga is what you can't see."

The benefits listed in the following asana descriptions are not exhaustive, but they will provide a guideline to help you to choose when to add a particular asana to your practice. If you wish to arrange your practice time around a particular area of the body or a particular organ that needs stimulation, the advice here may be useful. Combine this knowledge with the information provided on the affected joints, meridians and organs to structure your flow.

Contraindications should always be checked out before trying a posture for the first time. Remember, not all poses are for every body; know and respect your limits. If a certain pose is not right for you, don't worry about it; there are lots of other ways to work the same tissues. Choose another posture that is more appropriate for you. You will find some suggestions offered in the alternatives and options.

The recommended time to hold a pose is very subjective. There are guidelines offered, which you should completely ignore if they are not appropriate for you. Some students can remain in the asanas

---

[225] One of the first two Americans to learn the Ashtanga practice.

much longer than indicated; others must come out much earlier. Listen to your inner teacher and respect your body's unique needs.

When coming out of a pose there will be a natural sense of fragility – we have been deliberately pulling the body apart and holding it apart. The sense of relief is to be expected, and even enjoyed. Yes, despite some myths to the contrary, you are allowed to enjoy your practice! Smile when you come out of the pose! Laugh – cry even. Thank the Buddha, Jesus, Allah, Paul Grilley ... shout "Om Namah Shivaya!" Enjoy this moment.

One of the benefits of Yin Yoga is this experience of coming out of the asana. We learn what it will be like when we are ninety years old! We gain a new respect for our grandmother, and what she is going through, and we resolve to put off that inevitable day of decrepitude as long as possible. After a deep, long-held hip opener, it may feel like we will never be able to walk again – but be assured ... the fragility will pass. Sometimes, however, a movement in the opposite direction will help. This is a counterpose, a balancing posture that brings us back to neutral.

Many of these asanas will be familiar to experienced yoga students. However, these students will notice that the name is different in the yin tradition – this is deliberate. The pose may look the same, but the intention is different. The yin pose of Swan looks identical to the yang pose of Pigeon, but in Pigeon, as in most yang poses, the muscles are the targets. In a yang pose, we engage the muscles and stretch them. In the yin practice, we relax the muscles; we aim our intention into the joints and the deep tissues wrapping them, not the more superficial tissues of the muscles or skin.

There is no consensus in the world of yoga on naming asanas. Even in the yang tradition you will come across different names for the same postures and different postures sharing the same names. This is also true in the yin tradition; different names abound. The ones shown here are the names more commonly used but they are not universal. Where two names are common, both names are given, but we have not attempted to be exhaustive.

The Asanas

In this section we are going to explore a couple of dozen asanas (an exact count depends upon whether or not one wishes to include variations and options). This selection will suffice to work all the yin areas of the body normally targeted in a yin practice.

1. Anahatasana (aka Melting Heart)
2. Ankle Stretch
3. Butterfly
4. Half Butterfly
5. Camel
6. Cat Pulling Its Tail
7. Caterpillar
8. Child's Pose
9. Dangling
10. Deer
11. Dragons
12. Dragonfly (aka Straddle)
13. Frog
14. Happy Baby
15. Lying Twist
16. Saddle
17. Shavasana
18. Shoelace
19. Snail
20. Sphinx and Seal
21. Square
22. Squat
23. Swan
24. Sleeping Swan
25. Toe Squat

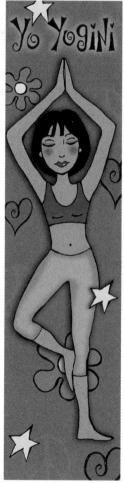

Yo Yogini AB

Anahatasana
(Melting Heart)

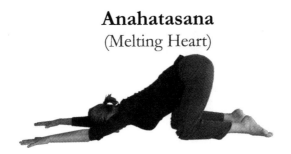

Benefits:

- Good stretch for the upper and middle back;
- Will also open shoulders;
- Softens the heart.

Contraindications:

- Be careful: if student has a bad neck, this could strain it.

Alternatives & Options:

- If shoulder pain prevents the arms going over head, move arms wider apart;
- Flexible students can bring chin to floor and look ahead, but this could strain the neck;
- If knees are uncomfortable here, place a blanket underneath them;
- Toes can be tucked under;
- Chest can be rested on a bolster (allowing the body to relax);
- Can do this pose with just one arm forward at a time, resting the head upon the other forearm.

Meridians & Organs Affected:

- Along the spine, the Urinary Bladder lines;
- The arm meridians, especially the Heart and Lung lines.

Joints Affected:

- Upper back (which is actually the scapula, not the thoracic spine);
- Mildly stresses the lower spine;
- Shoulder/Humerus joint.

Hold for How Long?

- Three to five minutes;
- If the student is resting chin on floor, the hold may need to be shorter … the student has to carefully watch the sensations in the neck.

Counterposes?

- Lying on stomach, or go back to Child's Pose.

Similar to?

- Half Down Dog (aka Puppy Dog).

Other Notes:

- It is nice to do this pose after a series of lower back bends;
- Could be used as a gentle warm-up before deeper back bends;
- If students feel pinching in the back of the shoulders, they may be reaching a compression point … abducting the arms (moving them farther apart) may release this. If this does happen here, it probably happens in Down Dog and the Wheel too, so they may be well advised to have hands wider in these poses.

Ankle Stretch

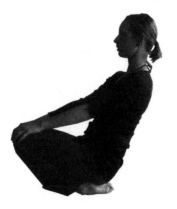

Benefits:

- Opens and strengthens the ankles;
- Strong stimulation of four meridians flowing through the feet and ankles;
- Great counterpose for squatting or toe exercises.

Contraindications:

- Any sharp pain in ankles, back off. Students can try a blanket or towel under the feet, to cushion them;
- Knee issues may prevent the student from sitting on heels: placing a rolled up towel, or other cushions, between the thighs and calves may reduce this.

Alternatives & Options:

- Leaning back on the hands is the first position, and is the least stressful, but beware of collapsing backward … keep the heart forward;
- After a few moments, the student can try to bring the hands to the floor beside the legs;

- Try not to lean away from the knees … keep the heart open, arching the back forward;
- Finally, the very open student can hold the knees and gently pull the knees toward the chest.

Meridians & Organs Affected:

- Stomach, Spleen, Liver, Gall Bladder lines are strongly stimulated.

Joints Affected:

- The ankle.

Hold for How Long?

- About one minute. This is relatively yang and shouldn't be held for a long time.

Counterposes?

- Pushup/Plank/Chaturanga, Crocodile or any posture that straightens the legs and tucks the toes under;
- Dangling or Squatting is also nice.

Other Notes:

- This is a nice counterpose for many poses that stress the feet, such as sitting on heels with toes tucked under, Squats, and sitting meditations.

Butterfly

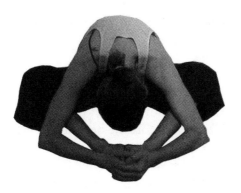

Benefits:

- A nice way to stretch the lower back without requiring loose hamstrings;
- If the legs are straighter and the feet are farther away from the groin, the hamstrings will get more of a stretch. If the feet are in closer to the groin, the adductor muscles get stretched more;
- Iyengar says this is good for the kidneys and the prostrate gland and highly recommends this pose for people suffering urinary problems;
- Iyengar also claims this removes "heaviness in the testicles and is a boon to women … to regulate periods, ovaries function properly and make delivery easier …"[226]

Contraindications:

- Seated forward bends are the hard on the pelvis and knees – they can aggravate sciatica. If a student has this condition, elevate the hips so the knees are below the hips. Beware of

---

[226] All quotations by Iyengar in this section are from his book *Light on Yoga*.

hips rotating backward while seated – we want the hips to rotate forward;

- Okay for pregnant women, as the legs are abducted, providing space for the belly;
- Avoid if the neck has suffered whiplash or has reverse curvature.

Alternatives & Options:

- Elevate the hips with a bolster or cushion;
- If neck is tired, support the head in the hands, resting elbows on knees or thighs;
- Could rest the chest on a bolster;
- Various hand/arm positions are possible: hold feet, hands on floor in front of student, or arms relaxed behind the body;
- Can do this lying down, keeping legs in butterfly.

Meridians & Organs Affected:

- The Gall Bladder lines on the outside of the legs as well as the Urinary Bladder lines[227] running along the spine in the lower back;
- If the feet are in close to the groin and a stretch is felt in the inner thighs, the Kidney and Liver lines are being stimulated.

Joints Affected:

- Hips and lower spine.

Hold for How Long?

- Three to five minutes;
- Can hold much longer if desired.

---

[227] These are the same as the ida and pingala nadis.

Counterposes?

- Sitting up, or a gentle sitting back bend;
- Lying on stomach, which is also a gentle back bend;
- Could do a spinal lift flow on the back or flow into Tabletop (aka Hammock);
- A seated twist.

Similar to?

- Baddha Konasana, but without the emphasis on a straight spine or the feet in tight to groin. In the Butterfly we want the back to round, allowing the head to drop to the heels.

Other Notes:

- Can be done after meals, as long as head does not touch the floor (which would place too much pressure in the abdomen);
- If the feet are closer in, tight adductors or lower back tightness may prevent student from folding forward. Move the feet farther away;
- Many students will automatically go into a tight butterfly, because of their yang training … encourage them to move the feet away, forming a diamond shape with the legs.

Half Butterfly

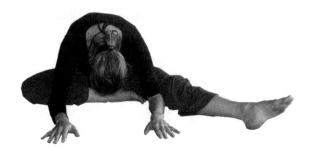

Benefits:

- A nice way to stretch lower back, without requiring loose hamstrings;
- The ligaments along the back of the spine are specifically targeted;
- Iyengar claims this stimulates the liver and kidneys and aids digestion (when folding over the straight leg).

Contraindications:

- Can aggravate sciatica – if the student has sciatica, elevate hips until the knees are below the hips, or avoid this pose entirely. Beware of hips rotating backward while seated: we want the hips to rotate forward;
- Beware of any sharp pain in knees … if knees issues are present, tighten the top of the thigh (quadriceps), which will close the joint, or reduce the angle between the legs;
- If the bent knee complains, place support under it, or move that foot away from groin;
- If the hamstrings protest, bend the straight knee and support the thigh with a blanket or block under it;
- Okay for pregnant women, because the legs are abducted, providing space for the belly.

Alternatives & Options:

- Can fold over the straight leg, which may stretch the hamstrings much more;
- Reach opposite arm to extended foot and/or lower that shoulder to emphasize the side of the spine;
- Add a twist to the spine by resting the elbow on the thigh and the head in that hand (or for more flexible students placing arm along side the straight leg) and the other arm behind the back, or over the head, and rotate the chest toward the sky. This deepens the emphasis along the side of the ribs and spine;

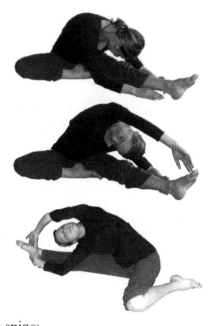

- Place the bent knee foot in Virasana (folded backward behind the buttock), but only if knee doesn't complain.

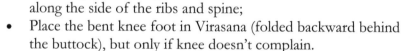

Meridians & Organs Affected:

- Urinary Bladder;
- If there is a lot of sensation in the groin and inner legs, the Liver and Kidneys are stimulated.

Joints Affected:

- Spine, especially the back and sides;
- Inner knees, although this is not as deep of a stretch for the inner knees as the Dragonfly.

Hold for How Long?

- This can be held up to five minutes, with the variations added after two or three minutes.

Counterposes?

- Sitting up or a gentle sitting back bend;
- Flow into Tabletop (aka Hammock);
- Windshield Wipers.

Similar to?

- Janusirsasana, but here we aren't trying to bring the head to the foot; rather, we are bringing the head to the knee. Allow the back to round;
- Paul Grilley calls the variation with the foot in Virasana, the Half Frog.

Camel

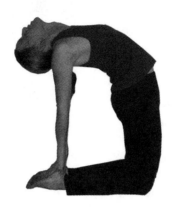

Benefits:

- Like Saddle pose, the Camel deeply arches the sacral/lumbar spine and opens the top of the thighs. There is less opening in the ankles than the Saddle, but there is still some opening there;
- Stretches the hips' flexors and opens the shoulders – Iyengar says this is excellent for people with drooping shoulders or hunched backs.

Contraindications:

- Iyengar claims that the elderly, or people with spinal injuries, can do this pose. However, to be sure this is safe, seek medical advice if you fit either category;
- Without support, the back can spasm, so people with weak backs may want to do only the gentle versions (see below);
- If you have any neck issues, do not drop head back – keep the chin to the chest.

Alternatives & Options:

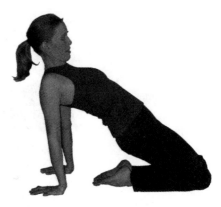

- There are two ways to go into this pose – by holding hands on the hips and keeping the hips forward as you arch back, or by having the hands on the floor behind you and walking the hands forward (as shown), until you have reached an edge;
- Dropping back may be unsuitable for people with back problems, because there is little support from the hands in this version. Do the hands on the floor version instead;
- Walking the hands on the floor toward the feet may be unsuitable for people with knee problems because there is more pressure in the knees in the early stages of this variation;
- Very flexible students may wish to bring their hands to the floor between the feet, or move the hands toward the knees;
- For less flexible students, the toes can be tucked under and the hands rested on the heels, or on a block between the feet.

Meridians & Organs Affected:

- Urinary Bladder, Kidney, Spleen and Stomach meridians;
- Sometimes the upper arms and shoulders are stressed, which stimulates the Heart and Lung meridians;
- The thyroid is stimulated, if the neck is dropped back.

Joints Affected:

- The spine, shoulders, and ankles.

Hold for How Long?

- One to two minutes at most.[228]

Counterposes?

- Child's Pose … Coming out slowly, lift chest forward, allowing the head to remain dropped back until the shoulders are over the hips, then bring the head forward and sit back into Child's Pose.

Similar to?

- Ustrasana (*ustra* means camel).

---

[228] This is a very yang-like pose and requires a lot of leg strength in the full posture, or if your hands are on your hips or lower back. In the supported pose, with the hands on the floor or on your legs or feet, you may stay longer, as you can rest on your arms.

Cat Pulling Its Tail

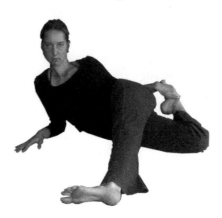

Benefits:
- This back-bending twist is useful as a nice counterpose to strong forward bends (such as the Snail);
- Compresses the lower back;
- Opens the quadriceps and upper thighs.

Contraindications:
- If student has lower back issues, this can still be performed, but go gently. Most students, in this case, will not be able to pull the foot away at all.

Alternatives & Options:
- Easiest version is to be propped up on one arm (as shown in the top picture);

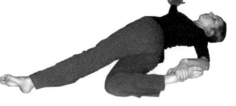

- The more challenging version is to recline, and look over shoulder to the bottom foot. This version becomes a reclining twist with a back bend. Emphasize pulling the foot away from the buttock (most students will not be able to do this).

Meridians & Organs Affected:

- Stimulates the Stomach and Spleen meridians (if the top of the thigh is activated) and the Urinary Bladder and Kidney lines (when the back is arched and twisted);
- If a twist is felt through the side of the rib cage, the Gall Bladder meridian is being stimulated.

Joints Affected:

- Mostly opens the lumbar/sacrum.

Hold for How Long?

- One minute, if doing as a counterpose to a forward bend;
- Can hold longer as a reclining twist – three to five minutes.

Counterposes?

- Hug the knees to the chest to release lower back in a gentle forward fold. Do this either while lying on the back or in Child's Pose.

Similar to?

- Jatharaparivartanasana, with a back bend.

Other Notes:

- If the student is actively pulling the foot away, the pose becomes yang-like in nature: in this case, she may shorten the time, or perhaps release the pressure after one minute.

Caterpillar

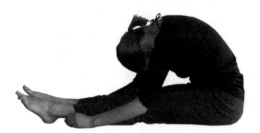

Benefits:

- Stresses the ligaments along the back of the spine;
- Compresses the stomach organs, which helps strengthen the organs of digestion;
- Stimulates the kidneys;
- Since the heart is below the spine, the heart is massaged;
- Iyengar claims this pose helps to cure impotency and leads to sex control.

Contraindications:

- Seated forward bends are the hard on the pelvis and knees – they can aggravate sciatica. If a student has this condition, elevate the hips so the knees are below the hips. Beware of hips rotating backward while seated – we want the hips to rotate forward;
- If the hamstrings are very tight, the knees should be bent and supported by a bolster, allowing the spine to round.

Alternatives & Options:

- Bend knees, and support them with a bolster, to allow the back to round fully;
- If neck feels strained by the weight of the head, students can support their heads in their hands, resting their elbows on the legs or a bolster;

- The student can rest the chest on a bolster, to help relax into the pose;
- Can also rest the legs up the wall (bend the knees and allow the feet to be flat against the wall);
- If knees are strained or weak, activate the quadriceps (but not all the time!).

Meridians & Organs Affected:
- The Urinary Bladder.

Joints Affected:
- The spine.

Hold for How Long?
- Three to five minutes or more.

Counterposes?
- Sitting up or a gentle sitting back bend;
- Lying on the stomach is a gentle back bend, as is doing a spinal lift flow on the back, or flow into Tabletop (aka Hammock);
- A seated twist.

Similar to?
- Paschimottanasana, but here we are not trying to lengthen the spine, or stretch the back muscles. Don't try to bring the head to the feet, but rather round the spine so the head comes to the knees.

Other Notes:
- Paul Grilley says this pose is excellent for balancing Chi flow, and preparing the body for meditation;
- Keep muscles relaxed, especially in the legs;
- Make sure the tops of the student's hips are tilted forward … if the student's hips are rotating backward, have her sit on higher cushions and bend the knees more.

Child's Pose

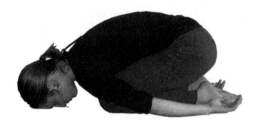

Benefits:

- A healing, restful pose – useful any time a break is needed;
- Gently stretches the spine – this is always a nice counterpose for back bends;
- Gentle compression of the stomach and chest is beneficial for the organs of digestion;
- Psychologically soothing when feeling cold, anxious, or vulnerable;
- Can relieve back and neck pain when the head is supported;
- Rocking gently side to side can help stimulate the flow of blood and lymph fluids in the upper chest and breast tissues.

Contraindications:

- Diarrhea or pregnancy;
- This can be uncomfortable just after eating;
- If knee issues exist, the student may need to place towel or blanket between thighs and calves, or avoid the pose altogether;
- While this is a gentle opener of the ankles, the student may need a blanket or other padding under her ankles to reduce discomfort on the top of the feet.

Alternatives & Options:

- Could be done with arms stretched forward;

- Some students cannot get their buttocks to their heels, which means the head will have a lot of weight on it. They can support the neck by placing the forehead on hands or on a bolster;
- Allow the knees to be as wide apart as is comfortable;
- Can do this as preparation for the Frog by spreading the knees farther apart halfway through the pose, but remain sitting on heels.

Meridians & Organs Affected:

- The Spleen, Stomach, Kidneys, and Urinary Bladder.

Joints Affected:

- The spine and ankles.

Hold for How Long?

- As long as the student wants;
- Used as a counterpose, hold for up to one minute;
- Used as a yin pose on its own, hold for three to five minutes. However, if student cannot get her head to the floor, five minutes may be too long.

Counterposes?

- A counterpose is not normally needed after this pose. Students can go directly to any other poses.

Similar to?

- Balasana or Garbhasana.

Other Notes:

- In Yin Yoga, this pose could be used as a preparation for Dragonfly pose, or for deeper forward bends like Snail.

Dangling

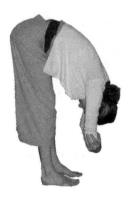

Benefits:

- Gentle stretch for the lower spine;
- Warms up the hamstrings and leg muscles;
- Compresses the stomach and internal organs;
- Diaphragmatic breathing is harder while in this posture – this pose builds strength in the diaphragm, while providing a massage for the abdominal organs;
- Cures stomach pain during menstruation;
- Heart rate is slowed and spinal nerves rejuvenated.

Contraindications:

- Avoid if student has high blood pressure;[229]
- If student has low blood pressure, to come out of the pose she should roll up to standing *slowly*, or go into squat, to avoid seeing the Yoga Faeries (feeling dizzy);
- If someone has a bad back, she must bend her knees a lot! She can also rest her elbows on her thighs.

---

[229] Poses where the head is below the heart can increase blood pressure.

Alternatives & Options:

- Bend knees more … this will strengthen the legs and release the back;
- Rest elbows against a table, a chair or on the thighs if the back feels strained;
- Caterpillar is an easy alternative;
- Really flexible students can hold wrists behind the legs, but we still want some rounding to the back in this yin posture.

Meridians & Organs Affected:

- Due to the intense stretch along the back of the legs and spine, the Urinary Bladder meridian is highly stimulated;
- Iyengar says this is great for the liver, spleen, and kidneys.

Joints Affected:

- Spine.

Hold for How Long?

- Three minutes can be pretty intense: sometimes this pose is done in two or more sessions of two minutes each, separated by two minutes of the Squat.

Counterposes?

- Squat or a gentle back bends.[230]

Similar to?

- Uttanasana – the emphasis here is not to stretch the hamstrings a lot, but rather to release the lower back. If the legs are straight, it is a nice stretch for the hamstrings, but

---

[230] For example, cat, lying on stomach, or, while sitting cross-legged with hands on the floor behind you, lift your chest and hips forward…

there is little muscular effort needed. If the knees are bent, it is a great strengthener for the leg muscles and allows the back to release more fully.

Other Notes:

- Ensure the arches of the feet are lifting;
- Balance the weight between toes and heels … can gently sway or wobble, but no bouncing;
- Straight legs will stretch the hamstrings;
- Bent knees will strengthen the thigh muscles;
- Better to bend the knees and receive a stomach massage too;
- Can intermix this and Squat – eventually hold both for four minutes, or more, in total.

Deer

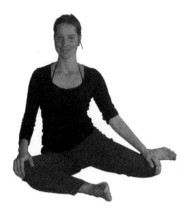

Benefits:

- A nice counterpose to hip openers or any external rotation of the hips;
- A balanced way to rotate hips, both externally (front leg) and internally (back leg);
- Improves digestion and relieves gas;
- Helps to relieve the symptoms of menopause;
- Reduces swelling of the legs during pregnancy (until the end of the second trimester);
- Therapeutic for high blood pressure and asthma.

Contraindications:

- If any knee issues exist, be careful of externally rotating the hip (front knee); keep that foot in closer to the groin. Could support the front knee with a bolster, or a folded blanket, placing it under the knee.

Alternatives & Options:

- The tendency here is to tilt away from the internally rotating hip of the back leg; make sure both sitting bones are firmly on the floor. This may require moving the feet more toward the core of the body;
- Very flexible students can begin to move their feet away from their hips;

- A nice stretch to the side body and the back thigh is to twist around towards the back foot by rotating to the opposite side. You may rest on your elbow here and try to bring your head to the floor.

Meridians & Organs Affected:
- If the front leg is firmly on the floor or if you are twisting, the Gall Bladder line is activated. Any inner groin sensations indicate that the Liver and Kidneys are benefiting. If the thigh is stretched, the Stomach and Spleen are activated.

Joints Affected:
- Hips.

Hold for How Long?
- Most students can't do this pose well enough to get a lot of benefit from it, so it is useful mostly as a counterpose. As a counterpose, just hold for up to one minute.

Counterposes?
- Since this pose is both an external and internal hip rotation, the best counterpose is to do the other side;
- Windshield Wipers are nice: they can be done lying down, sitting up, or reclining on elbows.

Similar to?
- This is a combination of Virasana (Hero Pose) and Padmasana (Lotus Pose).

Other Notes:
- Useful after long-held, external hip rotations such as Shoelace, Swan, or Dragonfly, where both legs were wide apart;
- Most students won't easily understand what the pose is about … they won't move their feet far enough away from the groin or hips, or they will tilt too much, allowing the internally rotated hip to rise off the floor. The teacher will have to inspect their efforts and offer guidance.

Dragons

Benefits:

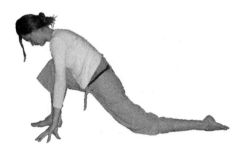

- Deep hip and groin opener … gets right into the joint;
- Also stretches the back leg's hip flexors and quadriceps;
- Many variations to help work deeply into hip socket;
- Can help with sciatica.

Contraindications:

- Can be uncomfortable for the kneecap or the ankle. If the student is stiff, the back thigh will be at ninety-degree angle to the front thigh, putting a lot of weight on the kneecap. Support the back knee with blanket under it, or place a bolster under shin, allowing the back knee to be off the floor.

Options:

- If back knee is uncomfortable, place a blanket under it, rest the shin on a bolster, or tuck the toes under and lift the leg off the floor;[231]
- If ankle is uncomfortable, place blanket underneath it, or raise knee by putting bolster under the shin;
- Press top of foot down firmly, emphasizing the little toe.

---

[231] Lifting the back leg off the floor is much more advanced.

Alternative Dragons:

- The first option is a simple low lunge, called the "Baby Dragon";
- The next option is to rest the arms or hands on the front thigh, and lift the chest – this increases the weight over hips. This is the "Dragon Flying High";

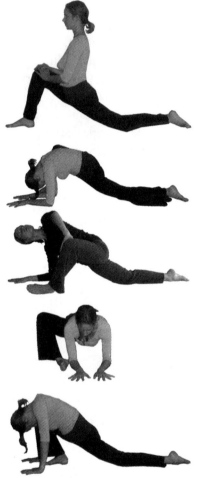

- A deeper option, Dragon Flying Low, is to place both hands inside front foot (ensuring the foot doesn't slide inward toward a Pigeon position) and walk hands forward, lowering the hips. For more depth the student could come down on elbows, or rest elbows on a bolster or block;
- "Twisted Dragon" – one hand pushes front knee to the side while the chest rotates to the sky;
- "Winged Dragon" – with hands on floor, wing out the knee a few times, rolling onto the outside edge of that foot, and then stay there with the knee low. Could come down on elbows or rest elbows on a block or bolster;
- "Overstepping Dragon" – exercises the ankle. From Baby Dragon, allow the front knee to come far forward and/or slide the heel backward, until the heel is just about to lift off the ground;

- "Dragon Splits" – the deepest stretch for hip flexors. Straighten both legs into the splits. Student can support the front hip with a bolster under the buttock, for balance and to release weight; this relaxes the muscles. Student can sit up tall or fold forward for different sensations;

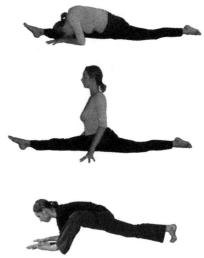

- "Fire-breathing Dragon" – in any of the above variations, tuck the back toe under and lift the knee up, lengthening the leg. This puts more weight into the hips, increasing the stretch.

Meridians & Organs Affected:

- Stomach, Spleen, Liver, Gall Bladder, and Kidneys (and even the Urinary Bladder in the Dragon Flying High or the Dragon Splits High).

Joints Affected:

- Hips and ankles;
- Lower back in the back bend options.

Hold for How Long?

- Could hold each variation for one minute and cycle through all of them or,
- Hold just one variation for three to five minutes.

Counterposes?

- A short Down Dog is delicious – take your puppy for a walk by bending one knee, lifting that heel and pushing the opposite heel down, and then switch sides repeatedly;
- Child's Pose feels really good after Down Dog and before switching to the other side of the Dragon.

Similar to?

- Low lunge (Anjaneyasana).[232]

Other Notes:

- Some people will not feel anything in the outer hip joint. If they are very tight in the hip flexor or quadriceps, that area will take all the stress. This is still a good pose for them, but to work their hips, other poses will be needed.

---

[232] Sometimes this pose becomes the "Pedicure Fixing Asana" due to the urge to fix up the pedicure. At these times, allow the urge to arise, but don't react to it!

Dragonfly
(Straddle-fold)

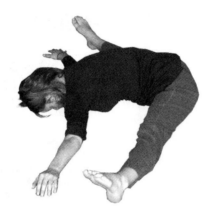

Benefits:

- Opens the hips, groin, and the back of thighs;
- Also provides a gentle opening to inner knees;
- Stimulates the ovaries.

Contraindications:

- Seated forward bends are the hard on the pelvis and knees – they can aggravate sciatica. If a student has this condition, elevate the hips so the knees are below the hips. Beware of hips rotating backward while seated – we want the hips to rotate forward;
- If the student has any inner knee trauma or issues, she should bring the legs closer together or tighten the top of the legs (the quadriceps) to engage the kneecaps.

Alternatives & Options:

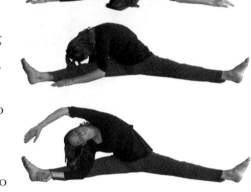

- Use bolster to raise hips;
- Could keep hands behind the back, or rest elbows on a bolster;
- Folding over one leg increases spinal and hamstring stretch. If knees feel bothered, tighten quadriceps to close knee joint, or bring legs closer together;
- If hamstrings feel too tight, bend the knee and place a bolster under the thigh;
- Legs can be ninety degrees apart to one hundred and twenty degrees for advanced students. The full split of one hundred and eighty degrees is not necessary;
- Advanced students can lie right down on stomach and rest arms to the sides;
- Use a bolster under the chest, if you are close to the floor;
- If head is too heavy for the neck, support the head in hands;
- For stiff students, bend the knees a lot! It is also okay to place the feet flat on the floor;
- Can come into a twist (like revolved Janusirsasana) by folding over one leg and rotating chest skyward (advanced students may hold the foot with both hands);
- Can also do a sitting up twist (helps to stimulate the upper body meridians under the scapula).

Meridians & Organs Affected:

- Urinary Bladder on back of legs and on the back, and the Liver and Kidney lines through the groin and the Spleen through the inner knees;

- The twisting version will stimulate the Gall Bladder along the side of the torso.

Joints Affected:

- Hips, lower back, and knees.

Hold for How Long?

- Three to five minutes;
- Often it is nice to spend half of the time in one variation, and then add the twist (bottom picture) for the last half of the pose.

Counterposes?

- Lean back on the hands to release the hips, and slowly bring legs together. Groaning is allowed.[233] Windshield Wipers are nice, or do a cross-legged, seated back bend;
- Tabletop (aka Hammock).

Similar to?

- Upavistakonasana.

Other Notes:

- Very frustrating for beginners: the adductor muscles tug on sitting bones, just like the hamstrings do, which causes the top of hips to tilt backward. Persistence is required! Sitting on a bolster helps;
- Keep weight forward on sitting bones – even tug the flesh away from the buttocks before folding forward.

---

[233] Groans coming out of Yin Yoga poses sound like "ommmm."

Frog

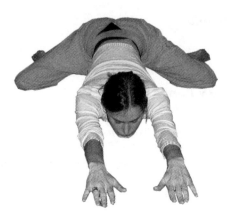

Benefits:

- Deep groin opener (especially the adductors);
- Provides a slight back bend, which compresses the lower and upper back;
- Aids digestion and relieves cramps.[234]

Contraindications:

1. Bad back;
2. Knees can be uncomfortable, so use padding under the knees;
3. If the neck is stiff, rest the forehead, not the chin, on the floor or on a bolster.

---

[234] Both menstrual cramps and cramps from eating.

Alternatives & Options:

1. Tadpole: From Child's Pose, separate the knees, but remain sitting on the heels;
2. Half Frog: Lift the hips higher, until the hips are in line with knees, keeping feet together;
3. Full Frog: separate the feet as wide as the knees.

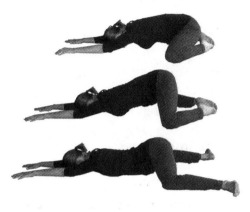

- Could extend just one arm at a time: this is safer. The other arm can be bent with the head resting on the forearm. Flexies (aka flexible students) can do both arms out at the same time;
- Allow the hips to come farther forward if the pressure in groin or hips is too severe;
- Alternately, keep toes together and allow hips to go backward;
- May rest the chest on bolster, to relax upper body;
- If the shoulders are uncomfortable, spread the hands wider apart.

Meridians & Organs Affected:

- The inner leg pressure works the Spleen, Liver, and Kidney meridians;
- When the arms are stretched forward, the upper body meridians are massaged, affecting the lines of Heart, Lungs, and Small and Large Intestines.

Joints Affected:

- Hips, lower back, and shoulders.

Hold for How Long?

- Three to five minutes;
- Could do first half of pose in tadpole, and then move to the full frog.

Counterposes?

- Child's Pose;
- Lying on the back, hug knees to chest, and rock side to side, or move knees in circles.

Similar to?

- Mandukasana or Bhekasana.

Other Notes:

- When the hips are in line with knees, gravity has maximum effect. Often students will move hips forward to avoid painful compression in the hips – that is okay;
- Can do this right after eating by resting on elbows … don't let the stomach rest on the floor though – allow it to hang – nice for digestion;
- A nice pose to do to begin a class, or if short of time;
- Flexies don't need to go deeper, just stay longer!

Happy Baby

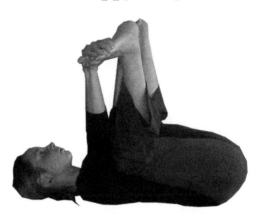

Benefits:

- A deep hip opener that requires arm strength, rather than letting gravity do the work. One of the few poses working with arm flexion (strengthening the biceps). A good yang pose for upper body strength, while being a good yin pose for the lower body;
- Releases the sacrum;
- Deep compression of stomach organs.

Contraindications:

- This can become a mild inversion: a student may want to avoid this posture if she is in her moon cycle, or if she has very high blood pressure.

Alternatives & Options:

- Half Happy Baby (like an upside down low lunge) holding one foot at a time;
- Very tight students may use a belt to hold the feet, or do this against a wall. It

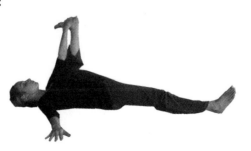

is like a lying down Squat, but with the feet pushing into the wall;

- Could hold the back of the thighs;
- Toes together – first stage, leave them near groin – later stage, bring toes to the nose;
- Eventually, feet go behind the head![235]

Meridians & Organs Affected:

- Urinary Bladder;
- Inner groin stimulation works the Spleen, Liver, and Kidneys.

Joints Affected:

- Hips and sacrum/lumbar.

Hold for How Long?

- Three to five minutes.

Counterposes?

- Gentle back bends (lying on stomach) or, while on the back, a mild spinal lift, coming up only halfway.

Similar to?

- Beginner's version of Yoga Nidra. Also called "window" or, in Los Angeles, "dead bug";
- Unlike in the yang style poses listed above, you may allow your tailbone to curl up to release, or decompress, the lower back.

---

[235] Eventually, not necessarily this lifetime.

Other Notes:

- It is easy for the student to get tired here and stop pulling. That is okay – by then the weight of the legs will add enough juice to make the pose work;
- There are two options to try here:
  1) Allow the tailbone to curve up in the air. Unlike the yang version, we do want to release the sacrum;
  2) Keep tailbone low to the ground. Notice the differences;
- This posture is the single, most important reason that video recording equipment and cameras are not allowed in yoga studios.

Reclining Twist

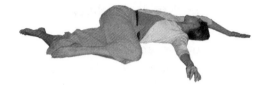

Benefits:

- Twisting at the end of the practice helps to restore equilibrium in the nervous system and release tension in the spine;
- Sarah Powers notes that bringing the bent knee more to the chest can relieve sciatica;
- Tones the stomach and cures gastritis.

Contraindications:

- If the student has shoulder issues (such as rotator cuff injuries), she may not want to raise arm to beside the ear or let it float. Arm can be bent or supported by a bolster.

Alternatives & Options:

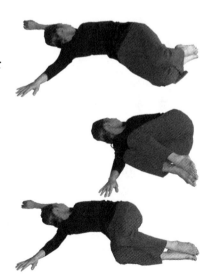

- Directing the knees lower, or higher, will affect where in the spine the stretch is felt. Knees high moves the twist to upper back, knees low moves twist more to lumbar/sacrum;
- If shoulder is off the floor, place a bolster under the bent knee to balance the body;
- Student can experiment with

the head turning to either
side – notice how the
sensations change;

- If the student has raised
  her hand alongside the
  ear, it could be resting on
  the floor or on a bolster;

- Twisted Roots – knees
  can also be crossed as in
  eagle pose (Garudasana);

- Top leg straight out to
  the side applies the most
  leverage, which helps to
  keep the hips fully
  turned.

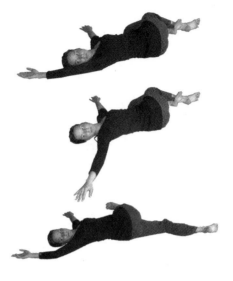

Meridians & Organs Affected:

- Twisting the spine stimulates the Urinary Bladder lines along
  the spine (the ida and pingala nadis);
- If arm is overhead, three meridians in the arms are stimulated
  – the Heart, Lung, and Small Intestines;
- Twists always compress the stomach. Also twisting through
  the rib cage stimulates the Gall Bladder meridians;
- Iyengar says this pose helps the liver, spleen, and pancreas.

Joints Affected:

- The shoulder joint, as well as all the tissues in the upper
  chest, breast, and shoulder are nurtured;
- The lower spine, especially the sacrum, if knee is at ninety
  degrees to the torso.

Hold for How Long?

- Three to five minutes.

Counterposes?

- Hug the knees and rock on back from side to side.

Similar to?

- Jatharaparivartanasana.

Other Notes:

- An excellent final pose of the practice, because it removes any kinks and knots;
- Student may want to slide right from this pose into Shavasana;
- If tingling occurs in the arms or hands, move them lower until the blood flows again;[236]
- Don't push into the twist – relax. Let gravity do the work.

---

[236] This is good advice for any yoga pose!

Saddle

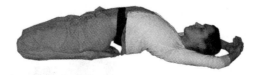

Benefits:

- A deep compression in the sacral-lumbar arch;
- Also stretches hips flexors and quadriceps – Iyengar says this is excellent for athletes and people who have to do a lot of standing or walking;
- The thyroid is stimulated, if the neck is dropped back;
- If the foot is, or the feet are, beside the hips, this becomes a good internal rotation of the hip.

Contraindications:

- Bad back, tight sacrum;
- Knees can be tested too much here;
- Ankles can protest as well;
- Any sharp or burning pain here, you must come out!

Alternatives & Options:

- If this is too deep for the lower back, do the Seal or Sphinx, or;
- Straighten one leg – this is also called "Half Saddle." Could bend the straight leg and place the foot on the floor (note pictures);
- Optionally, don't go back so far – just lean back on the hands, or on the elbows;
- Resting top of head on floor opens the neck;
- Arms overhead can open the shoulders;
- There are various places you may use bolsters – stack two crossways under the shoulders, or use just one, or place one lengthways under spine;

- A blanket or rolled up towel under the ankles can relieve pressure there;
- Flexies may want to lift hips even higher by placing a block between the feet and under the buttocks;
- If the thighs protest too much, bend one knee and place that foot on the floor. Very flexible students may want to hug the bent knee to the chest;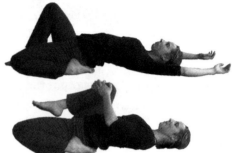
- Sarah Powers often adds a twist in the Saddle by bringing a hand behind the back and grabbing the inner thigh, which stimulates the shoulder lines. In this version, you won't lean back onto the head or the elbows – just arch back and remember to do both sides!
- Play with sitting *on* heels and *between* heels; the first emphasizes the lumbar more, and the second works the quads and hip flexors more.

Meridians & Organs Affected:

- Affects Stomach, Spleen, Urinary Bladder, and Kidney lines.

Joints Affected:

- Lower spine, knees, and ankles.

Hold for How Long?

- One to five minutes;
- Iyengar says up to fifteen minutes!

Counterposes?

- Coming out there are two choices: first, roll to one side and straighten the top leg, then the lower leg, and stay there for a while before rolling onto your back; or, second, push the elbows into floor, contract the stomach muscles, and sit up;
- After coming out, lie quietly for a few breaths with the legs straight, tighten kneecaps to release the knees. Finally, hug the knees in a gentle forward bend to release the lower back;
- Child's Pose: move into it slowly. Some folks may need to rest the head on the palms before coming into a full Child's Pose, to give the back a chance to release.

Similar to?

- Supta Vajrasana or Supta Virasana;
- Unlike the yang poses, don't tuck the tail bone (no "Cat tilt"), as we would do normally in back bends.

Other Notes:

- This is not a deep back bend for experienced yogis who are already very open in the lower back: the Seal may be more challenging for them. However, this pose does work three areas at once: thighs, ankles, and lower back;
- For beginners, this may be the deepest back bend, so it often follows the Seal;
- Can be done right after eating;
- If done at night before bed, legs feel rested in the morning.

Shavasana

Time to relax – time to rest the body so that the body becomes stronger and healthier. Time for the little death of *Shavasana.*[237] Shavasana symbolizes the end of your practice – a natural completion to the journey you have been on.

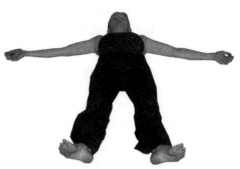

If you are practicing on your own, you may want to set a timer for your Shavasana. It is not uncommon for students to fall asleep. Falling asleep is okay, but most teachers prefer that you remain alert and aware while the body is relaxed. A timer will help rouse you at the end of the Shavasana. Decide how much time you need to relax. For an active yang practice, a good rule of thumb is to allow yourself about ten percent of your practice time. For the yin style, since the muscles were not used, a shorter period is okay – maybe five percent or eight percent will suffice. However, check in with your inner guide and see how much time would be right today.

Shavasana is not just a time to relax the body; in this quiet time the mind should remain alert, yet relaxed and aware of the body relaxing. Pay attention to the energies flowing. This is an ideal time to develop your ability to feel your energies. It is difficult to do this when you are in the postures. Practicing watching the energies during your Shavasana will assist you to feel energy flowing at other times. As you actively relax, watch the flow of Chi or prana into and out of the areas you worked in the asana practice. At first you may have to pretend, or imagine, you can feel these energies. Pretending will help you look closely at these areas. In time, you will notice the energy flow more easily.

There are many ways to perform Shavasana, and many teachers have their own unique and favorite methods. Collect several ways of relaxing by taking classes with several teachers. With a larger

---

[237] Which literally means the "dead posture."

repertoire, you can choose which way is best for any given day. The following suggestion is just one of the many possible options.

Preparing to Relax

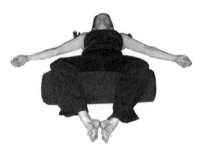

In a yoga studio, your teacher will make sure the surroundings are suitable for relaxation. If you are practicing by yourself, make your environment quiet: disconnect phones; turn off noises; open the windows to allow fresh air in, but stay warm; put any pets into another room; turn lights down, but not off completely – a completely dark room may encourage you to sleep – for the same reason you may want to avoid doing Shavasana in bed.

Begin by letting the body become open: take off glasses and watches; let your hair down; remove anything that may constrict the flow of energy. Also remove any metallic circles you have on – things like rings, bracelets, and body piercings can interfere with the flow of energy.[238] Ensure you will stay warm – put on socks, a sweater, and/or cover yourself with a blanket.[239]

Make yourself comfortable as you lie down on the floor. Bending the knees a little will allow the lower back to release to the floor. If

---

[238] As we discovered in Chapter Five: The Energy Body, electric generators and motors are possible only because metallic circles transform (or distort) energy flowing through them. In the yin practice, we are deliberately stimulating, and freeing, the flow of energy. We don't want it to be distorted now. In fact, it is a good idea not to wear metallic circles while doing your yoga practice. Remember, though, we are talking about completely closed circles; a bracelet or ring that doesn't quite form a circle is fine.

[239] If you are doing Shavasana after a sweaty yang practice, you may need to change your shirt to avoid getting too cold, but don't wipe off any sweat; allowing sweat to dry on the body is one of the yogic healing techniques. (In Yin Yoga you won't have to worry about any sweat!)

you do bend the knees, place a folded blanket or bolster under them so that the legs can relax. Allow the feet to fall outward. If you do not have the knees bent, separate the legs until the knees are hip-width apart or even farther. To really allow the sacrum to lie flat, slide your tailbone away from you. Next, let your arms lie beside you, palms face up and about a foot away from your hips. This will allow your shoulder blades to lie flat; snuggle them into the floor.

Lengthen the neck slightly by pointing the chin toward your feet. You can even roll your head from side to side a few times, until you find a comfortable position in the center. A pillow is nice.

Get all of your fidgeting over with; become still. Often, one or two deep breaths here with a loud sigh are delicious. Release your bones, let go completely – you are ready. Now close your eyes; time to relax.

Relax Completely

Scan your body slowly. Start with your toes and feet – allow your feet to relax. Feel them becoming heavy on the floor. Allow your awareness to rise up to the ankles, calves, and shins. Feel them melting into the earth; no effort is needed. Feel the space in the knee joints. Move slowly higher. Relax the thighs. Feel them become heavy, warm, soft. Notice your buttocks, hips, and groin relaxing; they too become soft and warm. If you have done a lot of hip work in your practice, linger here for a while feeling the openness, the flow of energy through the hips.

Now allow your awareness to come to the tailbone, Feel your sacrum and lower back release into the floor. Feel your lower back and stomach muscles relax. Allow this sensation to rise up the spine. Feel each vertebra – the space between them and their alignment. Allow the upper back muscles and the shoulder blades to sink into the floor. Relax your chest and all the muscles between the ribs. Come now to the shoulders, where we carry so much tension in our bodies. Let the shoulders release completely. Spend an extra moment here, and really soften. Feel the weight of the shoulders sink into the earth. Allow this sensation of softness to flow down the arms. Relax the upper arms, the elbow, and the forearms. Feel the space in the wrist joints. Feel the space around each finger and the energy in the palm of each hand.

Bring your awareness to your neck and throat, and release all tension there. Relax your jaw, lips, and tongue; relax your cheeks and eyes and all the muscles around the eyes and deep in the eye sockets; relax your forehead and your scalp. Allow your head to rest heavily on the floor.

Now relax your inner organs. Bring your awareness to the reproductive organs, and either feel or imagine them relaxing. Relax your prostate (if you have one), intestines, and kidneys. Imagine your liver, stomach, and spleen being filled with healing energies. Soften your diaphragm and lungs. Relax your heart. Let your heart become open ... vast ... undefended, and ... smiling.

Release the breath totally: let it be whatever it wants to be. Notice the breath – become aware of the short pauses between each breath. Relax your mind ... notice that the moment between each breath is the moment between thoughts. Enjoy those moments of complete silence and peace; feel this sense of peace growing deeper. Let this feeling of peace fill you; let it fill the space around you; let peace fill the room and beyond, touching everyone and everything.

Coming Out

When the time has come, the teacher is calling you, or your timer has beckoned, begin to return to life by allowing your breath to be deeper, longer. Bring some movement to your fingers and toes while you roll your head from side to side. Take a moment to move your wrists and ankles in circles: circle in both directions to stimulate energy flow again. When you are ready, hug your knees to your chest in preparation for making the body small and round. Take a deep inhalation, and on the exhalation bring your head and knees together, and squeeze. Make yourself as small and as round as you can – as small as a ten-pound turkey.[240] Release.

---

[240] Of course, being a yogi, this would be a tofu turkey.

Wake up by stretching out the whole body – this is a natural energizer, one that many people have forgotten to do when they wake up in the morning. Move any supports away, and stretch your legs out and arms over your head. Interlock your fingers and turn the palms away from you. Press your lower back down; flex your toes toward your nose. Now take a huge inhalation, fill your lungs – and stretch. Make yourself as long as possible; contract all your facial muscles, and make your face as small as possible. Push and pull yourself longer. Then release with a loud sighing "haaah."

Once more, flex the toes, flatten your lower back, and take a big inhalation. Stretch your body. This time, open your face, mouth, and eyes, as wide as you can; stick your tongue out; touch your chin – stretch! Reach! Exhale, and relax with a sigh.

Hug your knees once more into your chest, and roll to your left side; pause there a moment, and let the energy settle. Stretch out your bottom arm under your head, and use it as a pillow: enjoy how this feels.[241]

Don't linger too long here; coming back to life is like being reincarnated. Don't stay in the bardo state between Shavasana (your little death) and rebirth too long, or you may decide to stay there forever. When you are ready, spiral up to sitting and prepare for your final meditation or pranayama practice. If you still feel that you are not quite back to normal, you may want to end your practice with alternate nostril breathing to fully balance your energies.[242]

---

[241] Often teachers will ask students to end the class by lying on their right side to relax the heart. This is a great suggestion for ending a yang class. Lying on the right side helps to open the left nostril, due to a sinus reflex. However, the left nostril is the yin channel. After ninety minutes or so of yin practice, it is nice to balance the body by lying on the left side, allowing the right nostril, the yang channel, to open.

[242] See the section on Nadi Shodana to learn how to do alternate nostril breathing.

Shoelace

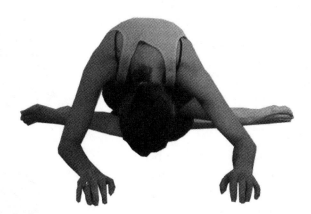

Benefits:
- A great hip opener, as well as decompression for the lower spine when folding forward.

Contraindications:
- Seated forward bends are the hard on the pelvis and knees – they can aggravate sciatica. If a student has this condition, elevate the hips so the knees are below the hips. Beware of hips rotating backward while seated – we want the hips to rotate forward;
- Pregnant women should not fold forward after the first trimester.

Alternatives & Options:
- If hips are tight, sit on a bolster to tilt the hips forward;
- If knees complain at all, the student can do the pose with the bottom leg straight. If that is still too hard, sit cross-legged and fold forward;
- Support the chest with bolster;
- Could support the head with the hands;

- Hands can be to the side or in front of the body, or stretch the arms back behind the body;
- Can rest elbows on a bolster;
- If sensations are too intense in the hips or the knees, remain upright, or take more weight into the hands and arms;
- Side bends or twists can be added here, which work the Gall Bladder meridian along sides of the torso;
- Other alternatives include Eye-of-the-Needle Pose,[243] Square Pose, or Swan.

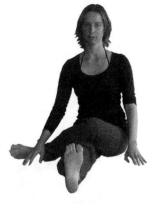

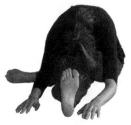

Meridians & Organs Affected:

- Liver and Kidney because these lines come through the inner groin, plus the Gall Bladder on outer legs. If folding forward, the Urinary Bladder line is stimulated and the stomach compressed.

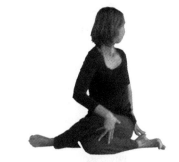

Joints Affected:

- Hips and lower spine.

Hold for How Long?

- Three to five minutes per side;

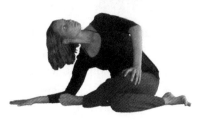

- Could do the first half of the time in a variation like side bend, or twist, and then fold forward for the remaining time.

---

[243] Lying on your back, cradle your shin in your arms.

Counterposes?

- Windshield Wipers lying down or sitting (to provide an internal rotation of the leg);
- Deer Pose;
- Tabletop (aka Hammock).

Similar to?

- Cowface (Gomukasana).

Other Notes:

- It is nice to follow this with the Swan or the Sleeping Swan, before doing other side;
- Could also do a sitting twist afterward;
- Start with most open hip first – whichever hip is more open, place that knee on top. This allows the energy to flow more easily, and aids in opening the tighter side;
- Keep weight back into sitting bones when you come forward – don't let the weight move into the knees;
- Keep hips even. There is a tendency for the top hip to be pulled forward.

Snail

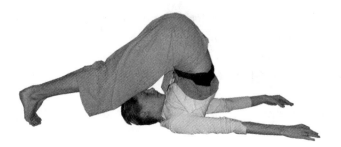

Benefits:

- One of the deepest releases of the whole spine;
- Compresses the internal organs, giving them a great massage.

Contraindications:

- This pose puts a lot of pressure on the neck; be cautious! Avoid if you have any neck problems;
- Because this is an inverted posture, this is not recommended for anyone with high blood pressure, upper body infection, vertigo, glaucoma, or suffering from a cold, or for women during their moon cycle;
- Do not do this posture if you have recently eaten or are pregnant.

Alternatives & Options:

- There are many intermediate stages to this pose. For beginners, or those not wishing to invert, replace this pose with a seated, straight leg, forward fold (such as the Caterpillar);

- There are three stages to the posture:

  1) Support the back with the palms;

  2) More challenging (but not shown) is to place palms under the feet, lowering feet to the floor, or rest the feet on a bolster;

  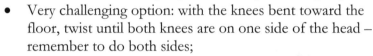

  3) Most challenging is to have the knees bent toward the floor (deepest rounding for the spine);

- Very challenging option: with the knees bent toward the floor, twist until both knees are on one side of the head – remember to do both sides;

- If legs are straight and the feet are touching the floor, the hands can come to the floor behind the back. Hands can be apart (easier) or

  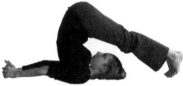

  together (if there are no shoulder problems), but be careful here; bringing the hands together could aggravate rotator cuff problems.

Meridians & Organs Affected:

- All internal organs are massaged and compressed. Each breath adds to the massage;
- Urinary Bladder lines are deeply stretched.

Joints Affected:

- The full spine.

Hold for How Long?

- Three to five minutes.

Counterposes?

- After coming out, lie down for a few breaths;
- Windshield Wipers, then a gentle back bend, such as lying on the stomach, or a mild spinal lift, coming up halfway only;
- A gentle fish, to release the neck (if the neck feels weak or tweaked, do an upward facing Cat);
- Child's Pose.

Similar to?

- Halasana (Plough) or Karnapidasana (Resting Pose or Ear Pressure Pose).

Other Notes:

- Because this is a deep forward bend, prepare the neck first by doing gentle forward neck bends;
- A nice alternative is Happy Baby;
- Unlike in the yang postures, we allow the spine to fully round. Do not try to keep the spine straight and the hips high;
- When coming out, you may hold hips with hands and roll out;
- You may let the chin stay on the chest, and let the head lift up as you roll out, and then support your head with the hands, and slowly lower the head down to the floor.

Sphinx & Seal

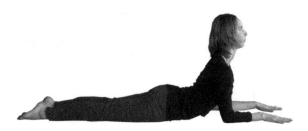

Benefits:

- This can be a very deep compression and stimulation of the sacral-lumbar arch;[244]
- The spine is toned;
- If the neck is dropped back, the thyroid is also stimulated.

Contraindications:

- Bad back, tight sacrum;
- Any sharp pain here, you must come out!
- Avoid pressing the belly into the floor if the student is pregnant (just do the Seal, not the Sphinx);
- Avoid if the student has a headache.

Alternatives & Options:

- For a gentle Sphinx, rest on the ribs, sliding the elbows away to reduce compression in lower back;
- Could use bolsters under the elbows, helping to elevate the chest and deepen the posture;

---

[244] Between the L2 and L3 is found the "Door of Life," where Jing energy is housed.

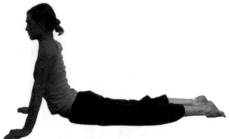

- Seal with straight, locked arms is the deepest pose; let the hands rotate outward a little. Student can slide hands away to lessen the intensity;
- Some students may feel the highest amount of compression in the lower back occurs if hands are not right under the shoulders, but slightly forward. This provides some pressure backward, into the lower back;
- Rather than have the arms in front, Paulie Zink likes to have the hands and arms straight out to the side, which makes this look more like a seal;
- Bend the knees for more compression in the sacrum;
- Some students like to spread legs apart, to deepen the sensations in the lower back;
- Other students prefer the legs together, to release the sacrum or make the sensations more even along the spine;
- Can place a bolster or blanket under pubic bone, to soften the pressure;
- Tightening the butt is okay! Sagging the shoulders is also okay;
- To arch the neck and stimulate the cervical spine, lengthen the neck, drop the head back, lift the chin, and open the throat;
- Flexies can try these postures with the legs in lotus.

Meridians & Organs Affected:

- Affects the Urinary Bladder and Kidney lines as they run through the lower back and sacrum;
- Affects the Stomach and Spleen meridians along top of legs;
- Iyengar notes that this stimulates the kidneys and adrenals through compression.

Joints Affected:

- Lower spine and the neck (if dropped back).

Hold for How Long?

- One minute, then lower down, rest, and repeat several times or;
- Up to five minutes;
- Eventually up for twenty minutes!

Counterposes?

- Coming out, just lie on the stomach, which is still a gentle back bend. Students could slide one bent knee up beside the chest to ease residual sensations;
- Cat's Breath: flow from the Upward Facing Cat to the Downward Facing Cat (aka Cat/Cow) but flow gently, in time with the breath. Don't make these your deepest Cats ever;
- Child's Pose: move into it slowly. Some folks may need to rest the head on the palms.

Similar to?

- Sphinx and/or Cobra.

Other Notes:

- Imagine the spine like a row of Christmas tree lights draping to the floor;
- If arms are straight, this pose is a deeper back bend than the Saddle; thus, this could be done after Saddle. If the arms are bent (as in Sphinx), this is not as deep as Saddle, so it may be done first;
- The Seal is nice and safe for pregnant students;
- Great pose for watching television!

Square

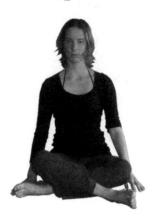

Benefits:

- Nice preparation for Lotus Pose;
- A deep opening of the hips, through strong external rotation;
- Decompresses the lower back, when folding forward.

Contraindications:

- Watch the pressure on the knees; if the hips are too tight, the pressure will go there.

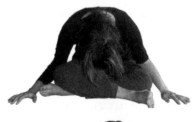

Alternatives & Options:

- Folding forward stretches the lower back and can intensify the stress in the hips. If the lower back rounds a lot, sit on cushion;
- A deeper option is to place one ankle over the opposite knee, and the other ankle under its opposite knee. But, if first knee is very high in the air, bring that foot to the floor in front of its opposite knee;

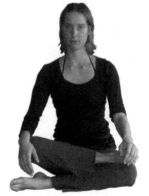

- More flexible students can try to slide knees closer together, allowing the feet go farther apart;
- Tight students, or anyone who experiences discomfort in the knees and if the knees are high off the floor, can place blankets or support under the knees;
- Other alternatives include Eye-of-the-Needle Pose, Shoelace, or Swan.

Meridians & Organs Affected:

- Liver and Kidneys, because these lines come through the inner groin; Gall Bladder line on outer leg; Urinary Bladder line if folding forward.

Joints Affected:

- Hips and spine.

Hold for How Long?

- Three to five minutes per side.

Counterposes?

- Deer, Windshield Wipers, Spinal Lifts.

Similar to?

- Double Pigeon.

Other Notes:

- Beginners tend to bring feet too close to groin: make sure this isn't simply a cross-legged sitting posture – we want to feel this in the hips.

Squat

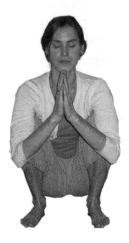

Benefits:

- Opens the hips and strengthens the ankles;
- Releases the lower back;
- Iyengar claims women suffering severe lower back pain, due to their moon cycle, will obtain relief.

Contraindications:

- If hips are too tight, this can torque the knees. Students with knee trauma should avoid this pose.

Alternatives & Options:

- If heels are raised, use a folded blanket or bolster under them – we want the body to relax;
- Can also widen the distance between the feet;
- Watch where the knees are pointing compared to where the feet are pointing – the knees should point in same direction as the feet. If not, spread the feet wider, or rest the heels on a folded blanket or on a bolster;

- A deep variation is to keep feet together with the knees wide apart and lean forward, wrapping arms behind the back, clasping the hands together;
- Another option is to place hands behind the head, and gently draw the chin to chest: this will add a stretch to the back of the neck.

Meridians & Organs Affected:

- The Liver and Kidney lines as they run through the groin and the Urinary Bladder lines on the back.

Joints Affected:

- Hips, knees, and ankles.

Hold for How Long?

- Two to three minutes at one time. However, you can revisit this pose a couple of times during the practice.

Counterposes?

- Dangling to release the knees and back;
- Ankle stretch or Vajrasana.[245]

Similar to?

- Malasana.

Other Notes:

- Elbows in front of knees can be used as levers to pull the chest forward, allowing tailbone to drop lower.

---

[245] In Vajrasana, keep the knees together and sit on the heels.

Swan

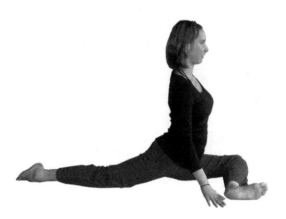

Benefits:
- A vigorous way to open the hips, allowing gravity to do the work. This is a strong external rotation of front hip (especially in the image shown). Will also provide a quadricep and hip flexor stretch for the side that has the leg back;
- A moderate to strong back bend, compressing the lower back;
- Iyengar claims this posture can control sexual desires due to lots of blood flowing through the pubic region.[246]

Contraindications:
- If you have bad knees (especially any problems with the inner meniscus), watch the pressure there; if hips are too tight, that is where the pressure will be. If this happens, bring the front foot back, more towards or under that hip.

Alternatives & Options:
- To protect the front knee, keep the front foot flexed;
- Try to move the hands closer to the hips, to increase the weight over the front hip;

---

[246] Recommended for boyfriends?

- Students leaning to one side can place a support, like a folded blanket, under the bent knee's hip to center themselves;
- Really flexible students may try to bring front foot forward parallel to the front of their mat and slide the bent knee more to the side: bring the foot beneath the sternum if possible;
- Other alternatives include Eye-of-the-Needle Pose, Shoelace, or Sleeping Swan. Could also do the Eye-of-the-Needle against a wall with the foot and buttocks touching the wall.

Meridians & Organs Affected:

- Liver and Kidney lines because these lines come through the inner groin; the Stomach and Spleen meridians (from the line on the top of the back leg); the Gall Bladder line on outer leg and the Urinary Bladder line through lumbar arch.

Joints Affected:

- Hips and lower back … make sure that the knees are NOT complaining!

Hold for How Long?

- This is a moderately yang posture, when chest is raised – hold one to three minutes.

Counterposes?

- Windshield Wipers (sitting or lying);
- Child's Pose;
- Quick Down Dog.

Similar to?

- Proud Pigeon (Rajakapotasana).

Other Notes:

- Come into the full Swan from the Sleeping Swan by walking hands back toward the hips;
- This is a deeper hip opener than the Sleeping Swan, due to more weight placed right above the front hip;
- A gentle back bend, but it can be deepened for really flexible students by raising arms overhead, or clasping hands behind the lower back and pulling them toward the floor;
- Classically, this is followed in the yang style by Down Dog, and this could be done here too if Down Dog is not held too long;
- The "Screaming Pigeon" is really a yang pose, but it can be tried at the end because those muscles won't interfere with the joints being targeted. Reach the hand of the same side as the back leg to that heel, and pull the heel to the buttocks.[247]

---

[247] Or until the screaming starts.

Sleeping Swan

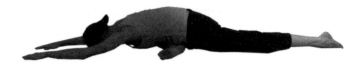

Benefits:

- A relaxing way to gently open the hips.

Contraindications:

- If you have bad knees (especially any problems with the inner meniscus), watch the pressure there; if hips are too tight, that is where the pressure will be. If this happens, bring the front foot back, more towards or under that hip.

Alternatives & Options:

- To protect the front knee, keep the foot flexed before coming forward;
- Keep the weight back into the hips as you come lower;
- Stay on the hands with arms straight, or come on to the elbows;
- Could lie on a bolster placed lengthwise under the chest;
- Students leaning to one side can place a support, like a folded blanket, under the bent knee's hip to center themselves;
- To increase the effect of gravity, you could tuck the back toes under and lift the knee off the floor, pulling the heel backward;
- Really flexible students may try to bring front foot forward, pull bent knee more to the side and lay chest on top of shin;
- An alternative is Eye-of-the-Needle Pose.

Meridians & Organs Affected:
- Liver and Kidney lines because these lines come through the inner groin; the Stomach and Spleen meridians (from the line on the top of the back leg); the Gall Bladder line on outer leg.

Joints Affected:
- Hips ... make sure the knees are NOT complaining!

Hold for How Long?
- Three to five minutes per side.

Counterposes?
- Reclining Windshield Wipers;
- Mild Spinal Lift or Supported Bridge Pose.

Similar to?
- Sleeping Pigeon.

Other Notes:
- Nice to do between sides of Shoelace;
- Can combine with full Swan, which adds a back bend as well;
- Another option is to skip this pose and do Eye-of-the-Needle while lying on back. This reduces gravity's effect and requires more upper body strength, but isn't so deep;
- The full Swan creates a lot of tension in the hip joint: the Sleeping Swan has less. The student can find a tolerable compromise position somewhere between the two extremes by remaining on her elbows or hands. Lying straight down is not the deepest version of this pose, but it is the most relaxing for most students;
- Sometimes a subtle adjustment of the legs can increase the sensation in the front hip, and reduce the stretch in the quadriceps of the back leg.

Toe Squat

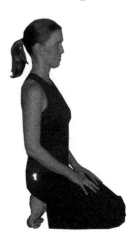

Benefits:

- Open the toes and feet and strengthens the ankles;
- The six lower body meridians begin or end in the toes: this pose stimulates all six lines.

Contraindications:

- Sitting on the heels may strain the knees;
- If ankles or toe joints are very tight, don't stay here long.

Alternatives & Options:

- Make sure toes are tucked under (including the little toes), and ensure that you are not resting on the tips of the toes: be on the balls of the feet;
- If the pose becomes too challenging, come up onto the knees, relieving most of the pressure on the toe joints;
- Don't stay if in pain;
- Can combine this posture with shoulder exercises, like Eagle arms or Cow Face arms;

- If the knees are uncomfortable, place a blanket under them, or place a cushion between the hips and the heels. Some students enjoy a rolled up towel behind the knees, which helps to release the knee joint.

Meridians & Organs Affected:

- All the meridians of the lower body get stimulated through the compression in the toes;
- The front of the ankle also becomes compressed helping to open the Spleen, Liver, Stomach, and Gall Bladder lines.

Joints Affected:

- Toes and ankles.

Hold for How Long?

- Two to three minutes.

Counterposes?

- Ankle Stretch or Child's Pose, or any pose that opens the ankles, such as Saddle.

Similar to?

- Seiza or Vajrasana, but with the toes tucked under.

Other Notes:

- This pose can become quite intense for most people fairly quickly – monitor the level of intensity. It is better *not* to stay in the pose if you are in pain;
- If doing shoulder work while holding the pose, take a break between sides. Do an Ankle Stretch, and then come back into the Toe Stretch and resume the shoulder work on the other side.

Chapter Fourteen:
Yang Counterposes and Yin Flows

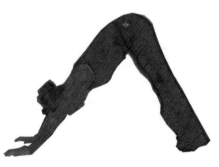

Between yin poses many teachers suggest a bit of yang movement. This feels nice and stimulates the flow of energy in the body before the next posture. Remember, you can do too much of anything. Too much yang leads to exhaustion and depletion – too much yin, however, leads to stagnation. Some yang between the postures helps keep stagnation from developing. Choose whatever yang movements would feel nice: let your body decide or pick something from the list below.

This list is not exhaustive and it is not the intention during this journey to understand yang asanas. You may have to find a teacher to offer you more yang options or more details on the postures suggested.

- Boat – while sitting, extend legs out in front of you and up in the air, holding the back of the legs, or for more challenge, extend the arms forward.
- Cat's breath – flowing from Upward Facing Cat to Downward Facing Cat.
- Crocodile – like a push-up but on elbows/forearms and held for a minute or less.
- Down dog and all its variations.

- Eye-of-the-needle – lie on your back with knees bent. Place the right ankle on the left knee. Reach the right hand through the triangular "window" formed by right leg and clasp the left hand on the top of the left knee (or underneath the knee if on top is not achievable). Pull the knee and ankle toward your left shoulder until you feel the stretch in the right hip. Remember to do both sides.

- Fish – but make it a gentle fish, sometimes done with legs in butterfly. Place your straight arms under your back as you lie down; hands can be right under the buttocks and elbows as close together as possible. Bend the elbows as you lift your chest. Relax the top of your head to the floor and rest on it gently.

- Hinge – while lying on your back, raise and lower the legs; knees bent is easiest, straight legs is harder. To support the back, place your hands, with palms down, under your buttocks.

- Locusts (aka Infant) – lie on your stomach and lift your arms, chest and legs up.

- Lie on your back and hug the knees to the chest and rock from side to side.

- Plank – full push-ups or hover above the floor in Chaturanga. For Chaturanga do the full push-up but lower a few inches toward the floor. Make sure you don't sink into the shoulders or let your hips sag. Your shoulders should not be lower than your elbows. You should be able to see your toes!

- Sun Salutations (recommended only at the end of a practice and done for at least ten minutes).

- Tabletop (also known as Hammock) or Slide – with hands behind you on the floor, lift your hips up. Feet can be on the floor with legs bent or legs straight (having the legs straight turns this into the Slide). Flow into this one by raising hips and lowering hips with the breath (up on inhale/down on exhale). After three or four cycles, hold the position for three or four breaths.

- Windshield wipers – sit with hands behind you on the floor and feet apart, drop knees from side to side. Can be done lying down too.

Sarah Powers and Paul Grilley have many excellent yang exercises you can choose from; check out their DVDs or Paul's book for more suggestions.

Yang movements between yin postures should be brief. If each style is performed for a long period (say over five minutes), the body can be confused by the constant shifting from yin mode to yang mode. If you want to include a lot of yang postures during a yin practice, group the yang asanas into a large segment of time. Allow at least fifteen minutes of constant yang practice or at least fifteen minutes of yin practice to unfold at the same time. Do not keep switching back and forth more quickly than that. Keep the yang counterposes brief between the yin postures.

Flowing

Knowing what the asanas are does not create a yoga practice. Before you attempt Yin Yoga you may want to consider why you are practicing and how you will practice. There are three things you could think about before hitting your mat:

1. How to begin the practice
2. How to choose the asanas and sequence them together
3. How to end the practice

We will visit each topic in turn. Once you have answers to these three questions, you can begin to flow. In fact, that is what the practice is often called: the flow. Learning how to create your own flows can be quite fun and rewarding, but it can also take a lot of experience to structure flows optimally. We will provide several example flows designed for specific themes or intentions. You can also find several well-designed, yin-style flows in the following sources:

> Biff Mithoefer's The Yin Yoga Kit
> Bryan Kest's CD *Long, Slow & Deep – Live Bootleg*
> Marla Ericksen's Yoga Inspired Functional Fitness
> Paul Grilley's book *Yin Yoga*
> Paul Grilley's DVD *Yin Yoga*
> Sarah Powers' DVDs – *Insight Yoga* and *Yin & Vinyasa Yoga*
> Sarah Powers' audio CD *Yin Yoga*
> Shiva Rea's DVD *Lunar Flow Yoga*

Now, let's go with the flow!

Beginning the Practice

Many students, faced with the challenge of practicing yoga at home, are defeated before they even begin. They feel overwhelmed by the possibilities of what they could do and are not sure how to proceed. Beginning teachers face the same quandary; what do I do to get started well? To reduce the size of this problem it is helpful to think, before you even start your practice, about your intention. Once you have your intention clear in your mind it becomes easy to choose the asanas you will do. We looked at choosing asanas in the previous chapter. Now let's look at intention.

Intention

Why are you going to do yoga today? You may never have asked yourself this question, and yet you still feel driven to practice. Why? There are no wrong answers to this question: anything 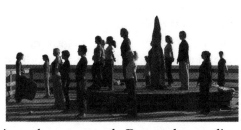 that brings you to your mat is to be respected. But understanding your inner drive will help you focus on your goal.

Reminding yourself of the reason you are doing yoga throughout your practice will help you achieve your purpose. For some students, the reason for doing yoga is to gain health. If this is your reason, remind yourself to feel your state of health as you practice, feel the healing energies flowing through you. You will heal faster when you remember this intention.

For others, the purpose of their practice is to strengthen the body or open it up. Maybe your intention today is to work on opening those stubborn hips. Perhaps in your yang practice you have gotten stuck in some pose, and no further progress has been coming. After years of effort in *prasarita-padottanasana*,[248] your head and the floor are still in two different time zones. Maybe your wheel is more like a sausage. What may be holding you back is not the flexibility of your muscles – it may be that your joints and ligaments are too tight. So your intention today may be to work deeply into those areas.

Perhaps you are going through a very hectic time in your life right now – you need to slow down. Yin Yoga will provide that balance, so that will become your goal today: balance. Some people do their yoga as part of a meditation practice. Many people do it just because they know they will feel better after they are finished. They like it.

---

[248] Wide-legged standing forward fold.

These are all perfectly valid reasons for doing yoga. But there can be more – we can set an intention beyond our own benefit. This can be done at the beginning of each and every practice. Certainly all the other physical, psychological, and emotional benefits will still be there but we can achieve even more than that. Prayer for centuries has been used in the same manner; we dedicate our efforts to a greater purpose than ourselves.

In the yoga texts, this is called "ishvara-pranidhana" – a surrendering of your efforts to something greater than yourself. As you sit or stand at the beginning of your practice, bring to mind someone or something that needs special assistance, attention, or gratitude. Dedicate your efforts during your practice to that person or thing. This dedication fills you with a resolve to actually do the practice with full *attention* along with the *intention*. As you practice, remind yourself why you are practicing. When a challenging time comes up in the practice (and it usually will), you will find the extra strength you need because of your dedication. Higher intentions allow the fruits of your practice to go beyond yourself. Paradoxically, this makes you even stronger, but that is not the point.

Invocation

Making an intention into a dedication is sending your energy outward. Sometimes this is not what you need. Sometimes what you really need ... is to draw energy inward. This can be done through an invocation. Invoking resources and support from outside ourselves is a common way to begin a yoga practice.

Invocations can be as simple as chanting "Om" once or thrice, and allowing the vibration to fill the body, and then linger. Longer chants can also be nice. Chanting is a wonderful form of pranayama, which not only stimulates energy to flow through us, but also has a calming, centering effect on the mind. Ashtangis use the *vande-gurunam* invocation.[249]

---

[249] An excellent rendition of this can be found on Richard Freeman's Web site www.yogaworkshop.com/Reading_details/ philosophy_chant_invocation.html

Many students recite chants from the growing amount of kirtan music available on CDs today, such as those by Deva Premal or Wah! and all the various Das brothers.[250] Deva has a couple of lovely versions of the Gayatri mantra, an invocation of the solar energy, which is recited daily in many India families.[251]

Not all invocations need to be chanted; you can invoke whatever symbols or energies you relate to. Simply ask in your mind for their support, strength, guidance, or whatever it is you feel you need right now. Your practice is your payment in return for this boon.

Meditation

Once you are clear in your mind why you are here today, you are ready to begin. Most beginnings are gentle. A period of meditation is nice. Sit, lie down, or sometimes stand in Mountain Pose – and meditate. Spend three minutes, or more if you are inclined, just to take inventory – note where you are starting from.

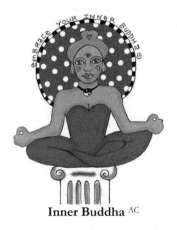

An inner inventory is very grounding. Begin by allowing your awareness to sink into your lower belly. From here notice the rhythm of

Inner Buddha [AC]

your own breath. Feel the rising and falling of each inhalation and exhalation. Do not try to change anything – accept the breath exactly the way it is; just notice it.

To remain focused, you may want to mentally say "in" and "out" with each breath, or note to yourself "rising" and "falling." Some people find it easier to follow the breath by noticing the movement of the air in and out of the body, the feeling of the air in the throat, or on the upper lip. Let your awareness linger wherever it is easier to stay with the sensation of the breath.

---

[250] Krishna Das, Bhagavan Das, …
[251] She has made the words and chords available on her Web site www.devapremal.com/pdfs/satsang_chords_lyrics.pdf.

After a few breaths, allow your awareness to broaden. Notice other feelings in your body: your weight on the floor, the temperature of the air against your skin. You may even choose to allow yourself to simply listen to the sounds around you; listening is a wonderful way to be present. We don't have to do anything to create the sounds; we just let them come to us – sounds from near or far, loud or soft. We just allow them in, without judging them as pleasant or unpleasant.

After a while, we bring our awareness higher, to the heart level. From here we check in with the state of our emotional body. This can be difficult; we are not well trained in our culture to notice or value our emotions. When asked, "What are you feeling right now," most people can't answer. They think they are feeling nothing. This is rarely so, but what is happening is that we are unaware of the state of our heart.

Emotions need not be big, dramatic feelings. Look closely and don't dismiss anything that appears. The emotion may be as small as … boredom. Perhaps there is a little bit of irritation about something that isn't quite to your liking; impatience is a common emotion during our practice. And contentment can also appear from time to time. The key is just to notice what is arising, without judging yourself for whatever is there. Don't criticize yourself for being bored or irritated; don't congratulate yourself for being content. Just notice what is happening right now. Watch it change. Watch it.

After another minute or so, allow your awareness to rise even higher – to that point right between the eyes; feel that point. From here, start to pay attention to the thoughts arising in your head. Don't try to stop the thoughts from coming; that is fruitless. Just watch each new one arise, notice it, and let it float away. Watch the next one come and go. Perhaps it will be helpful to label the thoughts. If so, just use a one- or two-word label such as "planning" or "remembering" or "imagining." Again, don't be judgmental about whatever thoughts do come up – just watch.

Beginning your practice this way is valuable because this is exactly what you will want to do during the asana practice. While you move into, and out of, and hold your postures – keep taking a new inner inventory. Notice how the practice affects you on the physical, emotional, and psychological levels. Accept whatever you find out. Just keep being curious. Begin to move your energy.

Yin Yoga removes the blockages deep in our connective tissues, allowing the Chi or prana to flow unhindered. But before the energy can flow, it has to be stimulated. In a yang practice we use movement to start this flow of energy, but that engages the muscles, which we try to avoid in the yin practice. To get the energy moving in Yin Yoga we can use other techniques. The chapter coming up on Moving Energy gives several ways to begin to move energy without engaging the muscles. If you plan to spend some time stimulating the energy flow, now is an ideal time – right after the opening meditation but before the first yin posture.

Once you have settled in for a few minutes, calmed the mind, and awoken your inner energy you are ready for the first asana. Now, we wonder – which asana comes first?

Sequencing

Are you going to work your spine today? Perhaps your hips are the area of interest. Maybe you want to focus on a particular organ. Is your liver feeling a little stressed from a hard weekend of partying? Knowing what you want to do makes it a lot easier to decide which postures to choose to use. In the section on Asanas you will find the benefits of the poses most commonly practiced in Yin Yoga. Pick out a few key poses that will help the areas you want to focus on and then you will be ready to link them together.

Not all asanas are equal. Before going deep into a back bend you will want to do a gentler back bend to prepare the body. The same advice applies to forward bends or twists. Open the body with easier postures before going to the deeper openings. It is for this reason that all yoga classes begin with warming up the body before the deeper work begins.

In Yin Yoga we are not actually trying to warm up; we want the muscles to remain cool, so that they are not taking up all the stress of the postures. When the muscles are cool, the stretch can go deeper into the connective tissues. But we still want to have a period at the beginning of the practice when we ease into the body. There are a few asanas that work well at the beginning of a practice to get us started.

Beginning Asanas

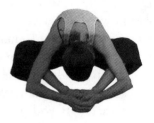

As we just saw, at the start of our practice we want to ease into the body. There are a few excellent beginning postures that we can use to help us open the body gently. These are:

- Butterfly – loosens up the spine for deeper forward bends
- Child's Pose – grounding and soothing
- Caterpillar – loosens up the spine for deeper forward bends
- Dangling – loosens up the spine for deeper forward bends
- Frog (aka Tadpole) – loosens up the hips and upper back
- Sphinx – loosens up the spine for deeper back bends

Each of these postures begins to work a specific area of the body and prepares it for the deeper postures to come. A very flexible student could start her practice with almost any postures if she remembers the first tattva of Yin Yoga: play your edges appropriately. However, there are a few asanas that definitely need preparation before attempting. Even the most flexible students will want to work up to asanas like Snail, the full Seal or the winged Dragon. Before the Snail, loosen up the neck. Before the deepest back bend like the Seal, do a gentler back bend. Before the deepest hip openers, start with milder versions.

Counterposes

In the yang styles of yoga, some sort of counterpose to release the tissues follows every deeply held posture. Counterposes move the body in the opposite direction of the previous pose. This may be as simple as doing the left side after doing the right side of a pose or doing a back bend after a long, deep forward bend. However, the counterpose should never be as deep as the original pose. This is good advice for a yang practice.

In the yin style, counterposes are also recommended; however, they do not need to occur right away. It is nice to do some gentle yang movements between postures to relieve any incipient stagnation and to get the energy flowing again. However, it is not necessary to do a counterpose immediately after any particular asana. Feel free to do all your forward bends before moving into back bends. Do all your hip work before moving on to the counterposes.

Counterposes are very logical. Back bends balance forward bends and vice versa. Right balances left. Internal rotation of the hips balances external rotations. Twists can be used to balance almost any pose involving the spine. By the time you have finished your practice, make sure you have done counterposes for all the deep postures you've held.

Let the body just rest between poses, especially if the pose was a very deep one. Your body will probably overrule any ego-driven urge to quickly move into another, more challenging pose. Respect the body's wishes and take your time between the postures.

Linking Asanas

Many asanas seem to beg to be paired with other asanas; Shoelace seems to flow naturally, organically into the Swan. Twists easily flow from one side to the other. Straddle folding over one leg (aka Dragonfly) easily invites folding over the opposite leg, and then a final fold right down the middle feels very natural.

Some yang poses seem to be made for when we come out of yin poses: Down Dog feels so good after the Swan. And if you never really cared for Down Dog before, after five minutes of playing with the Dragons, you will quickly learn why the Dog is a yogi's best friend. Down Dog after the Dragon can even cure atheism![252]

Shallow postures naturally precede deeper postures. For example, if you want to work on back bends or stimulate the kidneys, you may wish to start with Saddle Pose.[253] After the mild back bend of the Saddle, try the Sphinx for a few minutes. Then move into the Seal.

---

[252] You will sing, "Thank you, Jesus!" for letting you come out! Or maybe you will sing to Moses, Allah, or Shiva!

[253] If your knees allow it and your quadriceps don't make this the hardest pose of all for you.

Finish this sequence with Child's Pose for your forward bending counterpose.

Finishing Asanas

In the yang styles of yoga, the teacher will allow a significant amount of time at the end of the class to cool the body down. Again, in the yin practice this is not necessary. We never warmed the body up, but we still want to find a way back to neutrality, to balance. Any of the beginning asanas could work well at the end of a class, but the pose most often done is the reclining twist. This asana allows the body to fully relax and release. It is one of the most yin-like asanas of all.

The twist in the spine can be directly higher or lower to relieve whatever area was most worked in the practice. Moving the knees higher toward the armpit brings the twist more up the spine by curving the spine forward. Pointing the knees straight away straightens the spine, allowing the twist to be even along its length. Moving the knees downward arches the spine slightly, bringing the emphasis in the twist to the lumbar/sacrum.

Of course, twisting the spine can be done in many orientations. You can do it sitting up as well as lying down. And twisting the spine is not the only way to end your practice; but twisting does restore equilibrium to the nervous system and gets a lot of the residual kinks out of the system.

Other Considerations

For some students, one side of the body is definitely more open than the other side. Erich Schiffmann has a wonderful suggestion – start your asana on the more open side first. Dr. Motoyama agrees with this advice. Your closed side will watch with amazement at what is happening and will be inspired to open that much as well. Of course, if you don't know which side is more open, it really doesn't matter. But make sure you don't do the same side twice. You may end up with a limp. You laugh! But it happens. One way to make sure that doesn't happen to you is to always start with your right side.

That way you will always know that your next side will be the left side.

If you are short of time, do fewer postures instead of holding many poses for less time. It is those last few breaths that give you the most benefit in a pose. It is like that last push-up that strengthens you the most, or that last sugar-filled, creamy doughnut that puts on the most weight. Of course, there are no absolutes, so feel free to do the opposite too; do more poses for shorter holds if you have less time. But shortening the time in the poses moves us away from the real yin nature of the practice. If you have time for only one posture, do the Butterfly.

Finally, be aware of how much time you have allowed for your practice. The opening meditation and poses can take up to fifteen percent of this time, and finishing postures, including Shavasana, may be another fifteen percent or so. That leaves you seventy percent of the time for the key poses you really wanted to get into. Be aware of the time as you flow. Don't shortchange the ending because you got carried away with the fun postures in the middle of the practice. Shavasana is the most important part of the practice, as we will see next.

Ending the Practice

In the above section on sequencing, we looked at a few postures that fit nicely at the end of the practice. While in Yin Yoga we do not need to cool down, we do want to restore the body to neutrality. Once we have completed our last pose, it is time 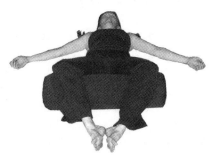 for rest, and then a transition back to the world we left behind. The rest period is called "Shavasana."[254]

There are two parts to any exercise: stressing the body and resting the body. Most teachers, trainers, and students spend a great deal of

---

[254] See Chapter Thirteen: Yin Yoga Asana for details on Shavasana.

time learning how to stress the body in a myriad of ways. And it is fun to do this. Equally important is Shavasana: the relaxation period at the end of the stressing period. Unfortunately, too many students are unaware of the need to balance stress with rest. They may skip their Shavasana, if they are practicing at home or by themselves. Or they may shorten it too much; better to shorten the other asanas and keep the full amount of time available for Shavasana.

Personal trainers know that if we work one area of the body today, we need to let that area recover for at least thirty-six hours or more, depending upon our age and the strength of the workout we just did. Tomorrow, the trainer will work a different area, allowing the first area to get the rest it needs. Rest is essential for optimal performance of the body. When we use an area and let it relax, the body naturally ensures that the area becomes more usable in the future.

Not all forms of rest are equal. One medical study[255] showed that effects of stress were reduced in significantly shorter time by Shavasana than by simply sitting quietly or lying down. Shavasana is an active form of relaxing, which sounds like an oxymoron on the surface, but Shavasana has been proven to be the most effective form of rest possible. Don't skip it!

Balancing Energy

When we have finished our practice, we should feel completely balanced. After Shavasana, or even just before it, some quiet pranayama or energy work is often done. Right after Shavasana you may find yourself in a deep, yin-like altered state. Performing some guided breath work can balance your yin and yang energies, and wake you up again. Nadi Shodana, also called "alternate nostril breathing," is a good way to balance yin and yang energies. Doing a couple of the Pawanmuktasana[256] exercises can also work well. Or, just do a couple of sun salutations to get the blood flowing again.

---

[255] In the October 1998 *Indian Journal of Physiology and Pharmacology.*
[256] See Chapter Fifteen: Moving Energy for this section.

Adverse **Reactions** to Shavasana – A Warning!

Several studies of the relaxation response have shown that, occasionally, relaxation can have adverse effects. These effects range from a feeling of being dissociated from your body or from reality, to feelings of anxiety or panic. Sometimes deeply repressed emotions start to surface. If these start to trouble you, remain calm, and resolve to watch whatever unfolds with the same dispassion with which you were watching the breath during your practice. Practice the A.W.A.K.E.N. process we learned in the first half of our journey. If conditions persist, seek assistance.

For some students, physiological reactions can occur; blood pressure can drop after deep relaxation, and a temporary hypoglycemic state can occur. If you are on medication, deep relaxation may intensify the effect of the drugs. Caution is advised for students taking insulin, sedatives, or cardiovascular medications. Check with your health care professional before beginning a yoga practice if you are on medication.

These occurrences are rare, but it is good to be aware that adverse reactions can happen. Don't be alarmed. If the situation warrants help, seek it.

Ending Meditation

After relaxing and balancing your energy, you may wish to conclude your practice with a brief meditation. This can mirror your opening meditation; you may wish to remind yourself of your intention for the practice and/or conduct an inner inventory once more. Compare the way you feel now, at the end of the practice, with the way you

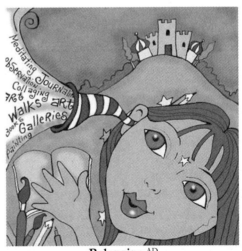

Balancing [AD]

felt at the start. Just note the differences, if any. Do not judge your practice as good or bad; just notice what it was like. And then – let it go.

You may wish to finish your practice with some sort of gesture of completion. Bring your palms together in prayer, leaving a bit of space between the hands to symbolize the space in your heart. Bow down to the floor.

When you rise you may wish to chant something brief. Chanting "Om" will suffice, or you can chant *"Lokah Samasta Sukhino Bhavantu."*[257] Or, simply end with saying *"namaste"* to all the teachers in your life who have guided you.[258]

For some dedicated yogis, the time after Shavasana is the time for a full meditation practice. The body is open and strong. Sitting may feel easier, the heart content. The breath is calm right now. It is a perfect time to train the mind.

Transition to Your Next Activity

When the practice is over, everyday life is waiting for you; don't just jump right back into it – savor the quietness for a while. Whatever your next actions are, do them with mindfulness. Allow this heightened awareness to linger throughout the rest of your day. Notice the openness in your body as you move. Smile often, and pause frequently. Take time to return to awareness; after all, this is what you were practicing – awareness. Enjoy it.

---

[257] Which means, "May all beings everywhere be happy."
[258] Namaste is an acknowledgement of the divinity in you and in others.

Yin Yoga Flows

There are only a couple of dozen Yin Yoga asanas. This is a very small number compared to the many thousands of yang asanas available.[259] The number of yang flows in which all of these asanas can be combined is virtually infinite. Despite the small number of yin postures, the number of possible yin flows can also be quite large, but fortunately not many are needed to work the key areas of the body.

The flows offered in this section are just a small sampling of what is possible, but they do provide a good representation of ways to work the main yin areas of the body. Feel free to experiment with them and change them around. Find out what works for you. There are eight flows offered:

- Three Beginner's Flows
- A Flow for the Hips
- A Flow for the Spine
- A Flow for the Kidneys
- A Flow for the Liver
- A Yin/Yang Fusion Flow

The last flow, the Yin/Yang fusion flow, is a combination of yin and yang poses woven together. There are many ways to create fusion flows. A simple way is to do the first half of your practice in yin mode, and the second half in yang mode. Or vice versa. These are just two individual, but short yoga classes combined together. More complex is to work yin and yang postures in between each other. Saul David Raye conducted the fusion flow offered here during one of his Advanced Thai Yoga Teacher Training classes. You can also experience a much more challenging fusion flow on Bryan Kest's CD *Long, Slow & Deep – Live Bootleg.*

Before doing any of these flows, it is useful to reread the descriptions of the asanas you will be doing, and to check the yang counterposes. These are all found in the section on Asanas.

---

[259] Krishnamacharya's teacher, Ramamohan Brahmachari, was said to have known eight thousand asanas!

Three Beginner's Flows

1) Time: Sixty minutes

This flow is a gentle one. Hold each posture for three minutes. Relax the body in any way that feels comfortable for thirty to sixty seconds between the asanas.

Opening Meditation

Butterfly
Dragonfly: fold over right leg
Dragonfly: fold over left leg
Dragonfly: fold down the middle

Sphinx
Child's Pose
Seal
Child's Pose

Half Shoelace with right leg forward
Half Shoelace with left leg forward
Happy Baby
Reclining Twist on right side
Reclining Twist on left side
Shavasana
Finishing Meditation

The above flow can be extended to ninety minutes by increasing the holds to five minutes per posture.

2) Time: Ninety minutes

Hold these poses for four minutes. This will make this flow more challenging than the first flow. Again relax the body in any way that feels comfortable for thirty to sixty seconds between the asanas.

Opening Meditation

Frog … tadpole for first two minutes
    … full frog for a second two minutes
Child's Pose for one minute
Sphinx
Child's Pose for one minute

Shoelace with right leg on top
Sleeping Swan with right leg back
Shoelace with left leg on top
Sleeping Swan with left leg back

Caterpillar
Dragon cycle with right leg forward:
Baby Dragon for first two minutes
Overstepping Dragon for last two minutes
Down dog for up to one minute
Child's Pose for one minute
Dragon cycle with left leg forward:
Baby Dragon for first two minutes
Overstepping Dragon for last two minutes
Down Dog for up to one minute
Child's Pose for one minute

Reclining Twist on right side
Reclining Twist on left side
Shavasana
Finishing Meditation

3) Time: Ninety minutes

This flow is more in the Paul Grilley style of shorter holds, but with repeated postures. It won't be necessary to relax as long between the postures here, but be guided by what your body is telling you. Notice how the experience of the Butterfly Pose changes each time you come back to it. Use a timer to make sure you are staying in the poses the right amount of time.

Opening Meditation

Butterfly for one minute
Swan with right leg back for one minute
Sleeping Swan for two minutes
Butterfly for one minute
Swan with left leg back for one minute
Sleeping Swan for two minutes
Butterfly for one minute
Dragonfly for three minutes
Butterfly for one minute
Sphinx, or Seal, for three minutes
Child's Pose for one minute

Dragon Cycle: right foot forward – one minute in each position
Baby Dragon
Dragon Flying High
Dragon Flying Low
Down Dog for one minute
Child's Pose for one minute
Dragon Cycle: left foot forward – one minute in each position
Baby Dragon
Dragon Flying High
Dragon Flying Low
Down Dog for one minute

Child's Pose for one minute with knees apart
Frog ... tadpole for two minutes
        ... full frog for two minutes

Child's Pose with knees together for one minute
Anahatasana for three minutes

Half Butterfly[260]
    with right leg straight to the side for three minutes
Hug knees to chest, while sitting, for one minute
Half Butterfly with left leg straight to the side for three minutes
Lie on the back and hug knees to chest for one minute
Twisted Roots on right side for one minute
Twisted Roots on left side for one minute
Shavasana
Finishing Meditation

Flow for the Hips

Time: Ninety minutes

This flow will get deep into the hips' sockets – it may be quite intense. Watch for any emotions that arise during the flow. Don't be alarmed, and don't stop … just watch the ebb and flow of feelings. Rod Stryker once asked his class, "If you have never cried, or laughed, during a yoga class, what are you waiting for?" Naturally, if it is a struggle to stay in the pose, if the body is tightening instead of releasing, you have gone too deep and will need to back off a bit.

Opening Meditation

Child's Pose with knees apart for one minute
Frog … tadpole for two minutes
    … full frog for two minutes
Child's Pose with knees together for one minute

Shoelace with right knee on top for five minutes
Swan with right leg back for one minute

---

[260] Paul Grilley calls this the Half-Frog.

Sleeping Swan for four minutes
Square with right foot in front of left knee for five minutes
Windshield wipers
    or Tabletop for one minute, as the counterpose

Shoelace with left knee on top for five minutes
Swan with left leg back for one minute
Sleeping Swan for four minutes
Square with left foot in front of right knee for five minutes
Windshield Wipers or Tabletop for one minute as counterpose

Sphinx for five minutes with,
    optionally, Seal at some point during this time
Child's Pose for one minute
Saddle for five minutes
Child's Pose for one minute

Dragon Cycle … right leg forward:
    Baby Dragon for one minute
    Dragon Flying High for one minute
    Dragon Flying Low for one minute
    Dragon Wing for one minute
Down Dog for one minute
Dragon Cycle … left leg forward:
    Baby Dragon for one minute
    Dragon Flying High for one minute
    Dragon Flying Low for one minute
    Dragon Wing for one minute
Down Dog for one minute

Twisted Roots on right side for up to three minutes
Twisted Roots on left side for up to three minutes
Shavasana
Finishing Meditation

Flow for the Spine

Time: Ninety minutes

Whenever you work the spine, be alert for any signals of pain; sharp, burning or electrical sensations are indications that you have gone too deep. Come out if you get to that point. Back bends, and long-held forward bends, can become addicting; beware of overdoing back work.[261]

Opening Meditation in standing position

Dangling for three minutes
Squat for three minutes
Dangling for two more minutes
Squat for two more minutes

Dragonfly: fold over right leg for five minutes
Windshield Wipers for one minute
Dragonfly: fold over left leg for five minutes
Windshield Wipers for one minute
Dragonfly: fold through the center for five minutes
Deer for one minute on each side
Caterpillar for five minutes
Tabletop
Sphinx for five minutes
Rest on your stomach or in Child's Pose for one minute
Seal for five minutes
Child's Pose for one minute
Lie on your back and hug knees to chest for one minute

Cat Pulling Its Tail for one minute, each side
Hinge for two minutes with head up,
	or support head with hands behind head

---

[261] If you start to feel achy or experience discomfort in the lower back between your practices, you may be overdoing the yin back bends. If this happens, stop doing them for a while.

Happy Baby for two minutes
Hug knees for one minute
Snail for three to five minutes
Mild Fish or upward facing Cat for a counterpose
Reclining Windshield Wipers for one minute

Reclining Twist on right side
Reclining Twist on left side
Shavasana
Finishing Meditation

Flow for the Kidneys

Time: Ninety minutes

The keys to stimulating energy flow to the kidneys are the Urinary Bladder and Kidney meridians. The Urinary Bladder lines run along the back of the legs and branch into two lines running up each side of the spine. The Kidney lines run along the inside of the legs into the groin, where they combine in the sacrum before rising up inside the body along the line of the spine. This is described in more detail in Chapter Six: The Daoist View of Energy. This flow includes forward and back bends that work these lines very well. Any flow focusing on the spine will be very effective at stimulating and nourishing the kidneys.

Opening Meditation

Butterfly for five minutes
Windshield Wipers for one minute

Dragonfly: fold over right leg for five minutes
Windshield Wipers for one minute
Dragonfly: fold over left leg for five minutes
Windshield Wipers for one minute
Dragonfly: fold through the center for five minutes
Tabletop for one minute

Seal (or Sphinx option) for five minutes
Child's Pose for one minute
Saddle Pose for five minutes
Child's Pose for one minute

Dragon with right leg forward:
    Baby Dragon for one minute
    Overstepping Dragon for one minute
    Dragon Splits for one minute
    Down Dog for one minute
    Child's Pose briefly
    Ankle Stretch for thirty seconds to one minute
Dragon with left leg forward:
    Baby Dragon for one minute
    Overstepping Dragon for one minute
    Dragon Splits for one minute
    Down Dog for one minute
    Child's Pose briefly
    Ankle Stretch for thirty seconds to one minute
Caterpillar for five minutes
Hug knees to chest, while lying down, for one minute
Happy Baby for two minutes:
    Toes to nose variation for one minute
Windshield Wipers lying down:
    knees drop from side to side for one minute

Reclining Twist on right side
Reclining Twist on left side
Shavasana
Finishing Meditation

Flow for the Liver

Time: Ninety minutes

The keys to stimulating energy flow to the liver are the Gall Bladder and Liver meridians. The Gall Bladder lines run along the outside of the leg and the outer hip. From there they zigzag their way up the front and sides of the ribs to the shoulder and face. The Liver lines come along the inside of the ankle, along the inside of the leg, and through the groin before going inside the body toward the liver.

To help activate the Liver and Gallbladder it is useful to activate the Kidneys too. The Kidneys support all the internal organs. The Kidney lines run along the inside of the legs into the groin, where they combine in the sacrum, before rising up inside the body along the line of the spine. This is described in more detail in Chapter Six: The Daoist View of Energy. This flow, and any flows, including hip openers stimulate the Liver and Gall Bladder lines very well.

Opening Meditation

Butterfly for five minutes
Come into Baby Dragon with right foot forward for one minute:
    Move into Twisting Dragon for two minutes
    Step back to Down Dog for one minute
Come into Baby Dragon with left foot forward for one minute:
    Move into Twisting Dragon for two minutes
    Step back to Down Dog for one minute
Dragonfly: fold over right leg for five minutes
Windshield Wipers for one minute
Dragonfly: fold over left leg for five minutes
Windshield Wipers for one minute
Dragonfly: fold through the center for five minutes
Tabletop for one minute

Sphinx (or Seal) for five minutes
Child's Pose for one minute
Sleeping Swan on right side for five minutes
Square on right side for five minutes

Sleeping Swan on left side for five minutes
Square on left side for five minutes

Cat Pulling Its Tail for one minute on each side

Twisted Roots on right side
Twisted Roots on left side
Shavasana
Finishing Meditation

A Yin/Yang Fusion Flow

Time: Ninety minutes

Saul David Raye, a wonderful yoga teacher and Thai Yoga Massage therapist and teacher, channeled this flow. It is a combination of yang and yin movements, which works well with a moderately bright CD playing in the background.[262]

Opening Meditation

Sit in Virasana (on your heels) for three minutes in meditation
Neck release: move your head in circles in time with the breath
    Circle left … one minute
    Circle right … one minute
Shoulder Circles:
    Move your shoulders in circles in time with the breath
    Up, back, and down … one minute
    Reverse directions … one minute
Heart Tapping[263] … one minute
    Use the tips of your fingers and
    tap up and down on your sternum

---

[262] He played Chinmaya Dunster's *Yoga on Sacred Ground* during this flow.
[263] Heart tapping will stimulate the thymus gland as well as open the heart chakra. Do *not* tap on the zyphoid process, that floating bit just below the sternum.

Sitting Side Bends while sitting cross-legged
    Place right hand on floor and left arm up in the air,
        lean to the right for one minute
    Switch sides: left hand to the floor, right arm in the air,
        lean to the left for one minute
Sitting Back Bend
    Place hands behind you,
        keep your knees low or on the floor and
        lift your hips forward/upward for one minute
Butterfly … for three minutes

Come to standing:
Uddiyana Bandha
    With empty lungs draw your lower belly in, up, and under
    your ribs.
Agni Sara
    With empty lungs, slowly pump your stomach in and out.
Pressing the Reset Button
    Make a fist with your right hand and stick out your thumb.
    Hold your right wrist with your left hand, and gently but
    firmly push your right thumb into the navel. Relax the
    stomach on the inhalations and push deeper. If pain occurs,
    stop.
Large Arm Circles … circle the arms in big circles crossing in
front of you.
    Circle in both directions for one minute each.
Hah Breath Drops
    With legs wide apart and bent slightly, raise arms up while
    inhaling deeply and shout "haaah!" as you drop the upper
    body and arms between the legs. Catch the wave and swing
    back up as you inhale, and repeat five times.

Squat for two minutes
Dangling for two minutes with knees very bent:
    chest and thigh together if possible
Squat two more minutes
Dangling two more minutes with legs straighter

Dragon Cycle ... right leg forward:
    Baby Dragon for one minute
    Dragon Flying High for one minute
    Dragon Flying Low for one minute
    Dragon Wing for one minute
Down Dog for one minute
Dragon Cycle ... left leg forward:
    Baby Dragon for one minute
    Dragon Flying High for one minute
    Dragon Flying Low for one minute
    Dragon Wing for one minute

Cat's Breath for one minute:
    Flow from Upward Facing Cat to Downward Facing Cat
        as you breathe
Squat for one minute (it should be much easier this time!)
Dangling for one minute
Roll up in Rag Doll to Mountain Pose (Tadasana)

Step feet apart three feet; turn feet outward
Squat down, lowering hips halfway to the floor,
    arms out to the side for one minute
Hands pull thighs apart for another minute
Side Fold (Parsvottanasana):
    Straighten legs, keep them apart and fold over right leg
        for one minute

Come up through center and fold over left leg for one minute

Wide Leg Squats:
    With feet wide apart, squat as low to the floor as you can go;
    place your hands on the floor. Walk hands and hips to the
    right, keeping feet on the floor if possible (especially the left
    foot). Walk to the left. Switch sides with each breath. After
    one minute, remain on one side for thirty seconds, and then
    go to the other side for thirty seconds.

Frog for three minutes
Reclining Windshield Wipers:
> With knees bent, feet on the floor touching the edges of your
> mat, drop your knees from side to side for one minute
Happy Baby for two minutes, holding both feet
Happy Baby, holding just right foot for one minute:
> Left leg straight on floor
>> (easier is to place left foot on floor with knee bent)
> Switch feet and repeat on the other side

Reclining Windshield Wipers for one minute
Sitting for one minute
Shoelace: right side for three minutes
Shoelace: left side for three minutes
Straighten both legs
Bounce the legs on the floor as fast and as hard as you can, for
one minute.
Bend knees and bounce the feet on floor, for one minute. Go
hard!

Hamsa Breath:
> Hear the word "*ham*" as you inhale and "*sa*" as you exhale.
> Slow the breath down so each inhalation and exhalation takes
> at least four seconds. Do Hamsa for two minutes.

Shavasana for seven or eight minutes
Finishing Meditation

Chapter Fifteen: Moving Energy

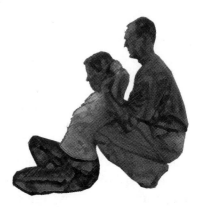

In Chapter Five: The Energy Body we introduced the concept of Chi and prana. Energy, as we defined it in Western terms, is the ability to do work. In Eastern terms, energy is that which provides breath and life. That which provides life is pretty important – without life, the practice of Yin Yoga would not be of too much interest to anybody, and Yin Yoga teachers would be out of work.[264] How to nurture and enhance this life giving energy is worthy of study.

Pranayama is the term often used to describe the practice of regulating our life force. However, pranayama is often used to describe regulating the prana flow by working with the breath. There are other ways to extend, and enhance, the flow of energy. Asana work itself stimulates energy flow. The Daoists invented similar movements as shown in Tai Chi, Qi Gong, and other practices. Massage does the same thing. In Thailand, a combined form of massage and yoga was developed out of the teachings of the Buddha. Thai Yoga Massage includes both practices in a very therapeutic way.

---

[264] In the last Yoga Journal survey very few dead people responded to the question, "Do you do yoga?"

In China, acupuncture and acupressure (which is also a form of massage) have been used for over two thousand years to stimulate Chi flow and remove blockages to its movement.

Just being with certain people can be beneficial for our energy body, while other people can be harmful to your energy health. Unfortunately, we have all experienced people who leave us feeling drained. Ancient masters have warned us to avoid those who are not good for us, and seek out enlightened company to benefit our energies. There are even ways to use our mind, our awareness, to enhance our energy body.

It is beyond the scope of our journey to visit all the myriad ways to free up, stimulate, and enhance energy. We will restrict our investigation to those methodologies most related to a Yin Yoga practice. Specifically we will cover:

Vinyasa ... gentle physical movement to regulate energy
Pranayama ... regulating energy through the breath
Meditation ... harnessing the mind to regulate energy

There is no best time to do energy work. Even though pranayama follows asana in the eight-limbed (ashtanga) methodology of the Yoga Sutra, this was not meant to say that we must do asana before pranayama, nor that we must do pranayama before meditation. These were called limbs (*angas*) for a reason. Just as limbs of a tree are not ordered in any sequence, it is possible to do any of these limbs at any time. It is always a question of what your objective is.

In the Yin Yoga practice, you may choose to stimulate the flow of energy at the beginning of a class, so that when we remove blockages to the flow, the energy can move right away. However, in this case, we may want to choose a way to free up the flow that will not overly warm up the muscles. Mild vinyasa work, or some forms of pranayama, would be good ways to move energy prior to the asana practice. We can equally attempt to move the energy while we are in the poses, or between poses. We could use other pranayama techniques, meditation, or brief yang vinyasas at these times. At the end of an asana practice, meditation is wonderful, but again some forms of pranayama are also excellent for bringing balance back to the body after the long yin emphasis.

There are many options – be creative. Try different ways to move energy and try at different times. See what works best for your body, but please respect the caution at the beginning of this section. Remember that you can do too much of anything. You can overdo a yin practice and become lethargic; you can overdo a yang practice and become exhausted; you can overdo energy development and suffer burnout and other traumas. If you plan to experiment with some of the procedures, go slowly and observe the results carefully. If you start to feel uncomfortable for any reason, stop. If you have any health concerns, do see your health care professional before beginning any energy work.

Vinyasa

Nyasa means "to place." This can refer to a physical placing of the hands in a specific way or a placing of attention to a specific area. *Vi* means "special." So vinyasa means to place in a special way. Often yogis will practice placing mudras in specific places on the body to improve the effectiveness of the mudra.[265] In the context of 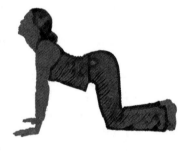 moving energy in the body, we will look at vinyasa as the physical practice of moving the body in a special and specific way.

There are many yang ways to physically stimulate prana to flow through the nadis; sun salutations are very effective and there are many variations to choose from. Full sun salutations are energizing, warming, engaging and wonderful for the muscles. They are very essence of yang: bright, hot, and dynamic. Just before a yin practice, however, they may be too stimulating for the muscles.

Never is never correct and always is always wrong … so there can be times when a vigorous round of sun salutations before a yin

---

[265] As we saw in the first part of our journey, a mudra is a seal or a circle made by the body. Generally it is done with the hands but it can be done with the whole body as well.

practice may be just what you need. An Alaskan morning in mid-December at 20 below may absolutely require it. But in general, the heating of the muscles that occurs in the sun salutation will increase the muscles' ability to absorb all the tension arising from the yin postures. This prevents the stretch from sinking into the deeper connective tissues where we want the tension to reside.

So what do you do when you still want to wake up the body, especially the spine, before beginning your yin practice? There are many vinyasas that will give you the openness you are craving, get your mojo moving, and yet still keep the muscles relatively cool. The moon salutation is one way; the variation offered here will also wake up the hips. If the moon is still too bright for you, other choices could include a mini-sun salutation, the cloud salutation or the least active of all, the Pawanmuktasana series of Swami Satyananda Saraswati. We will view all of these in the next sections.

A Moon Salutation

Everything is relative: the sun is yang relative to the moon. But, the moon is yang relative to the earth. Even the salutations to the moon can be too warming for the muscles at some times. However, on a cold winter morning when the muscles are very stiff and frozen, a few rounds of a moon salutation could be ideal just before a yin practice.

Just as there are dozens of variations of Sun Salutations, there are many versions of Moon Salutations. The offering below is based on the Kripalu tradition as adapted by the Ra-Hoor-Khuit Network. [266] You may find it a great way to prepare the hips for a yin session targeting the liver.

This *Chandra Namaskar* (Moon Salutation) begins in Mountain Pose (Tadasana), just like a Sun Salutation. From there the flow is quite different. Use your breath as the envelope for all movements – begin the breath before you begin the movement and end the movement before you end the breath.

---

[266] Additional information can be found at the Web site www.rahoorkhuit.net/library/yoga/hatha/kripalu.

1. **Anjali Mudra**: Stand in Tadasana. Root your feet, hug your thighs together, and lift your crown to the moon. Press palms together at elbow level in anjali mudra (prayer).

2. **Half Moon**: Lift arms overhead, interlacing fingers, and pointing index fingers upward in temple position. Root left foot and left hip, extending torso and bend to the right. Root right foot and right hip and, extending the torso, come back through center – bending to the left. Root left foot, return to center.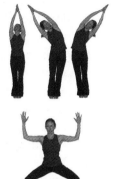

3. **Goddess**: Step to the right and point feet slightly outward. Soften knees and squat, lowering your sitting bones and your bent elbows downward, but raise your hands and fingertips upward.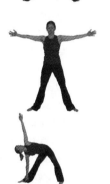

4. **Star**: Root feet and straighten legs, keeping feet wide apart. Hug thighs to the middle and lift your crown skyward. Extend fingertips and arms at shoulder level.

5. **Triangle**: Turn right toes to right, left heel to left, and press hips left, extending torso to right. Lower right hand as you raise left hand.

6. **Pyramid**: Lower both hands toward right foot, folding over the right leg. Rest your hands on leg, foot, or on the floor. Root your feet and tighten your thighs, lifting your kneecaps.

7. **Lunge**: Bend the forward (right) knee, bringing hands to floor on either side of front foot, and lower your back knee to floor (or optionally, keep the knee raised for more challenge). Root the right foot and top of the left foot into the floor.

8. **Wide Leg Squat**: Bring both hands to the inside of the right foot, and lower your tailbone as you pivot the right foot to face forward, rotating the left leg so that toes point upward (more challenging is to point left foot forward). Bring your hands together in anjali mudra. If that is too challenging, keep the palms on the floor.

9. **Squat**: Bring the right leg toward center. Root your feet, lowering your tailbone. If flexibility allows, bring palms together at your heart. If your heels are lifted, don't worry about it; you could try keeping the feet a little wider apart. Keep the knees and feet pointing in the same direction.

10. **Wide Leg Squat**: With hands once again on the floor, extend the left leg to the left. Slide your torso toward the left foot. Bring your hands together in anjali mudra. If that is too challenging, keep the palms on the floor.

11. **Lunge**: Pivot to face the left knee, with hands on either side of the left foot, rotating the right leg and bringing the right knee to floor (or optionally, keep the knee raised for more challenge). Root the left foot and top of the right foot into the floor.

12. **Pyramid**: This time fold over the straightening left leg. Rest your hands on leg, foot, or the floor. Root your feet and tighten your thighs, lifting your kneecaps.

13. **Triangle**: Sweep right arm upward and back, sliding left hand along the left leg toward the ground.

14. **Star**: Bring both arms to shoulder level, turning toes slightly outward. Root feet and straighten legs, keeping feet wide apart. Hug thighs to the middle and lift your crown skyward. Extend fingertips and arms at shoulder level.

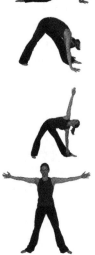

15. **Goddess**: Soften knees and squat, lowering your sitting bones and bend your elbows downward, but raise your hands and fingertips upward.

16. **Half Moon**: Straighten the legs and turn the toes forward. Step the left foot toward the right foot as you lift arms overhead, interlacing fingers and pointing index fingers upward in temple position. Root right foot and right hip, extending torso, and bend to the left. Root left foot and left hip, extending torso, come back through center – bending to the right. Root right foot, returning to center.

17. **Anjali Mudra**: Complete the cycle by coming back to Tadasana. Root your feet, hug your thighs together, and lift your crown to the moon. Press palms together at elbow level in anjali mudra. Repeat the moon salutation as many times as you feel necessary.

If you would like to view another version of a Moon Salutations you can check out Shiva Rea's *Lunar Flow Yoga* DVD. If the Moon Salutations are still a bit too vigorous for you, the mini-Sun Salutation that we are going to visit next may be more suitable.

A Mini-Sun Salutation

There are many variations that can be made to the mini-Sun Salutation flow offered here. After experiencing it once or twice, the student may naturally flow into new versions. The right music can enhance the flowing nature of this vinyasa.[267]

Just as was suggested for the Moon Salutation, when you flow, use the breath as an envelope for the movement. This is great advice for every asana practice: begin the breath, and then begin the movement – end the movement before you end the breath. This way, all your movements are done inside the breath. Watching this is a meditation all by itself.

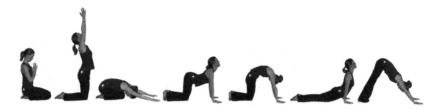

We begin the mini-Sun Salutation in Vajrasana, where we sit on our heels, hands folded in prayer at our heart. From this starting position we will flow in cycles. With each cycle, one new position will be added until the Down Dog is reached. After that, with each cycle one position will be subtracted until you come back to the beginning again. Note: if Vajrasana is not comfortable or possible for you, change your starting position to be the second posture; start from kneeling, and return to, and stop at, kneeling in each cycle.

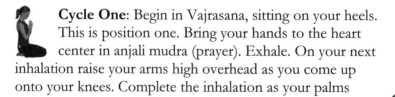

Cycle One: Begin in Vajrasana, sitting on your heels. This is position one. Bring your hands to the heart center in anjali mudra (prayer). Exhale. On your next inhalation raise your arms high overhead as you come up onto your knees. Complete the inhalation as your palms

---

[267] If you would like a very different musical experience, try Pink Floyd's Brain Damage and Eclipse from the *Dark Side of the Moon*. It works! For traditionalists, a wonderful CD to accompany your Yin Yoga practice is *Rosa Mystica* by Theresa Schroeder-Sheker.

touch. This is position two.

As you exhale return back to the starting position, sitting again on your heels with your hands in anjali mudra.

Cycle Two: Sitting on your heels, bring your hands to the heart center in anjali mudra. Exhale. On your next inhalation raise your arms high overhead, as you come up onto your knees. Complete the inhalation as your palms touch. As you exhale, lower your arms to the floor, reaching them way out in front of you while you sit back on your heels. This is the Salaam position (like being in Child's Pose but with your arms extended overhead on the floor). Complete the exhalation here. This is position three.

As you inhale, rise up again to standing on your knees with your arms reaching overhead. This is position three. As you exhale, return to position one.

Cycle Three: Come up to position two on the inhalation. Fold into Salaam, position three, on the exhalation. On the next inhalation, come onto your hands and knees into an Upward Facing Cat. Hide your spine deep into your back, as your tailbone and back of the head try to meet. Allow your belly to melt to the floor, but keep your hands actively rooting into the floor, shoulders high. Your toes may be tucked under to wake up the feet. This is position four.

As you exhale, fold, and sit back into position three, the Salaam. On the inhalation, rise again into position two, standing on knees. On the exhalation, return to Vajrasana, position one.

Cycle Four: Come up to position two on the inhalation. Fold into Salaam, position three, on the exhalation. On the next inhalation, come onto your hands and knees into an Upward Facing Cat, position four. On the exhalation, round your spine in the opposite direction into the Downward Facing Cat. The tailbone tucks under as you drop your chin to the chest. Lift the spine as high as you can, while maintaining the rooting action of the hands and toes. Shoulders remain high. This is position five.

As you inhale, round again into position four, the Upward Facing Cat. As you exhale, fold and sit back into position three, the Salaam. On the inhalation, rise again into position two, standing on knees. On the exhalation, return to Vajrasana, position one.

Cycle Five: Come up to position two on the inhalation. Fold into Salaam, position three, on the exhalation. On the next inhalation, come onto your hands and knees into an Upward Facing Cat, position four. On the exhalation, round your spine in the opposite direction into the Downward Facing Cat, position five. As you inhale, come into a straight-armed Cobra. Let your hips flow forward, as you move the chest up and between the arms. The arms remain straight, and your hips now lower to the ground. Your legs are straight behind you. Toes can remain tucked under or, for more challenge, point the toes away from you. Fill your lungs and open your heart. Look up. This is position six.

As you exhale, come back onto hands and knees into position five, the Downward Facing Cat. As you inhale, drop the spine again into position four, the Upward Facing Cat. As you exhale, fold and sit back into position three, the Salaam. On the inhalation, rise again into position two, standing on knees. On the exhalation, return to Vajrasana, position one.

Cycle Six: Come up to position two on the inhalation. Fold into Salaam, position three, on the exhalation. On the next inhalation, come onto your hands and knees, into an Upward Facing Cat, position four. On the exhalation, round your spine in the opposite direction, into the Downward Facing Cat, position five. As you inhale, come into position six, which is a straight-armed Cobra. Now, on the exhalation, flow into Downward Facing Dog. You may keep your knees bent for the first visit to the Down Dog. Lengthen the arms and the spine and turn the tailbone high in the air. Be a happy puppy – happy dogs always have their tails held high – wag your tail! Root your front paws deep into the earth. Linger here for a few breaths, if you like. Then, exhale completely. This is position seven.

On an inhalation, shift your hips forward, and come back into a straight-armed Cobra, position six. As you exhale, come onto hands and knees into position five, the Downward Facing Cat. As you inhale, drop the spine again into position four, the Upward Facing Cat. As you exhale, fold and sit back into position three, the Salaam. On the inhalation, rise again into position two, standing on knees. On the exhalation, return to Vajrasana, position one.

Repeating Cycle Six: Depending upon how much time you have, you may choose to do three or four more complete mini-Sun Salutation cycles. You can even add some variations to the Down Dog here, like lifting one leg in the air at a time.[268] Or, with a leg raised, bend that knee, and pretend you are a boy dog visiting a tree. On the other side, visit a fire hydrant.

Cycle Seven and beyond:

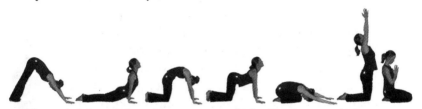

The mini-Sun Salutation now unwinds. Each new cycle removes one posture until we are back to the starting position:

Cycle Seven repeats Cycle Five.
Cycle Eight repeats Cycle Four.
Cycle Nine repeats Cycle Three.
Cycle Ten repeats Cycle Two.
Cycle Eleven repeats Cycle One.
Cycle Twelve … there is no Cycle Twelve … just sit in Vajrasana, close your eyes, and enjoy the feeling of energy flowing.

---

[268] Advanced students can lift both legs at once.

The Cloud Salutation

Any movement of the body releases energy. On some days, the world is shrouded in a damp fog of yin energy: vigorous movement just isn't in the cards. On some days you just want to be a cloud and float. Floating is still moving, and even while floating you can practice awareness. The Cloud Salutation is a wonderful way to move with the flow of life when it is quiet, or when you need to build some quiet into your life.

1.   **Beginning**: Come into mountain pose (Tadasana). Bring your feet together and root them into the earth. Hug your thighs together and lift your crown to the sky. Press palms together at elbow level in anjali mudra (prayer). To help with your balance throughout the flow, focus your eyes at eye level far in front of you on one spot that isn't moving, or at a spot on the floor. Exhale completely, and smile.

2.   **First Movement**: Begin to inhale, and then spread your arms wide like wings, raising them high over your head. Bring your palms together, and reaching as high as you can, complete the inhalation, pause … and smile again.

3.   **Second Movement**: Begin to exhale, and then slowly lower your palms down the center of your body, while at the same time lifting your right knee up to your chest. Empty your lungs as you pause briefly, with your palms just above your knee. Remember to lift the corners of your lips: it is called a smile.[269]

4.   **Third Movement**: Begin the next inhalation, and again spread your arms wide and up to the sky, while you lower your right foot slowly to the floor. Be aware that your foot will want to descend faster than your arms will lift: synchronize the movements so that the hands touch at the same instant your foot

---

[269] A grimace is not a smile.

touches the floor. Complete the inhalation, and pause slightly.

5. **Fourth Movement**: The other side now: begin to exhale, and then slowly draw your palms down the center of your body, while at the same time lifting your left knee up to your chest. Empty your lungs as you pause briefly with your palms just above your knee. This is challenging so keep smiling.

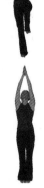

6. **Fifth Movement**: Begin the next inhalation, and then again spread your arms wide and up to the sky, while you lower your left foot slowly to the floor. Again, be aware that this foot will also want to descend faster than your arms will lift. Keep the movements equal. Complete the inhalation, and pause slightly.

That's all there is to this lovely salutation. Keep repeating the flow, alternating sides, and when you are done, return to your mountain; close your eyes, and feel the flow still moving inside you.

When you flow in the Cloud Salutation, move slowly, gracefully, like a cloud floating upon the wind of your breath. Once you have learned the graceful movements of the clouds, you can challenge yourself even more: move like the clouds move, with their eyes closed. Clouds don't look where they are going: they don't even care where they are going – they just go! Keep your breath calm, even if you begin to wobble. If the wobbling becomes too dramatic, open your eyes; come back to the original flow for a few cycles. This flow can become addicting. Enjoy it.

Pawanmuktasana

From the Bihar School in northern India and the great teacher Paramahansa Satyananda come the Pawanmuktasana sequences. This series of exercises is recommended as preparatory work before going into any other asana practice, either yin or yang. The series opens up the joints, relaxes the muscles, and promotes general health.

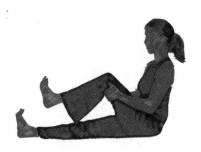

These exercises can be practiced by anyone: young, old, those in good health, and those in poor health. The exercises should be done in a relaxed state of mind; they are actually more mental than physical. As you will discover, these are not challenging postures, but they should be respected due to the great value they bring.[270]

Pawan means wind. *Mukta* means release. *Asana*, of course, means pose or posture. Thus, the Pawanmuktasana sequences are designed to release the flow of energy, and remove any blockages that prevent its free flow in the body, or in the mind. Continued practice of these sequences can prevent new blockages from forming. These movements are excellent for people suffering from rheumatic arthritis, high blood pressure, or for people with heart problems who are advised to avoid vigorous exercise.

Dr. Motoyama, in the book *Theories of the Chakras: Bridge to Higher Consciousness*, suggests that the Pawanmuktasanas be performed before any other asanas. He explains that they are part of the preparatory work of awakening the chakras.

In the book *Asana Pranayama Mudra Bandha* by Swami Satyananda Saraswati, we are given three series of Pawanmuktasanas. Dr. Motoyama basically follows the first of these, with some additional movements. We will be exploring his version in this section; however, interested readers can check out Satyananda's book.[271]

---

[270] The exception may be Crow Walking. You may find that a challenge.
[271] Or visit the Web site
www.healthandyoga.com/html/yoga/asanas/pawanmuktasana1.asp.

Dr. Motoyama recommends, before doing any of the Pawan-muktasana, one should begin with Shavasana. Paul Grilley also suggests this. Shavasana, before asana practice, relaxes the body and allows the energy to be more easily distributed and absorbed. If you are used to doing Shavasana only at the end of your practice, you may want to experiment with doing it at the beginning and the end, and even for a brief time between postures.

While you work your way through these movements, slow down. It is easy to move quickly, because they are so simple. Move with your breath, and breathe with awareness. Watching the breath will slow you down.

Lower Body Pawanmuktasana Sequence

The lower body cycle of Pawanmuktasana sequentially opens the joints, from the toes to the hips. People with poor circulation in the legs will benefit from this simple practice.

1. **Toe Bending**: The six lower body meridians all begin or end in the toes. This simple practice begins to awaken the flow right at the tips of the body. Sit with your legs extended and your hands behind you on the floor. (If you have tight hamstrings or sciatica, sit on a cushion.) Wave your toes back and forth ten times. Move slowly and hold the pose for a few seconds, keeping the ankles relaxed.
2. **Ankle Bending**: Remain with legs straight and flex the feet at the ankles, and then extend them. Move the feet back and forth ten times. We are now beginning to free up the ankle joints, through which all the lower meridians run. Again move slowly, and hold each position for a few seconds.
3. **Ankle Rotation**: Since some meridians run through the side of the ankles, simply bending the ankles doesn't remove all blockages. Now, we circle the ankles.

Keeping the knees from moving, and the feet apart, move the right foot in a circle: ten times in one direction and then ten times in the other direction. Do the same with the left foot. Next, bring the feet together and circle both feet, ten times, with both feet moving in same direction. Switch direction, and do ten more. Finally, separate the feet so the big toes can just touch, and rotate the feet in opposite directions ten times. Then switch and do the reverse direction for each foot ten times.[272]

4. **Ankle Cranking**: A deeper rotation for the ankles comes when they are cranked by hand. Bend the right leg and rest the ankle on the left knee. Use your left hand and take hold of the foot. Rotate the ankle ten times in each 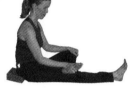 direction. A nice option is to interlace your fingers with the toes and spread them while you crank. Now, do the other ankle.

5. **Knee Bending**: Hold under the right thigh and lift the leg in the air. Alternately straighten, and 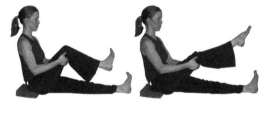 then bend the knee so that the heel comes close to the back of the thigh. Do this ten times. Repeat on the other side.

6. **Half Butterfly**: Rest the right foot on the left thigh, and hold it there with the left hand. Use the right hand to gently bounce the right knee down to the floor and back up. Do this ten times. Eventually you may be able touch the floor, but if you can't, don't be worried about it; you are opening your hip joints. Switch sides and do ten more.

---

[272] There is an old Daoist belief that if you rotate your ankles like this every day, you will never die of a heart attack. Just ask any old Daoist you come across if this is true. Saul David Raye relayed this story, but he isn't old.

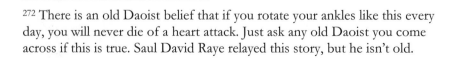

7. **Hip Joint Rotation**: Hold your right foot with your left hand and use your right hand to cradle your right knee. Flex your right foot to help protect the knee. Move the knee in big circles so that you can feel the hip joint being rotated. Do ten times in each direction. Switch sides and repeat.

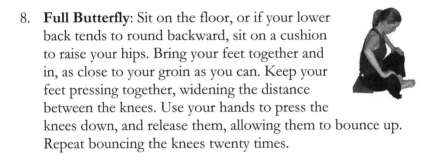

8. **Full Butterfly**: Sit on the floor, or if your lower back tends to round backward, sit on a cushion to raise your hips. Bring your feet together and in, as close to your groin as you can. Keep your feet pressing together, widening the distance between the knees. Use your hands to press the knees down, and release them, allowing them to bounce up. Repeat bouncing the knees twenty times.

9. **Crow Walking**: This is the most challenging action of the series. Squat with your feet either flat on the floor, or stay on your toes if you can't easily get your heels down. Now, keeping your butt near your heels, walk. Do this for a short time. As an option, you can try to touch your knees to the floor with each step. Crow Walking is an excellent preparation for the sitting meditation postures. Dr. Motoyama also mentions that Crow Walking can relieve constipation: drink two glasses of water, walk for a minute, drink another two glasses and walk for another minute. Your constipation should pass if you do this three or four times.

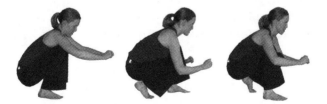

Upper Body Pawanmuktasana Sequence

The upper body cycle of Pawanmuktasana sequentially opens the joints from the fingers to the shoulders. Even if you cannot sense any energetic benefits from the movements, you are benefiting the joints. Fluids often accumulate in the joints, resulting in stagnation, inflammation, and stiffness that can lead to rheumatism and neuralgia. Pawanmuktasana is recommended for people suffering from these conditions because it helps to move the fluids.

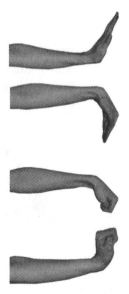

1. **Hand Clenching**: The six upper body meridians begin or end in the tips of the fingers. We will be awakening the flow of energy through these meridians. Sit with your legs extended out in front of you (or if that is uncomfortable, sit cross-legged or sit on a cushion). Extend your arms so that the hands are at shoulder level. Start with the palms open and facing each other. Now, close your hands with your thumbs inside the fist, and reopen them. Do this ten times. You are stimulating the energy at the tips of the fingers. Move slowly, deliberately.

2. **Wrist Bending**: With the arms still straight, open your palms, so they face away from you, fingers pointing up. Next drop the hands, so the fingers are pointing straight down. Wave the hands, ten times keeping the fingers straight. Do not bend the knuckles. You are now removing blockages to energy flow in the wrist joint. Go slowly.

3. **Wrist Rotation**: Begin with the right palm closed into a fist, facing the floor. The thumb should be inside the fist. If your arm is getting tired, support it with the free hand. Rotate the right wrist in a circle ten times in one direction, and then ten times in the other direction. Do the

same with the left wrist. Next, circle both wrists together, ten times in same direction. Switch direction, and do ten more. Finally do this again, but rotate the wrists in opposite directions ten times. Then switch directions, and do it ten more times.

4. **Elbow Bending**: Hold your arms out in front of you with the palms facing up. Bend at the elbows as you inhale, and touch your fingers to your shoulders. As you exhale, extend the arms again. Repeat this ten times. Next, do the same motion, but start with the arms stretched 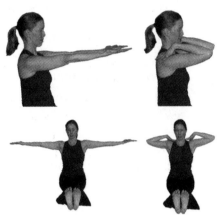 wide to the side. This practice removes blockages found in the elbow joints.

5. **Shoulder Circles**: Hold your right fingertips to the right shoulder, keeping your elbow at the same level as the shoulder. Your left hand rests on the left knee. Move the right elbow in large circles. Inhale as you lift up, and exhale as the elbow descends. Do ten circles in each direction, and then switch arms. After doing each arm individually, bring both hands to the shoulders and slowly trace ten large circles with the arms moving in opposite directions. Try to touch the elbows together as they come in front of you. After ten circles in one direction do ten more in the other direction. You have now opened the shoulder joints.

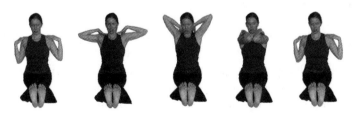

Pranayama

Caution: The performance of pranayama is not a practice to be undertaken casually. There have been many reports of adverse reactions to the practice, and it is always recommended that pranayama be studied only under the guidance of a knowledgeable teacher. For example, people suffering physical ailments, such as high blood pressure, should never forcefully hold their breath. People with psychological problems are similarly advised to avoid the practice, unless being taught by an expert. Hopefully, it is obvious that pranayama is not something that can be learned from a book, or a Web page. Seek personal instruction wherever possible. For more information on precautions before practicing yoga, please check the Before You Practice section.

As we discovered in the section The Yogic View of Energy, pranayama is made up of two words: prana, the ever-present life force, and ayama, which means to extend or release. Often students, and even some teachers, misinterpret this latter word to be yama, which means to restrict or control. Thus pranayama is sometime thought to mean the control, or restriction, of the breath. This confusion is understandable since, even with ayama, there is an element of control of the prana in this practice, but pranayama is not meant to restrict the flow of energy. Quite the contrary; pranayama is the stimulating, freeing, and then channeling of the life force within us.

Guidelines for Practice

Traditionally pranayama is done early in the morning. But, not everyone is a professional yogi, and realistically, getting up at 4 a.m. is not going to happen. Benefits can be obtained from the practice at any time, but it is suggested that you avoid strong, energizing pranayama practice in the evening, or you may find sleep hard to come by. Advanced students may schedule their pranayama practice in the afternoon and just do one long session of only pranayama, without adding any meditation or asana work.

You may wish to plan for your pranayama practice to occur between your asana practice and your meditation practice; however, some teachers use pranayama before the asana practice to help open up the nadis. Certainly, before commencing a Yin Yoga session, this may work well. Sometimes a brief Shavasana is nice as a transition from the pranayama practice to the asana, or meditation practice.

The stomach must be empty. The body should be healthy and free of toxins. This means that if you have been drinking alcohol recently (in the prior few days), or you have been binging on a lot of junk food, you may need to refrain from a serious pranayama session (anything over five minutes in length). Your diet should be pure. Do not practice pranayama when you are ill.

Choose a quiet, clean, uncluttered environment; the great outdoors is wonderful, especially in places that have a high concentration of natural Chi – high in the mountains, beside streams or the ocean, under a special tree. After a rainfall, or early in the morning, the air has more Chi than on a hot, dry afternoon.

Go slowly at first: never strain. The breath is always through the nose, unless otherwise indicated. Side effects that may arise from improper practice could include feelings of heat or coldness, itchiness, tingling sensations, and feelings of lightness or heaviness. If these symptoms continue, stop the practice and seek guidance. In fact, it is best to do pranayama practice under the watchful eye of a knowledgeable teacher.

Once you are ready to proceed with the practice, all that remains is to choose which kind of pranayama you are going to do – that depends on what you want to achieve. You can use pranayama to stimulate and increase energy, or to balance energy. We will look at three particular practices beginning with two energizers.

Kapalabhati and Bhastrika

Three great joys in the West are chocolate, coffee, and sex. In the East – there is no difference! The stimulating effects of all three sensual indulgences are legendary. Even better than chocolate, coffee, and sex is the stimulating effect of *kapalabhati* and *bhastrika*.[273]

Bhastrika

While similar in their nature, kapalabhati and bhastrika are distinct and quite different. Bhastrika is mentioned in the ancient Hatha Yoga texts, such as the Gheranda Samhita. Bhastrika means "bellows." Like a blacksmith trying to increase the flames of his fire, we use bhastrika to fan the flames of *Agni*,[274] the form of prana found in the abdomen.

To perform bhastrika, expand the belly outward, as the lungs fill with air. Now, the flow can begin: take quick strong breaths, actively pumping the air in and out, using your abdomen and diaphragm muscles. Do this pumping for twenty breaths. At the end of the twentieth breath, inhale, and retain the breath via kumbhaka.[275] After retention, release the breath slowly and sit quietly, watching the energy inside. If it feels safe to repeat this, do this whole sequence two more times. If any discomfort has arisen, do not do any more today.

Kumbhaka and Bandhas

Retention should never be forced: when the body needs to breathe again, breathe. You know you have held the breath too long if there is a gasping sound upon release. Another sign is a feeling of heat in the breath as it releases. Retention has a psychological purpose: the mind is still when the breath is still. Enjoy these periods of quiet mind. There is also a physiological benefit to retaining the breath after rapid breathing; it allows the blood chemistry to come back to normal.

When we breathe quickly, we increase the amount of oxygen in the blood, but we deplete the level of carbon dioxide. The body

---

[273] Well, better than sex anyway.

[274] Agni is also the name of the god of fire, who receives burnt sacrifices on behalf of all gods. Agni, in this guise, is the mouth of the gods.

[275] Kumbhaka means "pot": we hold the breath in the pot of the belly.

normally controls these two important levels through two sensing mechanisms,[276] one near the heart and the other in the brain. When we are low on oxygen, the heart sensor eventually notices this, and sends a signal to the body to speed up respiration.[277] If, however, the level of carbon dioxide is too low, the body also responds. A lowering of carbon dioxide affects the blood's acid balance and causes the small blood vessels in the brain to constrict, reducing the amount of oxygen going to this vital area. The sensor in the brain signals the body to slow down the breath, allowing carbon dioxide to build up again.[278]

There are two kinds of retentions of the breath (kumbhaka): the retention of the breath when the lungs are full (antar kumbhaka) and the shorter retention of the breath when the lungs are empty (bahir kumbhaka). These are often accompanied by *bandhas* or bonds[279] to keep the energies in the torso of the body, where they can be most effective. On the antar kumbhaka, the chin is dropped and the chest raised to prevent energy from escaping through the throat.[280] At the same time the perineum is engaged[281] to prevent energy from escaping to the lower body. On the bahir kumbhaka, a third bandha is added to the previous two, forming the *maha bandha* (the great

---

[276] Called chemoreceptors.

[277] There is a lag before the body notices and responds to this drop in oxygen levels in the blood.

[278] An interesting thing occurs at very high altitudes: if the body is not trained to live at high altitudes, the lungs don't get enough oxygen. The heart's chemoreceptor initially orders the body to increase respiration. However, carbon dioxide also is depleted at higher altitudes and by faster respiration. The brain's chemoreceptor orders respiration to slow down, despite the lack of oxygen in the blood. The brain's signals override the heart's signals, and the breath continues to slow down, sometimes to a dangerously, or even deadly low level. In these circumstances, conscious control is required to get enough oxygen into the blood. More information on the physiological affects of pranayama can be found in David Coulter's book *Anatomy of Hatha Yoga*, which every yoga teacher should not just read, but study.

[279] Also called valves, locks, or bridges.

[280] This chin lock is called "*jalandhara bandha*," named after the Hathi Yogi sage Jalandhari.

[281] This is called "*mula bandha*" or "root lock."

lock). This third bandha is performed by drawing the lower belly in, moving the navel to the spine, and lifting the abdomen up and under the ribs.[282] While the stomach is lifting up, consciously lower the diaphragm.

Antar kumbhaka is advised after bhastrika. While holding the chin lock, bring your attention to the ajna chakra, the third eye. After completing one round of twenty breaths and the kumbhaka, without concerns or difficulties, this can be repeated two more times. Again, if any straining is occurring, if irritation arises, a stitch develops … stop.

Kapalabhati

Kapalabhati means shining skull. Don't worry: this doesn't mean you will go bald performing the practice. There are two very different definitions of kapalabhati in the ancient texts. The Gheranda Samhita states that kapalabhati is one of the six cleanses[283], and thus is not a pranayama. In the Hatha Yoga Pradipika, kapalabhati is a breath exercise similar to bhastrika. This is the version we will look at.

Normally when we inhale, the diaphragm is active and lower than its resting position – we use muscular effort to draw in the breath. Exhaling is a passive relaxation of the diaphragm, which rises back to its shortened position just under the lungs, forcing air out. In kapalabhati this is all reversed; we actively exhale, and the rebounding effect results in a passive inhalation.

To do kapalabhati requires the stomach to be extended at the top of the inhalation, and drawn in at the end of the exhalation. This is not easy for many people. When we are born, our natural breathing rhythm is like this: watch a baby breathing while lying on her back – her belly rises on inhalation and lowers on exhalation. This natural movement is very healthy; each breath brings the diaphragm down onto the liver and stomach, compressing the abdominal organs. Each breath is a healthy massage. Unfortunately, almost one half of all people lose this natural breathing action and either reverse the movement of the stomach, or don't move the stomach at all when

---

[282] This is called "*uddiyana bandha*," which means the upward flying bridge.
[283] Called the "*shat kariyas*."

they breathe – instead, they move only the ribs (which is a much shallower movement). This deprives the organs of a regular massage sessions, and also restricts the amount of air that is drawn into the lungs.

If you are a belly breather, kapalabhati will be easy to start. If you are not, you will struggle with this practice. In either case, a beginner will find this much easier if she places one hand on her belly as she breathes. Focus on making a sharp inward movement with each exhalation. After the exhalation, relax the stomach and allow a passive intake of breath to happen. Go slowly until you can find a smooth rhythm. Sharply exhale through the nose, as if you had a mosquito stuck in there and you want to blow it out. Relax all your other muscles. Often beginners will contract and contort their whole body trying to get this exercise. You do not need to clench the facial muscles or jerk the torso; slow down and be more deliberate.

Do about thirty breaths, finish with a deep inhalation, and then exhale completely, bowing forward, squeezing the navel to the spine. Retain the breath on empty lungs, and straighten the body, engaging all three bandhas, performing the maha bandha. Bring your awareness to the muladhara chakra, the perineum. With lungs empty, you will not be able to retain the breath as long as when the lungs are full. Don't worry about it. When you need to breathe, breathe. If you have to gasp as you release, you are holding too long. After releasing, sit quietly and watch the energy inside. If you feel able, repeat this two more times.

Nadi Shodhana

Nadi means little river, and, as we have seen earlier in our journey, it refers to the channels through which prana flows. Nadis are equivalent to the meridians. *Shodhana* means purification. Thus, nadi shodhana is a cleansing of the energy passages. Other names for this practice are alternate nostril breathing or *anuloma viloma*.[284] The practice not only cleanses the nadis, it balances the energies on both sides of the body.

---

[284] Which means "against the grain."

The hand position is unique for nadi shodhana. The right hand is used, and the middle two fingers are either folded down to the palm or extended so they can rest on the spot between the eyebrows. The right thumb is used to press in on the right side of the nose, closing that nostril. The little finger and ring fingers are kept together, and are used to close the left nostril. Since the right arm will be kept lifted up during the practice, it may get heavy – students can use the left hand to support the right arm.

Basic Pattern

We begin with the left side: exhale, and then use the right thumb to press against the right nostril, closing it. Now inhale for a count of four through the left nostril, then release the right side while closing the left side, and exhale for a count of four. Complete the cycle by inhaling on the right side, close it and open the left side then exhale. Continue with a four count for eight to twelve cycles. When finished, sit quietly.

Adding Kumbhaka and Lengthening the Exhalation

A more advanced version of nadi shodhana keeps the same inhalation timing, but extends the exhalation for eight counts. When this is mastered, you may wish to add retentions. Between the inhalation and the exhalation, pinch both sides of the nose closed, and retain the breath for four counts. This is antar kumbhaka: retention with lungs full. As you gain experience, you may add bahir kumbhaka at the end of the exhalation, also for four counts.

More advanced, extended nadi shodhana practices are available after a few months of practice with these simple variations, if you experience no difficulties or side effects.

Extended Patterns

When the basic pattern of nadi shodhana is comfortable, the student can change the ratios of inhalations to exhalations. Initially the ratios are 1:1 – four count inhale: four count exhale or 1:2 – four count inhale: eight count exhale. When antar kumbhaka is added, the ratio can be 1:1:1, or 1:1:2. If the bahir kumbhaka is also added the counts can be 1:1:1:1 or 1:1:2:1. Once these ratios have been practiced and are comfortable, the ratio can be increased to 1:2:2:1, and then to 1:2:4:1. As always, this should never be forced. According to the Yoga Sutra, the breath needs to be even or calm (sukshma), while being long (dirgha).

Breathing in through the left nostril engages the energy along the ida nadi, which is the lunar or yin channel; breathing out relaxes that energy. Breathing in through the right nostril engages the energy along the pingala nadi, which is the solar or yang channel; breathing out relaxes that energy. Alternating the breath, through both channels, brings balance to the nervous system, and the mind becomes calm and still.

If one nostril is plugged, that nostril need not be completely closed. Generally you will find one nostril is more open than the other. This is normal, and nadi shodhana will even the flow in both sides. If both nostrils are closed, perhaps due to a cold or some other nasal infection or condition, pranayama should be avoided until the illness has passed.

Neti, another of the six cleanses listed in the Hatha Yoga Pradipika, can be used to clean the nose and facilitate nadi shodhana. In neti, warm distilled or filtered (non-chlorinated) water, with some sea salt added,[285] is poured into one nostril and drained out through the other nostril, or through the mouth. Other liquids can be used, such as milk or even warm ghee.[286] The professional yogis use a string threaded through one nostril and the mouth, gently pulling the thread back and forth, cleaning the nasal passage. Needless to say, these practices are not for the weak of stomach, and should be learned from a teacher.

Options

Nadi shodhana can also be used to open one side of the body. If a day has been quite yang-like, you may want to just breathe in and out through the yin channel. Close the right nostril, and breathe in

---

[285] To match the body's own salty nature. This should not be iodized salt.
[286] A butter-like substance.

and out through the left nostril; add the retentions if desired. The yin energy will be stimulated and will balance the yang energies.

On the other hand you may have had a day that is too yin-like, and you need to add some yang energy. In this case, close the left nostril and keep it closed, as you breathe in and out through the right side. This can also be done just after a yin practice, if you still feel you are in an altered state; engage your yang energies by closing the left nostril, and breathe for a while through the right side only.

Another way to manipulate and manage our energies, beyond vinyasa and pranayama, is by meditation. We will examine this practice next.

Meditation on Energy

There are four main ways to stimulate the flow of energy in the body: acupuncture, which relies upon needles inserted in special points along the meridians; acupressure, which again stimulates the tissues along the meridian lines (and, associated with this, are all the varieties of massage therapies and asana practices); simple awareness; and directed breathing.

Simple Awareness

Try this little experiment: look at your thumb, and imagine you can feel the energy inside of it. Notice how it begins to warm up, just by focusing there. Continue to focus, and feel the thumb for a full minute. The sensation of warmth is not imaginary.

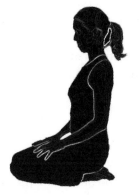

When we bring our attention to a specific part of the body, our parasympathetic nervous system is engaged. When this happens, our heart rate slows down, and the blood vessels dilate, allowing more blood and energy to flood the area. We can feel this happening. Simple awareness brings energy to where we concentrate. This is the reason we want to pay attention, during our yoga practice, to what we are experiencing in the body. We want to be focused, not distracted by thoughts. We want to enhance the flow of energy through the tissues being exercised, by feeling what is happening there.

Directed Breathing

In addition to feeling a particular area of the body, we can also send our breath there. This may sound strange to anyone who has not done this: how can we breathe somewhere beyond our lungs? But remember, the whole body is interconnected. Take a deep inhalation right now, and notice how your shoulders and abdomen move. This is movement beyond the lungs. When the diaphragm descends, it presses against the stomach and liver. The stomach and liver in turn press onto the lower organs; they also press into the pit of the abdomen. Blood pressure and pulse rate rise on the inhalation and fall on the exhalation. This effect is felt all over the body.

The breath affects every cell in the body, directly or indirectly. Initially, this is something that just happens – it is outside our conscious control. As we practice directing the breath, we can begin to feel the effect of the breath. Later, we can actually increase or enhance this effect deliberately. It is easiest in areas closest to the lungs. Feel the lower abdomen on your next cycle of breath: notice the tension ebb and flow there. Then begin to notice, not just the tension, but the transfer of energy too. This combination of both attention, which alone brings energy to the area being focused on, along with moving the breath to the region, doubly increases the energy moving toward the area.

Now we are ready to combine this bare awareness with the breath, and guide our attention deeper. We are now able to direct our energy.

Hamsa Mantra

On average, twenty-one thousand, six hundred times a day we chant the mantra *Hamsa*. "*Ha*" is the sound of the breath on our exhalations and "*sa*" is the sound of the inhalations. Some traditions reverse this, and the mantra is called "*So'ham*" – we hear "*hmmm*" on the inhalation and a sighing "*sa*" on the exhalation. Iyengar says they are actually combined; every creature creates so'ham on the inhalation (which means "He am I") and hamsa on the exhalation (which means "I am He"). This is called the "*ajapa mantra*."[287]

While we chant this barely audible mantra with each breath, we can feel energy moving within us. Close your eyes and notice the way your energy state is altered while you inhale and exhale. Experiment with hearing "ham" on the inhalation and "sa" on the exhalation. Does this feel energizing or calming for you? Next reverse it: hear "sa" on the inhalation and "ham" on the exhalation. Does this change the energetic feelings?

Many teachers will claim that hamsa is energizing and so'ham is relaxing. They teach that when we hear so'ham, prana is descending. On hearing hamsa, shakti (energy) rises. Other teachers claim the exact opposite. Of course, we are all different; half of us are natural belly breathers, half are chest breathers. It is not surprising that everyone doesn't respond the same way. You will need to experiment and find out which form of hamsa breathing energizes you, and which form calms you. Once you know, then you are ready to employ this tool in your practice. Preparing for a Yin Yoga class, you may want to use the calming breath. Preparing for a yang practice, you may want to use an energizing breath.

Of course, hamsa breathing can be used outside of your yoga practice too. We all have times in life when we are too stoked up and need to relax. The hamsa breath can be useful then. At other times, we need a quick boost of energy, and the opposite breath may be ideal. Instead of reaching, automatically, for that cigarette to calm you down, or that third cup of coffee or a cola to give you a pick-me-up, try working with the breath for a minute or two. You may be surprised at how effective it is, and it is a lot healthier.[288]

---

[287] Ajapa means "unpronounced," thus this is a silent mantra.

[288] There are two very interesting computer games produced by The Wild Divine Project (www.wilddivine.com) that helps people learn to calm and excite their own energy. The first game is called *Journey to the Wild Divine* and the second one is the sequel called *Wisdom Quest*. These games utilize computerized biofeedback sensors that are attached to three fingers. By controlling your breath and your energy levels, you navigate the imaginary

Now that we know how to stimulate or calm our inner energies, let's investigate how we can direct these energies.

Orbiting Energy

Ultimately, we would like the energy in our central channel (the sushumna nadi or governor vessel) to flow freely, unobstructed. Before this happens, we need the meridians flowing beside the central nadi to be open – the ida and pingala nadis. Nadi shodana is one way to open up both channels. Another way is to mentally circulate energy through these three channels, as we breathe and while we hold our postures. There are several ways to achieve this orbiting of our energy.

A Simple Orbit

A simple orbiting of energy begins by feeling the heart center. Sit comfortably and close your eyes – exhale. Start when the lungs are empty; as you inhale, feel or imagine energy flowing down your spine to the tip of the sacrum. As you exhale, reverse this, and follow the energy as it flows back to the heart space. Repeat this a few times. Slow the breath down to at least four counts for each inhale and exhale.

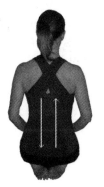

At first, there will be no sensation of anything flowing anywhere. That's okay. Don't be discouraged – this type of sensing takes practice. For now, just pretend you can feel it; if you could feel it, imagine what it would feel like. Maybe it would be helpful to imagine someone is running a finger along your spine – down from the heart on inhalations and back up to the heart on exhalations.

The direction the energy flows is the same direction that the diaphragm moves; if you get confused, just remember that. The

world, seeking wisdom. This game can help you learn to control your inner Chi.

diaphragm moves down as you inhale, so follow the flow in that direction. As the diaphragm rises, watch the energy rise too.

Once you can follow this flow, even if only in your imagination, add a short pause at the end of the inhalation. The energy now is in the muladhara chakra, at the base of the spine. Leave it there for a couple of seconds, but bring your awareness to the ajna chakra between the eyebrows. Just feel, or pretend to feel, energy there. After two seconds or so, exhale, following the energy back up to the heart.

Try this for a few cycles. If you can follow the energy without distraction for a few cycles, without losing the flow, add this final variation: continue to pause at the end of the inhalation, but add a short pause at the end of the exhalation as well. By the end of the exhalation, the energy will have returned to the heart space. Leave it there, but bring your awareness back to the muladhara chakra. Feel the perineum – notice the energetic lift there. Hold for just a couple of seconds, and begin the next inhalation by returning your awareness back to the heart.

When we allow energy to descend on the inhalation, we are joining the prana from the in breath to the apana in the lower belly. When we reverse this, we are joining the apana from the out breath to the prana in the upper body. Shakti and Shiva coming together is the objective of this practice. This simple work with the breath moves us toward this ultimate goal. We can do this while we hold the pose in a Yin Yoga practice, but we can also do this even in the most dynamic yang practice. All it takes is intention and attention.

Orbiting Energy While in a Pose

Back bends are naturally more energetic than forward bends; forward bends are naturally more calming than back bends. We can practice the simple orbiting of energy in any asana, but when we are in back bends, it feels more natural to pause only at the top of the inhalation, and bring awareness to the ajna chakra. When we are in forward bends, it feels more natural to hold the breath only at the end of the exhalation, and bring our awareness to the muladhara chakra.

When you come into back bends like the Seal, Sphinx, or Saddle poses, orbit the energy as discussed above, but only hold the breath at the end of the inhalation. Bring awareness up to the ajna. Pause for a few seconds and then complete the orbit. Do this for approximately half of the time you are holding the pose. For the second half, simply release and follow the breath's natural rhythm, or come to awareness of the predominant sensation in your body.

When you come into forward bends like the Butterfly, Dragonfly, or Snail poses, again orbit the energy, but this time, hold the breath only at the end of the exhalation. Bring awareness down to the muladhara. Engage your Chi bridge there.[289] Pause for a few seconds, and then complete the orbit.

In any other postures where you are in neither a forward bend nor a back bend, you can continue with holding the breath at the end of both inhalation and exhalation.

A Simple Variation

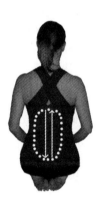

Now that you have mastered a basic orbit, you may choose to add the side channels. Here we draw the energy down, as before, on the inhalation, but as we hold the breath for a couple of seconds, we send the energy up the left side of the torso, through the heart space, and down the right side, back to the base of the spine. We just hold at the end of the inhalation; there is no retention at the end of the exhalation. On the next cycle, circle the energy up the right side, and down the left side, while you retain the breath. Cycling the energy through the left and right sides of the body stimulates and balances the flow of energy through the ida and pingala nadis.

In all these variations you may wish to add the hamsa or so'ham breaths.

There is a yang variation to the orbiting breath: breathe very *deeply* and hold on full lungs – this is energizing. In a yin variation, breathe

---

[289] The mula bandha.

much more quietly, shallowly, and hold only on empty lungs – this is calming.

The Microcosmic Orbit

The chakras are polarized. Recall, when we discussed the chakras in The Yogic View of Energy, we learned that Dr. Motoyama believes the chakras to be cones, with their roots on the spine and their open ends on the front of the body. Along with this third dimension, comes a yin and yang orientation to each chakra. The open end of the cone, on the front of the body, is the yin part of the chakra. The point on the spine is the yang part. So far, all the orbits of energy we have looked at were along the yang lines of the chakras. This touches only part of the chakras. The microcosmic orbit touches the yin and yang parts of the chakras, and circles the whole upper body.

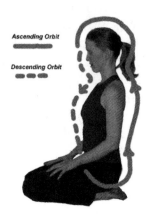

The term "microcosmic orbit" is a translation of the Daoist term for a full orbiting of energy through the front and back body. In Japan, it is called "*shoshuten*," which means a "circling of light." The microcosmic orbit is a way to gather, and channel, all the stray energies in the body, and raise them up from the muladhara to the ajna. An orbit is followed, beginning in the lower belly, circling down under the spine, up the back and over the crown of the head, ending at the ajna. This is the inhalation half of the orbit. On exhalation, the orbit is completed, as energy descends along the front of the body, back down to the lower belly. This activation of energy is a key preparation for many advanced Daoist practices. Through activating the microcosmic orbit, the reservoirs of the Governing Vessel and Conception meridians are refilled, which means this energy is available to all other meridians and organs. This is perhaps the best way to cultivate health and long life, while at the same time preparing the way to a deep spiritual understanding.

In the 1930s, Richard Wilhelm[290] described the benefit of the circling of light in his translation of the Secret of the Golden Flower, a Chinese Book of Life. This ancient text was transmitted orally for centuries before being written down in the eighth century. Wilhelm, a friend of Carl Jung's, wrote:

> If the life forces flow downward, that is, without let or hindrance into the outer world, the anima is victorious over the animus; no "spirit body" or "Golden Flower" is developed, and, at death, the ego is lost. If the life forces are led through the "backward-flowing" process, that is, conserved, and made to "rise" instead of allowed to dissipate, the animus has been victorious, and the ego persists after death. It is then possessed of shen, the revealing spirit. A man who holds to the way of conservation all through life may reach the stage of the "Golden Flower," which then frees the ego from the conflict of the opposites, and it again becomes part of Tao, the undivided, Great One.

It was Wilhelm's work that turned Jung in the direction of alchemy, which the Daoists had been practicing for thousands of year. The circling of light is an alchemical or transforming process. When the light circles long enough, it crystallizes and the body is transformed. We attain the natural spirit-body, and this body is formed "beyond all heavens." The sages claim in the Secret of the Golden Flower that the only tool we need to master is this concentration of thought on the circling light.

Circulating energy through the microcosmic orbit can be done at any time: prior to asana practice, just before meditation, during the long holds in the yin poses, or even at the beginning of Shavasana as we lay on our backs.

In Shavasana, bring your awareness to the second chakra, on the front of the body. This is the svadhisthana, which is about halfway between your navel and pubic bone. Feel, or imagine you feel, energy there. Exhale completely. As you inhale, follow a flow of energy down the midline of your body, under the pubic bone to the tailbone, and then upward, along the spine, the back of the neck, over the top

---

[290] Called the Marco Polo of the inner world of China.

of your head, and right to the ajna point between the eyebrows. Pause here at the top of the inhalation for two or three seconds. As you exhale, slowly feel the energy descend inside the face and throat. Continue to follow the midline of the body down to the sternum, to the navel, and right back to the svadhisthana again. Pause here for two or three seconds before beginning a new orbit.

As you orbit the body, touch each chakra on both the yin and yang sides (front and back) of the body; feel the energy at those points. Two or three minutes of orbiting the energy should be sufficient. When you have finished, release the effort, and let the breath be whatever it wants to be. Watch closely how you feel, without reacting to anything.

There is an orbit beyond the microcosmic called the "macrocosmic orbit." It is not considered as important as the microcosmic loop. The macrocosmic orbit extends the journey of energy down, and back up, the legs as well.

An orbit is a closed, circular path that is repeated over and over. The journey along an orbit never ends. Our journey together down the Yin River is nearing completion … but it too is not ending. While the time has come to leave you, we leave you to continue on with your own journey … perhaps with new guides who will help take you closer to the universal ocean.

The Journey Continues

We have drifted on the Yin River far from the dock where we boarded our little ferry, with the question on our lips, "What is Yin Yoga?" We have seen the history of yoga displayed before us. Our ferry took us into the waters of the physical body, the energy body, and the mind body. We were shown how the Eastern views compare to those in the West. Many small lakes through which we passed, invited us to linger and learn more. Perhaps you responded to a few of these invitations: the sights along this river are compelling.

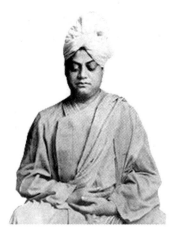

As different streams having their sources in different places all mingle their water in the sea, so, O Lord, the different path which men take through different tendencies, various though they appear, crooked or straight, all lead to Thee.
Swami Vivekananda AE

Most of the time, we trusted the river, and just went with the flow. We were shown *how* to practice Yin Yoga and *what* to practice. We heard the warnings of rapids and extreme white waters awaiting us, should we follow certain streams. These warnings advised us to seek an experienced guide, before braving the treacherous waters. We also discovered that, at times, floundering is just another part of the journey; when we travel a river, we should expect to get wet now and then.

The journey is not finished by any means ... and that is okay. The destination is still ahead, and the river will take us ever onward. After all, it is the journey itself that is most important. Still to be discovered are the waters of deeper yoga – we have only floated around the outer edges of the lakes of the vijnanamaya and anandamaya koshas. The serious traveler will want to find a pilot to take her safely to, and through, those deep waters.

The Buddha once said, "Place no head above your own." He warned us that the spiritual path has to be traveled; staying at home and reading about it is not a substitute. Hearing tales from others who have gone before you will be of absolutely no value, unless you make the journey yourself. You must experience for yourself the truth of any teaching. But this does not mean you need to make the journey alone; guidance through white waters is absolutely necessary in order to survive.

Plan the rest of your journey with care. Seek out those whom you can trust and whose wisdom your respect. Don't overplan though – that is often an excuse for not doing. Your plans will never be one hundred percent complete or perfect. Don't worry about it; there is boldness in beginning any endeavor.

Just do it … Go!

And remember to smile …

Source of Selected Images

All pictures provided by James Oschman are from his book, *Energy Medicine – The Scientific Basis*, copyright Elsevier Limited, 2000, and are with the kind permission from Elsevier and James Oschman.

Yang Mountain – Yin River courtesy of Louise LeBlanc.

A   This image is from the of the 20th US edition of Gray's Anatomy of the Human Body, originally published in 1918.

B   Russian Doll images are courtesy Wikipedia
     http://en.wikipedia.org/wiki/Image:JapaneseNestingDolls.jpg.

C   This montage of the muscles is courtesy Wikipedia
     http://upload.wikimedia.org/wikipedia/commons/c/c0/
     Skeletal_muscle.jpg

D   This illustration of the muscles is courtesy Wikipedia
     http://upload.wikimedia.org/wikipedia/commons/c/c0/
     Skeletal_muscle.jpg

E   These two images are courtesy of Ron Thompson.

F   Image courtesy of the Visible Human Project.

G   Reprinted from Gray's Anatomy, 38th Edition ...
        The Anatomical Basis of Medicine and Surgery,
        copyright by Pearson Professional Limited 1995,
        and with their kind permission.

H   These two images are from the of the 20th US edition
        of Gray's Anatomy of the Human Body, originally published
        in 1918. These images are in the public domain because their
        copyright has expired.

I   This collagen image is courtesy of Matthew P. Dalene and
        the Rensselaer Polytechnic Institute.

J   These images are courtesy of James Oschman.

K   This image is from the of the 20th US edition of Gray's
        Anatomy of the Human Body, originally published in
        1918. This image is in the public domain because
        its copyright has expired.

L   Drawings courtesy of Wikipedia
     http://en.wikipedia.org/wiki/Image:Gelenke_Zeichnung01.jpg

M   From the 19th century Tibetan sage Ratnasara.

N   Image courtesy of Wikipedia
    http://upload.wikimedia.org/wikipedia/
        en/c/c6/Illu_endocrine_system.jpg.

O   Image courtesy of Wikipedia
    http://en.wikipedia.org/wiki/Image:Lao_Tzu_-
        _Project_Gutenberg_eText_15250.jpg.

P   Aurora courtesy of Wikipedia
    http://en.wikipedia.org/wiki/Image:Aurora2.jpg.

Q   Image courtesy of James Oschman.

R   Image courtesy of Wikipeda:
    http://en.wikipedia.org/wiki/Image:Electromagnetism.png.

S   Image courtesy of Wikipedia
    http://en.wikipedia.org/wiki/Image:Biological_cell.png.

T   Image courtesy of James Oschman.

U   Image courtesy of Dr. Christoph Ballestrem.

V   Image courtesy of Violette www.violettesfolkart.com.

W   This image is from NOAA's Project Vortex – 99.

X   Image courtesy of Violette www.violettesfolkart.com.

Y   Image courtesy of Wikipedia
    http://en.wikipedia.org/wiki/Image:Yantra-tripura-sundari.jpg.

Z   Image courtesy of Wikipedia
    http://en.wikipedia.org/wiki/Image:MayaDream.JPG.

AA Image courtesy of Violette www.violettesfolkart.com.

AB Image courtesy of Violette www.violettesfolkart.com.

AC Image courtesy of Violette www.violettesfolkart.com.

AD Image courtesy of Violette www.violettesfolkart.com.

AE Image courtesy of Wikipedia
    http://en.wikipedia.org/wiki/Image:Vivekananda.png.

Bibliography and References

Acupuncture Imaging by Mark Seem
The Alchemy of Yoga by Tim Miller
American Family Physician – April 1998
Anatomy of Hatha Yoga by H. David Coulter
The Anxiety and Phobia Workbook by Edmund Bourne
Asana Pranayama Mudra Bandha by Swami Satyananda Saraswati
Autobiography of a Yogi by Paramahansa Yogananda
Awakening of the Chakras and Emancipation
    by Dr. Hiroshi Motoyama

Breath by Breath by Larry Rosenberg
Buddha by Karen Armstrong
Buddhism Without Beliefs by Stephen Batchelor
Buddhist Bible by Dwight Goddard
Buddhist psychology: A review of theory and practice by Silva Padmal

Chinese Acupuncture and Moxibustion published
    by the Shanghai University
Cognitive Therapy and the Emotional Disorders by Dr. Aaron Beck

Dao De Ching by Lao-tzu
Dreams by Carl Jung, translated by R.F.C. Hull

Energy Medicine: the Scientific Basis by James Oschman
Energy Medicine in Therapeutics and Human Performance
    by James Oschman
Essence CD by Deva Premal
The Essence of Jung's Psychology and Tibetan Buddhism
    by Radmila Moacanin
Everyday Zen by Charlotte Joko Beck

Frogs into Princes by Bandler and Grinder

Gheranda Samhita
Gospel of Saint Thomas

Hatha Yoga Pradipika by Swami Swatmarama
The Heart of Yoga by T.K.V. Desikachar

Identifying and challenging unhelpful thinking
    by Chris Williams and Anne Garland
Indian Journal of Physiology and Pharmacology, October, 1998 –
    effect of shavasana on stress
Insight Yoga DVD by Sarah Powers
Issue at Hand by Gil Fronsdal

Journey to the Wild Divine by The Wild Divine Project

Light on Life by B.K.S. Iyengar
Light on Yoga by B.K.S. Iyengar
Long, Slow & Deep -- Live Bootleg CD by Bryan Kest
Lunar Flow Yoga DVD by Shiva Rea

Measurements of Ki Energy, Diagnosis, & Treatments
    by Dr. Hiroshi Motoyama
Mind Over Mood by Dennis Greenberger and Christine Padesky

Nothing Special by Charlotte Joko Beck

Peace is Every Step by Thich Nhat Hanh
Philosophies of India by Heinrich Zimmer
The Power of Now by Eckhard Tolle

Realities of the Dreaming Mind: The Practice of Dream Yoga
    by Swami Sivananda Radha
Rig Veda

Satsang CD by Deva Premal
The Science of Flexibility by Michael Alter

The Secret of the Golden Flower by Richard Wilhem
The *Shambhala Encyclopedia of Yoga* by Georg Feuerstein
Shat-chakra-nirupana by Purananda
Shiva Samhita
The Structure and Dynamics of the Psyche by Carl Jung

Taittiriya Upanishad
Tantra, the Path of Ecstasy by Georg Feuerstein
Taoism by Eva Wong
Theory of the Chakras by Dr. Hiroshi Motoyama
The Three Pillars of Zen by Philip Kapleau
Tibetan Book of the Dead
Transformation of Myth Through Time by Joseph Campbell
Two Essays on Analytical Psychology by Carl Jung

Unlimited Power by Anthony Robbins

The Web That Has No Weaver by Ted Kaptchuk's
Who Dies? by Stephen Levine
Wisdom Quest by The Wild Divine Project

Yin Yoga by Paul Grilley
Yin Yoga DVD by Paul Grilley
Yin Yoga CD by Sarah Powers
Yin & Vinyasa Yoga CD by Sarah Powers
The Yin Yoga Kit by Biff Mithoefer
Yoga Inspired Functional Fitness DVD by Marla Ericksen
Yoga Mala by Pattabhi Jois
The Yoga Matrix by Richard Freeman
Yoga on Sacred Ground CD by Chinmaya Dunster
Yoga Sutra

Zen Mind, Beginner's Mind by Shunryu Suzuki

Index

Asanas (poses) are in **boldface.**
Page numbers followed by "n" indicate footnotes.
Numbers in *italics* indicate photos or illustrations.

A

abhinivesah (fear of death), 165, *165,*
166
acceptance, 227, 232–233, 252
acting, 235–236
action and karma Daoism, 85–86
active imagination, 220, 221
active listening, 209–210
acupressure, 386
acupuncture, 386
aging
    changes in muscles as we age,
      32–33
    of connective tissues, 44–45
Agni, 380n
agni (fire), 75
ahamkara (I-maker), 154–155, 160
ahimsa (non-harming), 168, 180
ajapa mantra, 388
ajna chakra, 76, 78
akasha (space), 76, 209
alabdhabhumikatva
    (lack of perseverance), 164
alasya (fatigue or sloth), 164
alchemy, 219, 393
    internal, 86

allowing, 232–233
alternate nostril breathing,
    342, 383–386
alternative thoughts, 229
AMA. *see* American Medical Association
ama, 47n
American Medical Association
    (AMA), 70n
AMI (Apparatus for Meridian
    Identification), 142
anahata chakra, 75, 78
Anahatasana (melting heart),
    261, 261–262
ananda (bliss), 148, 172, 223
anandamaya kosha, 24, 148n
Anapanasati Sutra, 200–201, 203–205
anavasthitatva
    (instability or regression), 164
anicca (impermanence), 193
anima, 173
Anjali Mudra, 363, *363,* 365, *365*
anjali (prayer) mudra, 177, *177*
ankle bending sequence, 373, *373*
ankle cranking sequence, 374, *374*
ankle rotation sequence, *373,* 373–374
Ankle Stretch, *263,* 263–264
annamaya kosha, 24, 25–26

B

Z

About the Author

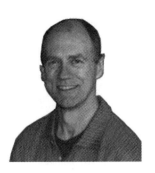

Bernie Clark has been teaching yoga and meditation since 1998. He has a bachelor's degree in science from the University of Waterloo and combines his intense interest in yoga with an understanding of the scientific approach to investigating the nature of things. His ongoing studies have taken him deeply inside mythology, comparative religions, and psychology.

All of these avenues of exploration have clarified his understanding of the ancient Eastern practices of yoga and meditation. His teaching, workshops, and books have helped many students broaden their own understanding of health, life, and the source of true joy.

Bernie's yoga practice encompasses the hard, yang-styles, such as Ashtanga and Power Yoga, and the softer, yin-styles, as exemplified in Yin Yoga. His meditation experience goes back to the early '80s when he first began to explore the practice of Zen meditation. During those days, while he struggled with the conflict between practice and theory, Bernie also worked as a member of the executive team of one of Canada's oldest and largest hi-tech companies, assisting it to become a world-renowned leader in its field. He has two children who have launched successful careers of their own.

Contact Information:

Web: www.yinyoga.com
Email: BernieClark@yinyoga.com
Studio: Semperviva, Vancouver, B.C.
       www.Semperviva.com

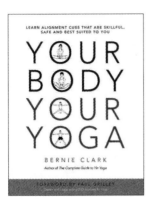

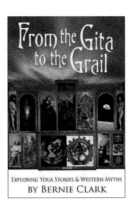

Your Body, Your Yoga

Learn Alignment Cues That Are Skillful, Safe, and Best Suited To You

Your Body, Your Yoga goes beyond any prior yoga anatomy book available. It looks not only at the body's unique anatomical structures and what this means to everyone's individual range of motion, but also examines the physiological sources of restrictions to movement.

"*Your Body, Your Yoga* is a fascinating, provocative, and scientifically-informed look at the inner workings of the body as it affects the practice of asana. Bernie Clark challenges much dogma in the modern postural yoga world, including a few heretofore sacrosanct principles of alignment, to demonstrate that a healthy and effective yoga practice should be adapted to each individual's unique needs, abilities and anatomy. Required reading for yoga teachers and yoga therapists, and highly recommended for avid practitioners."
—*Timothy McCall, MD, author of Yoga As Medicine; U.S.A.*

From The Gita to The Grail

Exploring Yoga Stories & Western Myths

Learn what the myths of yoga mean to those of us who grew up in Western culture and with Western stories.

"In this insightful book, Bernie reminds us that we have a choice in how we live our lives; we can hold tight to our beliefs, allowing them to dictate our reality, or we can invite every story (or even encounter) to be a gateway into the poetic, multifaceted dimensions of truth, and the fluid nature of reality."
—*Sarah Powers, author of Insight Yoga and founder of the Insight Yoga Institute*

"Bernie's book covers mythical territory any student of yoga should be aware of. Diving into both unfamiliar and familiar stories of creation and the path of the hero, Bernie's readable style is like the voice of an Elder. If you could record Joseph Campbell and Carl Jung's conversation over a game of chess, it might sound something like this."
—*Daniel Clement, founder of Open Source Yoga*